OXFORD MEDICAL PUBLICATIONS

SPORTS INJURIES

SPORTS INJURIES

RECOGNITION AND MANAGEMENT

Second Edition

Edited by

M. A. HUTSON

Orthopaedic and Sports Physician,
Park Row Clinic, Nottingham
and
London Bridge Clinic, London

Oxford New York Tokyo
OXFORD UNIVERSITY PRESS
1996

Oxford University Press, Walton Street, Oxford OX2 6DP

Oxford   New York
Athens   Auckland   Bangkok   Bombay
Calcutta   Cape Town   Dar es Salaam   Delhi
Florence   Hong Kong   Istanbul   Karachi
Kuala Lumpur   Madras   Madrid   Melbourne
Mexico City   Nairobi   Paris   Singapore
Taipei   Tokyo   Toronto
and associated companies in
Berlin   Ibadan

Oxford is a trade mark of Oxford University Press

Published in the United States
by Oxford University Press Inc., New York

First edition published 1990
Second edition published 1996

© Oxford University Press 1990, 1996

A catalogue record for this book is available from the British Library

Library of Congress Cataloging in Publication Data
Sports injuries, recognition and management /edited by M. A. Hutson.—2nd ed.
p.   cm.—(Oxford medical publications)
ISBN 0–19–262676–0 (hbk).—ISBN 0–19–262675–2 (pbk.)
1. Sports injuries.   I. Hutson, M. A.   II. Series.
[DNLM: 1. Athletic Injuries—diagnosis.   2. Athletic Injuries—therapy. QT 261 S7647 1995]
RD97.S72   1995
617.1′027—dc20
DNLM/DLC
for Library of Congress   *95–17108*
                                                       CIP

Typeset by
EXPO Holdings, Malaysia
Printed in Great Britain by
The Bath Press Ltd, Avon

FOREWORD
HRH, The Princess Royal

As a competitive horse rider I have spent a great deal of time and effort worrying about the physical condition of my horse and trying to prevent injuries from either happening or getting worse. My own problems seemed less important. However, it is an inevitable consequence of sport, or recreational activity, that physical injury will intervene from time to time. Whatever the source of injury, the overall effect is to increase the demands made upon the medical profession.

Dr Michael Hutson has a background of general practice in which he developed his knowledge in orthopaedic and sports medicine and became medical officer to professional soccer and cricket teams in Nottingham.

Dr Hutson clearly understands the need for a greater background of knowledge of sports injuries by medical practitioners, particularly by physicians of first contact—the general medical practitioner and the Accident and Emergency doctor. Only by disseminating such knowledge into the general body of the medical profession will the requirements of the sporting populus at large be satisfied.

Fortunately, he is not alone as there are contributions from consultants in other medical disciplines who describe the recognition and management of more specialized problems.

The theme that underlines the purpose of the book is a *practical* approach to the problems of sports injuries. It should provide a valuable addition to the understanding of this increasingly important discipline, and it is a pleasure to be associated with it.

ANNE

PREFACE

The discipline of Sports Medicine has progressed, albeit in a haphazard way, to a considerable degree over the last decade or so. The development of exercise physiology, for instance, has been such that there are a number of texts of excellence available to the sports physiologist and clinician alike in his pursuit of a basic understanding of fitness and the body's response to various energetic sports and recreational exercise. However, the needs of the medical practitioner, who is concerned principally with the recognition and management of *injury* sustained during or as a result of sport, have been less well served. His overall requirement, notwithstanding the need for a satisfactory background knowledge of basic sciences, is for a greater clinical appreciation of the athlete's problems so that he may undertake both a principal and coordinating role. Inherent in these responsibilities is an awareness of the importance of early assessment of the severity of the pathological process in order to achieve maximal influence on healing, the relationship of the injury to the athlete's expectations regarding his future participation in sport, and recognition of the benefits of expert rehabilitation.

This book is not an encyclopaedia of medical conditions associated with sport. It is primarily designed for the clinician who requires a method of learning a suitable approach towards the musculoskeletal problems encountered in sport. Diagnosis, treatment, and rehabilitation of the most common, yet often inadequately treated, injuries are considered in some depth. Aetiological factors, particularly in overuse injury requiring some knowledge of biomechanics, are given due emphasis. A guide is given to the timely referral for further advice and to the role of the consultant in certain specialized fields. An attempt is made to define objectives for the sports physician and to outline aspects of his educational, managerial, and advisory responsibilities to the community.

The purpose therefore is for the text to be essentially a means of reference to complement the development of the practical skills required by the general practitioner with limited resources and facilities, the traumatologist in the hospital casualty department, and the already established sports physician who requires greater in-depth information. Since the future specialists in sports injuries will come largely from the ranks of general practitioners, the more so as postgraduate educational degree courses in Sports Medicine are now available, it is understandable that the author has general practioners in mind. However, both physicians and surgeons who have already developed specialist skills in disciplines such as orthopaedic surgery and rheumatology should find that the text provides information on those soft-tissue problems arising from sport that lie outside their principal field of interest or experience.

The 1990 text has been fully revised and updated. Basic principles will stand the test of time. However, over the last five years there have been a number of improvements in investigative techniques and in some management strategies, and these have been incorporated in this edition. In particular, a more comprehensive section on MRI scanning is now included and the latest advances in specialized fields such as anterior cruciate deficiency are outlined.

1995   M.A.H.

ACKNOWLEDGEMENTS

The following are gratefully acknowledged for permission to reproduce figures.

Figs. 1.1. and 1.8, T. Bailey Forman Newspapers Ltd, Nottingham; **Figs. 1.2a, 1.5, 3.7 a and b, 4.8b, and 5.10b**, B. Thomas, 19 Charnwood Ave, Northampton; **Fig. 1.2b**, The Associated Press Ltd, London; **Fig. 1.9**, T. Duffy, 83 Sutton Heights, Surrey; **Fig. 2.7**, Thomas Bond (Optometrist), 130 Melton Road, West Bridgford, Nottingham; **Fig. 4.2**, E. D. Lacey, 16 Post House Lane, Leatherhead; **Figs. 4.5, 5.3**, and 5.*10a*, Supersports Photographs, Baslow, Derbyshire; **Fig. 6.9**, *The Times*, London; **Fig. 4.17**, Stark, H., Jobe, F. W., Boyes, J., and Ashworth, R. R. (1977). Fracture of the hook of the hamate in athletes. *J. Bone Jt. Surg.*, **59A**, 576; **Fig. 4.24**, Henderson, J. J. and Arafa, M. A. M. (1987). Carpometacarpal dislocation. *J. Bone Jt. Surg.*, **69B**, 213; **Figs. 4.25, 4.27, 4.28, 4.38, 4.40, and 4.42**, Watson Jones (1982). *Fractures and Joint injuries*, 6th edn, (ed. J. N. Wilson). Churchill Livingstone, Edinburgh (Figs. 4.27 and 4.28 modified from, London, P.S. (1967). *A practical guide to the care of the injured*. Churchill Livingstone, Edinburgh); **Fig. 4.41**, Stack, H. G. (1968). Mallet finger. *The Hand*, **1**, 85; **Fig. 6.21(c)**, T. Bailey Forman Newspapers Ltd. Nottingham; **Fig. 13.1**, The Resuscitation Council (UK).

CONTENTS

List of contributors   vii

1 Introduction
M. A. HUTSON   1

2 Head injuries
J. L. FIRTH and N. R. GALLOWAY

Intracranial injuries *J. L. Firth*   17
Ocular sports injuries *N. R. Galloway*   25

3 Injuries to the shoulder
W. A. WALLACE and M. A. HUTSON   31

4 Injuries to the upper limb
M. A. HUTSON and N. J. BARTON

Overuse injuries *M. A. Hutson*   51
Injuries to the hand and wrist *N. J. Barton*   60

5 Spinal injuries
M. A. HUTSON and F. R. I. MIDDLETON

Soft tissue injuries *M. A. Hutson*   79
Injuries to the spinal cord *F.R.I. Middleton*   94

6 Pelvic injuries
M. A. HUTSON   103

7 Injuries to the knee joint
M. A. HUTSON   115

8 Injuries to the ankle and foot
M. A. HUTSON   131

9 Lower limb muscle and overuse injuries
M. A. HUTSON AND M. J. ALLEN

Muscle injury *M. A. Hutson*   141
Overuse injuries of the knee *M. A. Hutson*   145
Shin pain *M. J. Allen*   151
Overuse injuries of the ankle and foot
M. A. Hutson   155

10 Investigations
M. A. HUTSON AND D. B. L. FINLAY

Non-radiological investigations *M. A. Hutson*   167
Radiological investigations *D. B. L. Finlay*   169

11 Prevention of injury
M. A. HUTSON   183

12 Treatment and rehabilitation
M. A. HUTSON   203

13 First aid in sport
M. A. HUTSON   225

Epilogue: whither sports injury services?
M. A. HUTSON   229

Index   231

CONTRIBUTORS

M. J. ALLEN
Consultant in Sports Medicine
Leicester General Hospital
Leicester

N. J. BARTON
Consultant Hand Surgeon
University Hospital
Nottingham

D. B. L. FINLAY
Consultant Radiologist
Leicester Royal Infirmary
Leicester

J. L. FIRTH
Consultant Neurosurgeon
University Hospital
Nottingham

N. R. GALLOWAY
Consultant Ophthalmic Surgeon
University Hospital
Nottingham

M. A. HUTSON
Specialist Orthopaedic and Sports Physician
Park Row Clinic
30 Park Row
Nottingham

F. R. I. MIDDLETON
Consultant in Rehabilitation and Disability Medicine
Spinal Injuries Unit
Royal National Orthopaedic Hospital
Stanmore

W. A. WALLACE
Professor of Orthopaedic and Accident Surgery
University Hospital
Nottingham

1 Introduction

M. A. HUTSON

Basic concepts

The primary requirement of medical practitioners needing to advise those patients injured during, or as a result of, sport is the establishment of an accurate diagnosis. Even when a specific diagnosis has been made, full assessment requires a knowledge of the aetiological factors associated with the development of injury, behavioural aspects, including motivation, and the standard of performance achieved. When underpinned by an appropriate level of knowledge of pathoanatomy and biomechanics, management of injury may incorporate varying treatment modalities in proceeding to rehabilitation of the patient to a satisfactory level of fitness.

The theme throughout the text will therefore be one of *assessment and management*.

Assessment: history
                  aetiological factors
                  specific diagnosis
Management: treatment
                  rehabilitation

It is unfortunate that within the clinical curriculum of the medical student there is a very limited amount of time devoted to an introduction to the extensive field of orthopaedics and rheumatology. A paradox exists in that, although soft tissue problems of all kinds, encompassed by the specialities of orthopaedic medicine and sports medicine, represent a high proportion of the work-load of doctors in general practice and in traumatology departments, there is little opportunity to prepare them for examination of the musculoskeletal system. Examination procedures will therefore be described in some detail in this book. In the past the author has relied heavily on those basic procedures as laid down by, amongst others, James Cyriax in his *Textbook of Orthopaedic Medicine* (Cyriax 1982). Expansion in some directions, modification in others, and the addition of techniques such as ligament stress testing make it possible to build from basic orthopaedic medical principles in an orderly fashion, thus reducing the likelihood of diagnostic error from inadequacy of musculoskeletal examination.

Assessment

A basic knowledge of the biomechanical forces involved in 'normal' participation in specific sports is required. Track athletes run anti-clockwise both in their events and during training, so that asymmetrical forces are continually being applied to their lower limbs in particular. Javelin throwers may have an overhead style, or tend to sling, in which case different forces are applied to their shoulders and elbows (Fig. 1.1). Tennis players may use a single-or a two-handed backhand, imposing different stresses upon the trunk and upper limbs (Fig. 1.2), and so on. Numerous examples are given throughout the text. These technical factors are particularly relevant when considering overuse injury.

An assessment of joint mobility some distance away from the site of injury is also included in the categorization of relevant aetiological factors. A squash player with a limited range of hip rotation, owing to early degenerative disease, may develop low back pain when excessive rotational stress is repeatedly transferred to the lumbar spine. Weakness or tightness of one group of muscles acting about a joint may similarly result in injury elsewhere. Tight hamstrings for instance may be responsible for low back problems, or for muscle injury in compensating muscle groups.

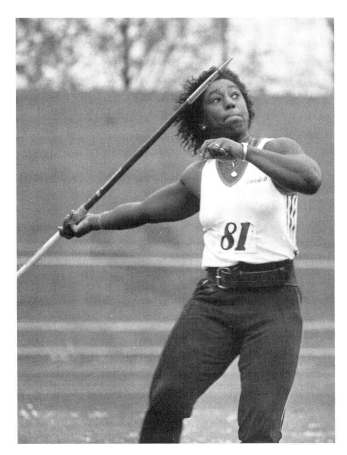

FIG. 1.1 Javelin throwers may have an overhead style or tend to sling: different forces are applied to the shoulders and elbows.

(a)   Fɪɢ. 1.2 Tennis players may use a single- or two-handed backhand, thereby imposing different stresses upon   (b)
the trunk and upper limbs: (a) single-handed backhand; (b) two-handed backhand.

These are simply a few of the factors that require identi-fication for full assessment of the nature of the injury, and they will be explored in greater detail in the individual chapters which follow. Training schedules, behavioural tendencies, particularly the behavioural aspects of pain perception, indi-vidual motivation, and ambition also need study. Although 'holistic' medicine enjoys much popularity at the moment, it has surely always been incumbent upon medical practitioners to develop a breadth of vision which includes every patient—a facet of their skills that they are trained in from the first weeks of the clinical curriculum in medical school. Sports injuries need no less perspicacity than other illnesses that are recogniz-ably 'stress' related. When injuries in children are considered, the interrelationship between ambition on the part of the patient, parents, coaches, and teachers becomes even more important.

The history given by the patient is often revealing. When injury is acute, particularly when extrinsic forces are involved, the direction of the externally applied forces should be estab-lished if possible. When injury is of a more chronic nature ('overuse injury', see pp. 5–6) the history is quite different, as exemplified by the phases of discomfort experienced during the development of tendinitis:

(i)   discomfort (+ stiffness) after activity;
(ii) discomfort during the initiation of activity, subsequently improving ('run off') during further activity, and worsening afterwards;
(iii) discomfort worsening during activity, associated with func-tional impairment;
(iv) discomfort sufficient effectively to prevent activity.

Following the extraction of a symptom history and relevant background information, the establishment of a satisfactory diagnosis requires the application to the musculoskeletal system of examination techniques which previously may not have been extensively used by the majority of doctors. An appreciation must be gained of the importance of an examination routine that is founded upon sound orthopaedic principles, so that an *assessment of function* may be made. The moving parts require clinical appraisal according to the following code.

1. Observation.
2. Active movements.
3. Passive movements.
4. Resisted—i.e. isometric—muscle contraction (selective tissue tension).
5. Palpation.
6. Neurological and vascular examination.

The passive movements offer information on joint function and the integrity of the periarticular structures, and may be further subdivided into

● range of motion (around physiological axes)
● 'joint play' (movements not under voluntary control)
● stress testing for ligamentous competency.

The only compromise to this orthopaedic *medical* system of examination should be when, as a result of a history of acute trauma and the disposition of the patient or of the injured area, a fracture is suspected: gentle handling of the injured site may be followed by early X-ray, prior to more extensive examination procedures if appropriate (thereby conforming to the orthopaedic *surgical* system).

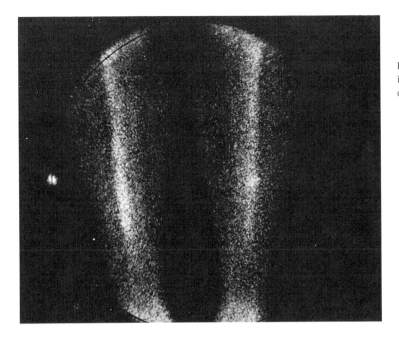

FIG. 1.3 Scattered increased uptake, representing recurrent physical stress, may be seen on bone scans in the lower limbs of long-distance runners.

Further investigations such as X-rays, arthrography, ultrasound scans, bone scans, CT scans, MRI scans, haematology, etc., should be considered where relevant. Full assessment relies on an understanding that, just as there is a wider range of ECG changes in an athlete than in the non-sporting population, so 'abnormal' findings, such as are seen in X-rays of 'footballer's ankle' (marginal osteophytes and avulsion fragments (see Fig. 9.16, p. 155) or on bone scans of long-distance runners (scattered increased uptake in the bones of the lower limbs (Fig. 1.3) are simply a manifestation of recurrent physical stress. Interpretation must therefore be made with due care.

Management

Management of athletic injury requires substantially more than 'treatment' of an injured area. Patients need advice on a number of other aspects, including maintenance of overall fitness during recovery, and require a suitable prognosis. If physical treatment is desirable it is necessary to have some knowledge of therapeutic modalities, and preferably a sound professional working relationship with the therapist of choice. It is erroneous to assume automatically that ice and ultrasound, for instance, cure all soft tissue lesions; more critical evaluation of the options is required before prescribing specific therapeutic regimes. A good physical therapist needs, above all else, a diagnosis, following which he/she will probably have more experience in the usefulness of modalities such as effleurage, friction massage, laser therapy, etc. than the referring practitioner. However, it is incumbent upon the referring doctor to offer guidance, and thereby encourage suitable feedback of information on patients' progress.

Depending on the type, severity, and duration of the injury, it may be necessary for the patient to progress from the therapy room to the rehabilitation area, where progressive strengthening exercises and flexibility exercises may be performed. Isotonic, isometric, and isokinetic exercises all have their place; they should be combined with suitable stretching schedules. With a greater availability of gymnasia and health clubs, in which sophisticated equipment such as the Nautilus range is commonly available for both training and rehabilitation, it is increasingly important for progress to be monitored by the practitioner and for prescriptive exercises to be specific to both the injury and the sport. It is often forgotten that strengthening exercises which are primarily performed for specific muscle groups may impose stresses on other parts of the body—this is particularly relevant to the prevention of spinal injury during the rehabilitation of an injured limb.

Liaison with the coach or trainer should be considered to be an important aspect of both assessment and management. The coaches of athletes, particularly those in the younger age groups with considerable aptitude, may well be able to furnish useful information regarding the cause of injury which has not otherwise been disclosed; conversely they need guidance on the reduction of specific forms of stress during the subsequent resumption of training. Occasions frequently arise when a telephone call to the coach of an up-and-coming tennis starlet, for instance, reveals the existence of abnormal biomechanical stress associated with faulty serving technique. Hyperextension of the spine on a tennis service (Fig. 1.4) or excessive forearm rotation on the forehand are not uncommon. Unless such information is presented to the physician, and flawed technique identified and corrected, recurrence of injury is to be expected.

Overall, the patient needs reassurance, whenever possible, regarding the likelihood of a satisfactory outcome, as his worst fears are not always overtly expressed. The parents of an adolescent with Osgood–Schlatter's disease often need a positive statement that the 'lump' is not a tumour, and likewise the patient with a thigh swelling from a rectus femoris tear (Fig. 1.5). These and other considerations will be more fully explored in subsequent chapters. In this branch of medicine, in which the frustration of injury is often compounded by a psychological 'low' secondary to inactivity, sympathetic understanding is required. Too many patients inappropriately receive a bland prescription for absolute rest, or an unhelpful reaction such as, 'I am not surprised that you have leg pain if you run seventy miles a week.' Patients, quite rightly, expect advice for injuries that have occurred in an era when recreation and sport are encouraged, not least by government-backed 'Sport for All' and 'Exercise for Health' campaigns. The abrogation by some members of the medical profession of

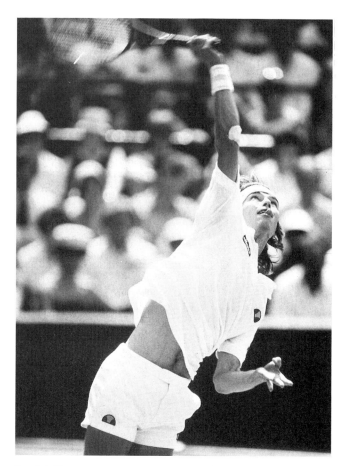

FIG. 1.4 The tennis serve may give rise to shoulder or spinal injuries if technique is faulty. In this illustration the server avoids spinal hyperextension, having thrown the ball up correctly in front of his body.

FIG. 1.5 Patients may need reassurance that a previous rectus femoris tear is not a tumour.

their responsibility to provide a caring service on the grounds that sports injuries are 'self-induced' is quite intolerable. Despite the reluctance of central government to release funding for Sports Injury Clinics or for postgraduate medical education in sports medicine, increasing expectations on the part of patients are likely to be a major stimulus to the development of a greater awareness of the need for the advancement of sports medicine within the medical profession. It is hoped that funds from the National Lottery will be a further stimulus to the development of regional centres of excellence in Sports Medicine. However, doctors of first contact will take the brunt of an increasing workload.

Features of soft tissue breakdown and repair

Acute inflammatory phase

When injury is sustained to the soft (connective) tissues, whether as a result of acute trauma or of repeated microtrauma, localized cellular damage results. In the early inflammatory phase chemotactic agents are released from platelets and mast cells. These agents stimulate the migration of polymorphs (which are particularly active against pathogens) and monocytes (which develop into macrophages having a phagocytic function upon tissue debris). Degradative enzymes are released from a range of inflammatory cells. The concentration of the chemotactic agents appears to be dependent, in part, upon a raised intracellular level of calcium ions. Vasodilation and increased capillary permeability occur, mediated (at least in part) by prostaglandins (Anderson and Ramwell 1974). Interstitial oedema and frank bleeding into the tissues from the larger blood vessels are features of this early phase. During the inflammatory phase over the next few days, in the continued presence of macrophages, further chemotactic factors are released from within their granules: such factors stimulate the development of undifferentiated connective tissue cells into fibroblasts and endothelial and other mature cells.

If sufficiently severe, the inflammatory phase is responsible for the clinical features of erythema, heat, pain, crepitus, swelling, and dysfunction. The physical modalities of treatment described in Chapter 12 help alleviate the symptoms and the extent of the inflammatory process. Prostaglandin synthesis is inhibited by non-steroidal anti-inflammatory drugs (NSAIDs). Although it is conventional to think in terms of 'anti-inflammatory' treatment for acute soft tissue injury, the inflammatory phase is nevertheless essential to normal repair. Therefore modalities such as ultrasound may more accurately be considered to be 'pro-inflammatory' by stimulating mast cell activity, and *accelerating* the normal repair process (Dyson 1987). In chronic inflammatory conditions, however, it is more appropriate to remove the (overuse) inflammatory stimulus before the use of specific therapeutic modalities. However, despite relative, or even 'complete', rest, some chronic inflammatory conditions (such as plantar fasciitis and lateral epicondylitis) appear to be self-perpetuating. Stress reduction may then need to be combined with the more powerful anti-inflammatory activity of the injectable corticosteroids.

Proliferative phase

Within a few days of injury the proliferative phase commences, thereby overlapping the late inflammatory phase. Fibroblasts form a connective tissue matrix and endothelial cells develop into blood vessels; the resulting highly cellular and vascularized tissue is known as granulation tissue. It is essential at this stage that the collagenous matrix is allowed to proceed to relative maturity without the imposition of excessive stress. In more chronic conditions, particularly in poorly vascularized tissue such as tendons, it may be useful to stimulate therapeutically the development of endothelial cells into capillaries. Extensive tissue destruction from the inflammatory phase or excessive fibrosis may sometimes develop, for example in chronic subacromial bursitis and Achilles paratendinitis, thereby creating the risk of permanent dysfunction.

Remodelling

The process of collagen maturation continues for some weeks and months thereafter. Collagen turnover is maximal in the early stages, when linear thickening may be palpable. The orderly deposition of maturing fibres is presumably dependent upon numerous factors, not least of which are the mechanical stresses to which they are subjected. Initial deposition may be somewhat haphazard, yet improved—that is, fibres are laid down in parallel—if the healing tissue is subjected to gentle stress, and is allowed to undergo a restricted amount of normal function. Noyes *et al.* (1974) have demonstrated the increase in wound strength related to mobilization rather than immobilization. Thus early gentle mobilization after connective tissue injury is desirable, and immobilization techniques are best eschewed unless absolutely necessary.

Categorization

Injuries can be classified according to their nature or aetiology into

(1) trauma (acute)
(2) overuse (chronic).

Trauma

Traumatic incidents occur suddenly, and can be considered to be *direct* (extrinsic) or *indirect* (intrinsic) in type. Examples of the

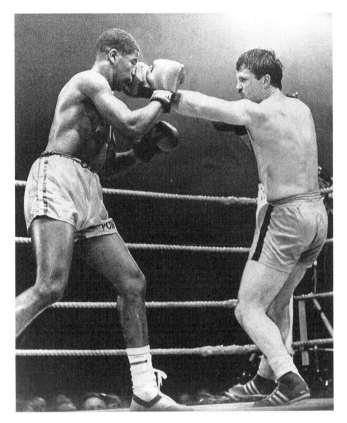

Fig. 1.6 Punching results in direct (extrinsic) trauma.

former are direct blows to the body, for instance from the force of a cricket ball or as the result of an opponent's punch in boxing (Fig. 1.6), or direct confrontations with immovable forces, for example falling heavily to the ground. Injury to either the hard (osseous) or soft tissues may occur, and may present to the attendant medical officer, general practitioner, or traumatol-

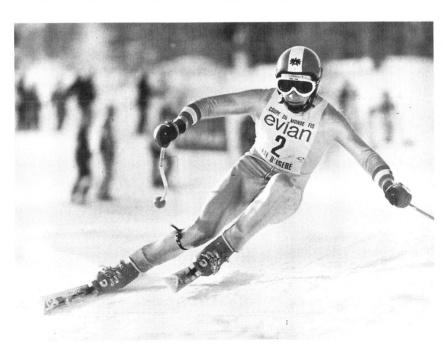

Fig. 1.7 The application of stress some distance from the injured site results in indirect (intrinsic) trauma: injury to the medial collateral ligament of the knee may occur while 'edging' during downhill skiing.

ogist in the local Accident and Emergency Department. In-depth analysis of fractures will generally not be undertaken in this book, though emphasis will be placed upon their recognition. Certain fractures—for example those to the wrist and hand—*will* be given further consideration, as early diagnosis and appropriate management, if necessary by referral for an expert opinion, are often required for good functional results.

Indirect trauma indicates the application of stress some distance from the site of injury, or not involving direct body contact (Fig. 1.7). The tissues involved may be muscular (rupture or 'pull'), tendinous (tendinitis, partial or complete rupture), ligamentous (sprain, partial or complete rupture), osseous (fracture), or cartilaginous. The latter may be further divided into injuries to articular cartilage (chondral), or to fibro- and hyaline cartilage, for example intervertebral disc injury.

Overuse

When describing the nature of overuse injury to patients an analogy may be useful. Non-biological materials, such as aeroplane wings, have a fixed stress point, and if they are subjected to a defined number of flights fatigue fracture will inevitably result. Biological materials and organisms, on the other hand, may, with carefully graded incremental increases in stress, withstand the most enormous loads—for instance the reputed forces as high as ten times body-weight in the Achilles tendon during running. Nevertheless if the application of submaximal stress has not been carefully graded, or there are adverse biomechanical stress factors, subsequent breakdown of the tissues results in *stress or overuse injury*. This may occur in any tissue, from bone (stress fracture) to bursa (chronic bursitis).

Whatever the cause or type of injury sustained, the response of the tissue is the development of inflammation. In some rheumatological conditions the causative factor is known: bacteria, uric acid, and pyrophosphate crystals for instance. Tissue breakdown products resulting from repeated microtrauma are probably responsible for inflammation in overuse injury.

Tissue injury

Muscle

The musculotendinous unit comprises a contractile element (muscle) and a non-contractile element (tendon). Muscle fibres (muscle cells) contain hundreds of thousands of myofibrils, each composed of approximately 1500 myosin filaments and twice that number of actin filaments. The myofibrils lie in parallel, and are responsible for the striated appearance of muscle: contraction results from these filaments gliding past each other.

Muscle fibres are not homogeneous; several fibre types have been identified using histochemical and physiological techniques. Red type I (slow twitch or ST) fibres are well endowed with mitochondria, and thus with oxidative enzymes: they fatigue slowly, and are found in muscles with predominantly antigravity or postural function, such as the soleus muscle. White type II (fast twitch or FT) fibres are principally anaerobic, using creatine phosphate and anaerobic glycolysis for release of energy; they fatigue quickly, and are found in muscles requiring fast propulsive activity, such as the hamstrings and gastrocnemius muscles. Further analysis reveals that some type II fibres have relatively high potentials for oxidative metabolism, and

FIG. 1.8 Myositis ossificans may result from direct (extrinsic) trauma. (a) In this instance the proximal thigh muscles have been involved. (b) In this lateral radiograph of the femur an area of myositis ossificans is well defined and contains bony trabeculae.

(a)

these are labelled type II-A; others have a relatively low content of oxidative enzymes, and are called type II-B.

In addition to being a contractile unit, muscle acts as a shock-absorbing system; this is perhaps best illustrated by the automatic flexing of the knees that absorbs the shock through the legs when landing from a jump. Loss of shock-absorbing capacity (as in fatigued muscles) predisposes to injury (Chapter 11).

Muscle is capable of storing energy when preloaded by stretching. Muscle efficiency is enhanced when eccentric contraction (preloading) precedes concentric muscle contraction; viscoelastic energy is initially stored, and then released in this process, which is known as the 'stretch-shorten cycle'. The basis of athletic performance is the reliance upon eccentric contraction, with its inherent energy-storage characteristics. Thus activities such as running, jumping, racket sports, throwing, and kicking utilize the stretch-shorten cycle. By contrast other types of exercise, such as swimming, rowing, and cycling, despite the fact that muscle groups are used rhythmically, do not have a phase of eccentric contraction; the recovery phase is passive (Shorten 1987). Storage of energy also takes place in tendon, which is a more compliant material and thereby has a much greater storage capacity. Overall the capacity for elastic energy storage is greatest in muscle groups with long tendons.

Most muscle injuries result either from an excessive sudden demand for concentric contraction following eccentric contraction, or from excessive stretch during preloading. Sometimes unexpected (external) resistance to muscle contraction—for instance, kicking the ground or an opponent instead of the ball in soccer—is a causative factor. Although injury may occur anywhere in the contractile unit, the musculotendinous junction is a common site. A relatively minor injury may be referred to as a muscle 'pull' or 'strain'; more severe injury, in which capillaries are ruptured and intramuscular bleeding occurs, is known as a 'tear' or 'rupture' (partial or complete). Predisposing factors are as follows.

(i) *Immobilization*. Following disuse there is a gross deterioration in the essential contractile and elastic properties, as well as in strength. Proprioception is also adversely affected, as the normal mechanism is to a considerable extent dependent upon normal function of the ST fibres in postural muscles. Casting is thus eschewed as a therapeutic option as far as possible.

(ii) *Muscle imbalance*. This is particularly relevant to sprinters if the hamstring-quadriceps power ratios are disturbed. As a consequence of explosive hip flexion the muscle antagonist (hamstrings) may be injured. Imbalance of the muscle components of the rotator cuff around the shoulder joint may be responsible for subacromial injury or glenohumeral instability.

(iii) *Inadequate fitness*. Poorly trained muscles are prone to early fatigue, with loss of shock absorption. Statistics reveal increased incidence of injury in the last quarter of games such as rugby football as a result of muscle fatigue. Furthermore, training prolonged into fatigue may promote muscle imbalance. Flexibility is essential for the development of viscoelastic energy, and to allow efficient biomechanical joint function.

(iv) *Inadequate warm up*. Increased temperature should be achieved by graded 'limbering up' exercises which include long

(b)

slow stretches. Amongst the effects on metabolism of raised temperature is an increased rate of muscle enzyme activity. Of additional significance in patients with established coronary artery insufficiency who undertake recreational (or therapeutic) exercise, a raised temperature delays the onset of ST depression.

'Warm down' and post-exercise stretching prevent over-rapid cooling. Removal of lactic acid is best achieved at 40–60 per cent of the previous level of activity.

Muscle may be injured by direct contusion (extrinsic trauma), or by overload when excessive tension is applied to a contracting muscle (intrinsic trauma). At a microscopic level the initial biomechanical failure may occur in the interstitial muscle collagen lattice, although this view is conjectural (Medoff 1987). Fibre disruption occurs, with associated bleeding. Torn ends contract, and the defect fills with blood, subsequently becoming a clot invaded by fibroblasts and macrophages. If a complete tear occurs, dysfunction rather than pain is the predominant feature, and bleeding extravasates into the surrounding tissues. Partial tears may create a greater problem, as the developing haematoma may be 'intramuscular' (that is, retained within an intact fascia) instead of 'extramuscular' (when it escapes through a torn fascial lining, and is revealed as subcutaneous bruising, often some distance away). An intramuscular haematoma is more painful, and results in more prolonged rehabilitation. Occasionally it becomes cystic and requires surgical drainage.

During organization the intramuscular haematoma is gradually replaced by scar tissue. Although scar tissue remains inelastic, it may contract somewhat and become surrounded by hypertrophied muscle fibres, thus reducing the residual functional disability.

One complication of a severe contusion by direct trauma is the development of myositis ossificans (Fig. 1.8). Ectopic ossification may manifest itself radiologically within ten days, the most common site being the quadriceps femoris, though it does occur elsewhere whenever muscle is deep and adjacent to underlying bone. Numerous theories have been proposed for the development of bone within muscle haematoma, including the migration of cells through damaged periosteum and crystalline calcification in necrotic tissue, leading subsequently to ossification. Whatever the cause, it appears to be a reaction by 'irritable muscle' to trauma, subsequently requiring a period of several months' rest to allow the bone to mature and contract. Of greater importance is the recognition of the risk of myositis ossificans, so that appropriate measures may be taken to prevent its onset (see Chapter 9: quadriceps injury).

Clinical assessment of muscle function involves four of the examination procedures previously described.

(i) Observation of wasting.
(ii) Passive stretching, invoked by passive movement of the joint(s) over which the muscle acts.
(iii) Resisted (isometric) contraction, thereby imparting information on muscle strength and additionally (when contraction is painful) on torn fibres. Strength may be graded 0–5 on manual testing (see Chapters 2 and 5).
(iv) Palpation—specifically for tenderness, the presence of a defect, or a swelling.

The more significant muscle tears are dealt with in individual chapters.

Following an acute incident the patient's subjective awareness of pain on movement, and the resulting relative disability, are usually effective in stimulating early rest. Reduction of bleeding

and stimulation of the repair phase are mainstays of treatment. However, there is often inadequate realization of the importance during rehabilitation of the two Ss: *stretching* the inelastic scar formation, and *strengthening* the weakened muscle unit. The main reason that muscle injuries such as hamstring tears have such a bad reputation for recurrence is that training is resumed before 100 per cent elasticity and 90 per cent of muscle strength (compared with the normal leg) have been regained. Inadequate elasticity may have pre-existed and been a primary cause of the injury; muscle imbalance (either between the ipsi- and contralateral limbs, or between the involved muscle and its antagonist) should be detected and subsequently remedied during rehabilitation. An isokinetic dynamometer is a useful tool for such assessment (see Fig. 11.11, p. 193), and for use during the later stages of rehabilitation.

Tendon

Tendons connect muscle to bone, and are composed of blocks of collagen and elastin. These collagen fibres are highly ordered; their function is to withstand the distractive force associated with muscle contraction. Tendon is able to withstand approximately half the tensile strength of cortical bone, and twice the tensile strength of the associated muscle (thus muscle ruptures are more common than tendon ruptures). The basic pathophysiological cause for breakdown is the repetitive application of tensile forces beyond the biomechanical yield strength of the tendon (Medoff 1987). Although many *tendinopathies* are the result of overuse, some injuries, such as complete or partial rupture, are acute. Even so an acute-on-chronic situation may arise. It is recognized that middle-aged sedentary males are at risk of rupturing their Achilles tendons when undertaking a sudden or unexpected burst of running; it is not always so readily appreciated that chronic stress in the experienced athlete may so undermine the tensile properties of tendon as to result in a likelihood of rupture. Sudden contraction of an already stretched musculotendinous unit may be the final provocative stress. The tensile strength of tendons may also be reduced by steroid injections, which should never be given into weightbearing tendons (see Chapter 12).

Since the musculotendinous unit acts as a united contractile structure the clinical examination procedures in tendon injury are the same as for muscle injury. Although tendon may heal with conservative measures, there are circumstances (which are identified in the text) when a surgical approach is desirable, not least to allow more accurate approximation of the ruptured ends by evacuation of haemorrhage or granulomatous tissue.

Enthesitis is the term applied to a lesion that occurs at an enthesis—i.e. the teno-osseous junction. Examples of enthesopathies are lateral epicondylitis (tennis elbow), chronic adductor longus strain, and patella tendinitis (jumper's knee) (Fig. 1.9).

A *tendinitis* is normally secondary to overuse. It may occur in a tendon that is essentially healthy in other respects, or in one in which a central or focal degenerative process has taken place. Repetitive submaximal loading leads to recurrent microtrauma in the presence of a poor blood supply. Occasionally calcium hydroxy-apatite crystals are deposited in a degenerative tendon: the resulting calcific tendinitis may be acutely painful (Fig. 1.10).

If the tendon has a sheath, a *tenosynovitis* may result from overuse: occasionally this may be crepitating, as in intersection syndrome of the forearm. If the tendon has a paratenon,

a

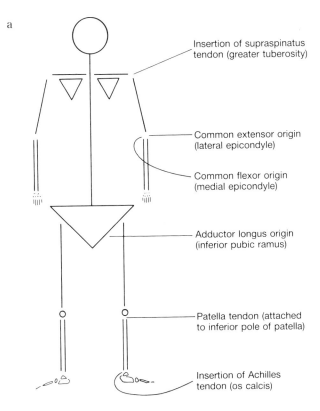

Insertion of supraspinatus tendon (greater tuberosity)

Common extensor origin (lateral epicondyle)

Common flexor origin (medial epicondyle)

Adductor longus origin (inferior pubic ramus)

Patella tendon (attached to inferior pole of patella)

Insertion of Achilles tendon (os calcis)

FIG. 1.9 The common sites of enthesopathies.

FIG. 1.10 Calcific tendinitis (of the flexor carpi radialis) may be acutely painful.

paratendinitis—for example Achilles paratendinitis—may develop secondary to an underlying tendinitis, or be caused primarily by friction from extrinsic causes. A complication is the development of chronic paratendinitis, when the paratenon becomes progressively thickened, and may require surgical excision.

Ligament

Ligaments are composed primarily (70–80 per cent) of bundles of collagen, demonstrating a greater 'weave' pattern than tendons which have a similar structure. Ligaments are the 'static' stabilizers of joints, though the presence of elastin (3–5 per cent) allows some elongation under stress. At a certain stress level—the yield point—deformation of collagen fibres becomes excessive, with the formation of microtears and the loss of previous resting length. Frank rupture then occurs. Assessment of ligamentous competence is by stress testing in various positions of the joint. The clinical aspects of ligament injuries are considered in greater detail in the relevant chapters, as they are often inadequately assessed and therefore commonly mismanaged. Important factors to appreciate following ligament injury are as follows.

1. Joint stability is created by ligaments (the primary or static stabilizers) and muscles (the dynamic stabilizers). A significant degree of ligament rupture may give rise to mechanical instability, incurring the risk of permanent functional instability—for example, ankle and knee ligament tears. Ligament injuries can be divided into three grades:

(a) sprain (grade I), in which there is no macroscopic discontinuity;

(b) partial tear (grade II), in which some degree of joint laxity secondary to ligamentous insufficiency is recognized;

(c) complete tear (grade III), in which dislocation or substantial disruption of the joint occur (Fig. 1.11).

2. The proprioceptive reflex is usually profoundly deranged as a result of disturbance to or disruption of the articular mechanoreceptors found in the joint capsules and ligaments (Wyke 1972). Specific rehabilitative exercises are required for restoration of function.

3. The capsule of the joint may be irritated, causing capsulitis or synovitis. Such a traumatic synovitis may resolve spontaneously, but it is sometimes prolonged, again requiring specific treatment.

4. Capsular disruption may occur, resulting in substantial soft-tissue bleeding and oedema.

5. Intracapsular bleeding (that is, bleeding within an intact capsule) may take place—for instance, rupture of the anterior cruciate ligament, in which situation the resulting haemarthrosis must be recognized and dealt with by aspiration or washing out so as to reduce the severely irritating effect of blood on the synovium. A haemarthrosis may be suspected when a joint swells substantially within a couple of hours of the injury. A serous effusion, on the other hand, normally takes twenty-four hours to arise, and thus is usually recognized by the patient the

Fig. 1.11 A complete (grade III) tear of the lateral ligamentous complex of the knee is demonstrated on a varus stress test.

following day. A haemarthrosis may develop in any joint; beneficial results of aspiration may be expected in such joints as the ankle, the elbow, and the interphalangeal joint of the hallux, as well as the knee. The immediate injection of steroid in appropriate dosage, once fracture or osteochondral injury has been excluded, should be considered. For aspiration it is essential to have a sound knowledge of topical anatomy.

6. Disorganization of the parallel alignment of collagen fibres and bundles in ligaments occurs after immobilization (for instance in the management of ligament tears). Akeson *et al.* (1987) have summarized the *biomechanical and biochemical* effects as follows.

Biomechanical (a) increased deformation with a standard load (greater compliance);
(b) failure at a lower load and reduced energy-absorbing capability of the immobilized bone-ligament complex (at which destruction of fibres occurs).

Biochemical (c) effects on collagen: reduced mass, increased turnover, increased degradation rate, increased synthesis, increased reducible collagen, and crosslinks.

Management strategies that are consequent upon exact diagnoses are outlined in the relevant chapters: the accepted procedure for grade I sprains is *early mobilization*, so that adequate function may be restored rapidly, often inside ten days. An important distinction in ligament injuries is between joint stability and instability, thereby determining the need for functional support during healing. The use of cast-bracing (hinged cast) techniques may be appropriate in the management of certain grade II/III lower-limb ligament injuries.

Joint

The capsular pattern

The soft tissue components of a joint are the synovium and capsule (strengthened by ligaments that have a close anatomical relationship). When a joint is injured or inflamed from whatever cause its movements are restricted, initially from involuntary muscle spasms, in a *capsular pattern*. Capsular patterns vary from one joint to another, though are identical from one person to another, and are described in the relevant chapters. The same pattern is produced by different provocative stresses—for example, synovial irritation from a haemarthrosis, rheumatological conditions such as rheumatoid arthritis, crystal arthropathies, or osteoarthrosis (OA). In some conditions, such as adhesive capsulitis of the shoulder, the restricted movements are due to capsular contracture. If the passive movements are restricted in a *non-capsular pattern* the possibility of intra-articular derangement arises; otherwise the periarticular structures are at fault.

Synovitis. A synovial reaction may be secondary to injury such as a ligament tear or a meniscus tear when it is associated with a serous effusion. Alternatively a serous effusion, accompanied by synovial thickening, may be due to a rheumatological condition. Rheumatological screening is described in Chapter 10. Synovial irritation *per se* gives rise to the capsular pattern of restriction of movement. However, if synovitis is secondary to a mechanical derangement, such as a prolapsed meniscus or an intra-articular loose body, the signs resulting from the locked joint (a non-capsular pattern) will prevail.

Osteoarthrosis (OA). Degenerative joint disease should be included in the differential diagnosis when the capsular pattern exists from the fourth decade onwards. The hips and knees are predominantly affected following years of competition in contact sports such as soccer. Although less common, OA of the upper limb joints may be secondary to previous fracture, or due to repeated joint-loading—for instance, from weight-lifting (see Fig. 4.5, p. 55).

Hypermobility

Although several terms are used in an interchangeable fashion, it is conventional to accept the following:

flexibility refers to a joint's range of motion—that is, it is principally a function of muscle/tendon tightness;

laxity refers to joint distraction and shear—that is, it is a function of ligamentous competence;

hypermobility refers to generalized joint laxity (Fig. 1.12).

Hypermobility may be associated with connective tissue disorders such as Ehlers–Danlos and Marfan's syndromes. Even with no connective tissue disorder it is clear that some individuals have an inherited joint laxity. Although, at first sight, this

FIG. 1.12 Generalized joint hypermobility is associated with an increased incidence of injury and osteoarthrosis in later life.

would appear to be beneficial in, for example, gymnastics and dance disciplines such as classical ballet, there is an increased incidence of injury and osteoarthrosis in later life (Bird *et al.* 1978; Nicholas 1970; Scott *et al.* 1979). Increased flexibility, resulting from training, may be best demonstrated by the ability to flex the spine and place the palms of the hands on the floor. Other hypermobile joints (for example, 'back-knee' and hyperextension of the elbows) would not appear to be due to training, and only result from genetic disposition or in some cases injury.

The Beighton and Horan (1970) modification of the Carter and Wilkinson (1964) index is often used (a score of 4 points or more indicates hypermobility):

1. Passive dorsiflexion of the little finger beyond 90°—2 points.
2. Passive apposition of thumbs to flexor aspects of the forearm—2 points.
3. Hyperextension of elbows beyond 10°—2 points.
4. Hyperextension of knees beyond 10°—2 points.
5. Forward flexion of the trunk with knees extended so that the palms rest flat on the floor immediately in front of the toes— 1 point.

(Total = maximum = 9 points)

Hypomobility

The majority of acute traumatic incidents of all types give rise to local (or segmental) restriction of movement of the nearest joint: differentiation into articular and periarticular (soft tissue) lesions is made by the examination routine already described. The joint-play movements (Zohn and Mennell 1976)—that is, movements that are not under control of the voluntary muscles—perform a particularly useful role in the diagnosis and rehabilitation of spinal dysfunction. Peripheral joint dysfunction—that which is secondary to trauma or immobilization, for instance—also gives rise to loss of joint play.

Subluxation and dislocation

When distortion of the alignment of the opposing joint surfaces results from stress applied to a joint, subluxation occurs. Often this is transient, though it indicates weakness of the surrounding structures or abnormal biomechanical stress and therefore may be recurrent. When gross distortion of alignment takes place dislocation occurs. This inevitably indicates rupture of the joint capsule, and possibly of the reinforcing ligaments. Apart from the sternoclavicular and acromioclavicular joints (in which reduction of subluxation and dislocations in not usually undertaken) manual relocation is necessary for a dislocated joint that does not spontaneously reduce. If ligaments have been disrupted, these must then be treated.

Bone

The application of force to a joint or limb may give rise to *osseous* injury, either at the point of impact or some distance away; hence the fractures that occur around the ankle on rotating the leg on a fixed foot, fracture of the scaphoid on forced dorsiflexion of the wrist, and fracture of the clavicle on falling on the outstretched hand. Although management of major fractures lies within the province of the orthopaedic surgeon, the simpler fractures, often not requiring fixation, are described here in the relevant chapters. Guidance is also offered concerning the timely referral of injuries, such as hand fractures, which require particularly good functional results.

In children fractures often occur at the *epiphyseal* (growth) *plate*, which is responsible for longitudinal growth of the bone, and is weaker than both ligaments and tendons. Of course, the presence of angulation suggests the presence of a fracture, possibly epiphyseal, and indicates the need for referral; the possibility of epiphyseal fracture should also be considered in the absence of significant deformity when a dislocation or even a sprain is diagnosed. Fractures involving the epiphyseal plate have been categorized into five types of Salter and Harris (1963). Separations usually heal satisfactorily unless there is vascular disturbance (for instance, at the upper femoral epiphysis, when avascular necrosis may occur). Fractures across the plate need careful assessment by an orthopaedic surgeon, as premature fusion and a shortened limb may result.

Traction injuries, sometimes termed traction osteochondroses, occur at the *apophyses*. These are a particularly common type of stress injury in the adolescent—for instance, at the tibial tubercle (Osgood–Schlatter's disease) and os calcis (Sever's disease): they result from overactivity. At some sites around the pelvis—for example, the anterior superior iliac spine, the anterior inferior iliac spine, the lesser trochanter, and the ischial tuberosity—the injury to the apophysis may be due to acute (indirect) trauma. Fracture separation of the apophysis takes place, and the injury behaves effectively as an acute muscle tear, which is its counterpart in the adult (Fig. 1.13). Rarely, a similar injury occurs at the shoulder, for example avulsion of the subscapularis attachment to the lesser tuberosity (Fig. 1.14).

Stress fractures result from the application of repetitive stress to bone. During endurance activities bone increases in strength by constant remodelling. This response to loading may become inadequate, however. Two theories are propounded. In one it is suggested that, as muscles fatigue during repeated endurance activities, the subsequent loss of shock absorption results in the application of increased stress to bone. In the other, it is thought that repeated muscle activity itself creates increased stress on

bone. Examples in weightbearing bones are commonly quoted—for example, femur, tibia, fibula, and metatarsal (Fig. 1.15; see also Fig. 10.10, p. 174). Stress fractures may also occur in non-weightbearing bones, such as the humerus in baseball pitchers and the ribs in rowers. They may also occur at epiphyseal plates—for instance, at the distal radius in gymnasts (Fig. 4.7, p. 57).

Bursa

Bursae are synovial lined sacs whose function is to reduce friction between tendon and bone, or between skin and bone. Direct, particularly repetitive, trauma may give rise to inflammation (bursitis) in the more superficial bursae—for example, olecranon bursitis, prepatellar bursitis ('beat knee'), and postcalcaneal bursitis ('pump-bump'). Alternatively, overuse of the overlying tendon (or tract) may result in a chronic bursitis due to excessive friction—for example, trochanteric bursitis and iliotibial tract syndrome. In some situations the aetiology of bursitis may be multifactorial—for instance, the effects of rotator cuff degeneration and attrition under the coracoacromial arch on the development of subacromial bursitis (see Figs. 3.7 and 3.8, p. 35). Bursae are also a common site of soft tissue inflammation in such rheumatological conditions as gout or Reiter's syndrome.

Cartilage

The articular surfaces of joints with a wide range of movement are composed of hyaline cartilage. Intervertebral discs and intra-articular menisci contain fibrocartilage. *Chondral injury* (involving articular cartilage) or *osteochondral* injury (also involving the adjacent subchondral bone) occurs after jarring or compression. Common sites are the ankle, knee, and elbow. There may be a history of acute trauma when an initial haemarthrosis (which may be unrecognized as such) is followed by recurrent pain and swelling as one articular surface impinges on another; there is a further possibility of loose body formation resulting in temporary locking of the joint (Fig. 1.16). An acute jarring injury to the ankle may cause an osteochondral fracture of the dome of the talus. During patella dislocation an osteochondral fracture involving the posterior surface of the patella is to be expected (see Fig. 10.16, p. 173). Although there is dispute over the aetiology of *osteochondritis dissecans*, this condition, which commonly occurs in the teenager, may be due to recurrent compression trauma resulting in osteochondral fragmentation and separation. Frequent compression secondary to valgus strain is responsible for osteochondritis of the capitellum at the elbow in gymnasts and baseball pitchers (see Figs. 4.3 and 4.4, pp. 52 and 54).

Articular cartilage is nourished by synovial fluid, which appears to be dependent upon joint motion for normal function. Degenerative changes, including erosions, may be seen in articular cartilage following prolonged immobilization.

Prolapse of an intervertebral disc occurs when the gelatinous nucleus pulposus herniates through a ruptured annulus. Previous stress changes will probably have already occurred at the disc, manifesting as small radial tears, so that the provocative traumatic incident may be apparently trivial or even not recorded at all ('the straw that breaks the camel's back').

Meniscus injury at the knee is considered in Chapter 7. The menisci which are present in other joints—for instance, the acromioclavicular and radiocarpal joints—may also be deranged by trauma.

FIG. 1.13 Fracture separation of the ischial apophysis in an adolescent is equivalent to a hamstring muscle tear in an adult.

FIG. 1.14 Avulsion of the subscapularis attachment to the lesser tuberosity of the humerus is shown on this teenager's X-ray.

FIG. 1.15 Stress fracture of the distal fibula: a common type of overuse injury in the leg.

Nerve

Nerve entrapment may result from overuse. Both the sensory and motor components of the larger-diameter myelinated fibres in peripheral nerves may be damaged by compression. A potentially reversible neuropraxia is the type of neuropathy found in the carpal tunnel and tarsal tunnel syndromes, in which entrapment occurs beneath an inflexible retinaculum. In other situations, such as compression of either the radial or median nerves

in the proximal forearm of weight-lifters and rowers, entrapment results from muscular hypertrophy. Alternatively, direct pressure may be responsible for such conditions as 'handlebar palsy' (compression of the ulnar nerve in Guyon's canal at the wrist) and acute compartment syndromes in the lower leg, affecting either the deep or superficial peroneal nerves. Spinal nerve roots may suffer entrapment due to HNP (herniated nucleus pulposus), from spinal canal ('bony') stenosis or from an inflammatory reaction within the spinal canal that is secondary to trauma or overuse (see Fig. 5.6, p. 84).

Aetiological factors in overuse injury

Overuse aetiological factors *must* be determined, and can be categorized as follows.

1. Inadequate training schedules:
   (a) intensity;
   (b) frequency;
   (c) overall loading;
   (d) associated physiological fitness characteristics.
2. Training surfaces, for example tarmac, tartan, flooring (sprung or otherwise), canted, uneven.
3. Equipment, for instance the suitability of footwear or protective devices.
4. Biomechanics:
   (a) technique;
   (b) joint mobility;
   (c) musculotendinous balance and adequacy;
   (d) inequality of limb length;
   (e) malalignment.
5. Growth factors in children, such as size by size rather than age by age matching in contact sports, bone-muscle length ratios.

Examples are legion, and will be described in the subsequent chapters. Liaison with parent, coach, or trainer is often necessary. Repeated reassessment may reveal clues not evident on the patient's first visit. Other evidence—derived, for example, from video recording or treadmill running—may be required. Examination of footwear or equipment, as well as the patient, is advisable. Examination of those parts of the musculoskeletal system some distance away from the injured site is mandatory; an obvious example in distance running, for instance, is the study of foot biomechanics (pronation etc.) when faced with a presentation of low back or limb pain. Finally it must be remembered that slowly progressive pain may indicate a more serious pathology. From time to time osteoid osteoma presents in a similar fashion to a stress fracture (see Fig. 10.14, p. 172); metastatic deposits may present as restriction of joint movement.

A 'philosophy'

An adequate history is important in orthopaedic and sports medicine. Cyriax taught that many diagnoses should be strongly suspected from the history alone. To balance this view it is not unusual for atypical presentations to occur—perspicacity is required. Furthermore, the subjective description of pain has little discriminative validity: behavioural responses are a better guidance. Frustratingly, in many overuse injuries there may be a paucity of physical signs; re-examination of the patient when the

FIG. 1.16 A loose body in the elbow joint may give rise to recurrent pain, swelling (effusion), and locking.

affected area is placed under stress—for instance, measurement of compartment pressures in the lower leg immediately after exercise—may be required to establish the diagnosis. More refined investigations, such as CT or MRI scanning, may be necessary.

That there is an art to learning and to the practical application of knowledge is not an original concept. However, it is as applicable to assessment of sports injuries as it is in other fields. Just as the medical student attempting final MB understands the need for a sound written and practical examination technique to provide the examiner with evidence of his clarity of thought, so the practising physician requires the logical application of functional anatomy and biomechanics (allied to sports techniques) for the purpose of correct diagnosis and management. All too often these basic principles are forgotten. When the physician is faced with a history of localized pain, 'hands-on' palpatory techniques in the painful area are too often and too rapidly employed without due attention either to history (the patient often supplies both diagnosis and aetiological factors if given the chance) or to the functioning both of the structure containing the lesion and of the musculoskeletal system adjacent to the lesion. Using by way of illustration the distribution of C5 pain, this is felt in the upper arm, particularly in the region of the deltoid insertion, and often radiates to the radial border of the wrist. Deltoid lesions may be incorrectly diagnosed (they are extremely rare), and useless injections given to the site of the pain. However, functional assessment of the cervical spine and shoulder will reveal the real *site* of the lesion, which may be found, for instance, in the neck, causing nerve-root pressure, or in the shoulder joint, causing referred C5 dermatomal pain. Given the opportunity, the patient may recall the neck stiffness and pain which had been temporarily forgotten when the presentation was of persistent arm pain. The pathological lesion may then be treated appropriately.

Furthermore, problem solving should relate to the likely sequelae if an injury should be misdiagnosed or mistreated. The simple (stable) ankle sprain, involving the lateral collateral ligament of the ankle, may give rise to greater problems from an overcautious approach that incorporates immobilization, thus increasing proprioceptive deficit, than from early mobilization; a discriminating functional assessment is a prerequisite (see Chapter 8). Although functional stability, provided by external or internal splintage, is required when acute bony or ligamentous instability is identified, early joint mobilization is still desirable. Bone has an excellent blood supply and therefore may be expected to heal well. However, management of the less well-vascularized soft tissues, particularly ligaments and tendons, requires sensitive judgement. The capsule, articular cartilage, and surrounding muscle react adversely to immobilization, while ligament requires suitable apposition if ruptured. Ligament heals in a more physiological fashion—that is, with parallel rather than haphazard collagen deposition—if the joint is allowed some degree of natural movement *during* healing: hence the frequent reference to cast-bracing techniques for the weightbearing joints of the lower limbs. In this way muscle tone and articular cartilage nutrition are also maintained.

Overall, whatever tissue has been damaged, the desired primary objective is restoration of normal joint function.

The responsibility of the sports physician in advising and assessing potential participants in different sporting activities receives special attention in subsequent chapters. The popularity of certain endurance activities practised for aerobic fitness, such as long-distance running, is directly proportional to the incidence of overuse injury. The injuries sustained, however, are usually only temporarily disabling, and as far as is known do not appear to cause those degenerative joint conditions in the lower limb associated with years of participation in sports, such as soccer, which involve greater shearing forces. Endurance events such as marathon runs and competitive squash games place substantial demands on competitors' cardiovascular and other physiological resources: screening procedures, although considered contentious because of their time-consuming and often financially unrewarding nature, should be invoked whenever possible. Furthermore, sports physicians, in conjunction with sports associations, should be prepared to advise individuals and sports clubs on the inherent dangers relating to their particular sport. This responsibility extends to the provision of suitable first-aid facilities, and early management of injury advice to teachers, coaches, and trainers (see Chapter 13).

Prevention of injury is a major topic, which is explored in detail in Chapter 11.

References

Akeson, W. H., Amiel, D., Abel, M. F., Garfin, S. R., and Woo, S. L. Y. (1987). Effects of immobilisation on joints. *Clin. Orthop. Relat. Res.,* **219** (June), 28–37.

Anderson, N. H. and Ramwell, P. W. (1974). Biological aspects of prostaglandins. *Arch. Intern. Med.,* **133**, 30–50.

Beighton, P. H. and Horan, F. T. (1970). Dominant inheritance of familial generalised articular hypermobility. *J. Bone Jt. Surg.,* **52B**, 145–7.

Bird, H. A., Tribe, C. R., and Bacon, P. A. (1978). Joint hypermobility leading to osteoarthrosis and chondrocalcinosis. *Ann. Rheum. Dis.,* **37**, 203–11.

Carter, C. and Wilkinson, J. (1964). Persistent joint laxity and congenital dislocation of the hip. *J. Bone Jt. Surg.,* **46B**, 40–5.

Cyriax, J. (1982). *Textbook of orthopaedic medicine* Vol. I: *Diagnosis of soft tissue lesions* (8th edn). Baillière Tindall, London.

Dyson, M. (1987). Mechanisms involved in therapeutic ultrasound. *Physiotherapy,* **73(3)**, 116–20.

Medoff, R. J. (1987). Soft tissue healing. *Ann. Sports Med.,* **3(2)**, 67–70.

Nicholas, J. A. (1970). Injuries to knee ligaments, *J. Am. Med. Assoc.,* **212**, 2236–9.

Noyes, F. R., Torvik, P. J., Hyde, W. B. *et al.* (1974). Biomechanics of ligament failure II. An analysis of immobilisation, exercise and reconditioning effects in primates. *J. Bone Jt. Surg.,* **56A**, 1406–18.

Salter, R. B. and Harris, R. (1963). Injuries involving the epiphyseal plate. *J. Bone Jt. Surg.,* **45A**, 587–622.

Scott, D., Bird, H. A., and Wright, V. (1979). Joint laxity leading to osteoarthrosis. *Rheum. Rehabil.,* **18**, 167–9.

Shorten, M. (1987). Muscle elasticity and human performance. In *Medicine and sports science,* Vol. 25, *Current research in sports biomechanics,* pp. 1–18. Karger, Basel.

Wyke, B. (1972). Articular neurology—a review. *Physiotherapy,* **58(3)**, 94–9.

Zohn, D. A. and Mennell, J. McM. (1976). *Diagnosis and physical treatment: musculoskeletal pain.* Little, Brown, Boston, MA.

2 Head injuries

J. L. FIRTH AND N. R. GALLOWAY

Intracranial injuries

J. L. FIRTH

With the exception of pugilism, head injury is not an intended objective in sport. Indeed, as man is his brain, deliberate brain injury cannot reasonably be described as 'sport'. Head injury in sport is therefore both unnecessary and unacceptable. A primary objective in sport must be to eliminate or minimize the opportunities for head injury. To achieve this requires an understanding of its nature.

Head injury mechanisms

Head injury may be defined as the injurious application of energy to the head. The key factor in head injury is brain injury. Brain injury requires the injurious transfer of that energy from head to brain. The three common mechanisms are head penetration, deformation, and acceleration.

Penetration

Penetration of the skull by missiles or sharp objects causes laceration of the meninges that cover the brain and the brain itself, together with their blood vessels.

Deformation

Deformation of the skull by compression, causing injury or mechanical distortion, distorts the brain itself and causes skull fracture and meningeal tears. Skull fractures may be 'undisplaced' or 'depressed'—bone being driven into the head, reducing the overall intracranial volume and producing local brain and meningeal disruption, with potential laceration of meningeal and cerebral or cerebellar blood vessels and laceration/obstruction of the intradural venous sinuses. Tearing of these vessels leads to haemorrhage and blood clot formation between the dura and the skull (extradural haematoma). Such bleeding can cause a significant space-occupying lesion—a large expanding intracranial mass (see Fig. 10.21, p. 176). Haematomas produce local cerebral distortion and displacement, as well as an overall rise in intracranial pressure. Brain distortion, displacement, and raised intracranial pressure (RICP) disturb cerebral blood flow. The consequent increase in local cerebral blood flow is due to loss of auto-regulation in the cerebral terminal arterioles—the phenomenon of auto-regulatory failure or 'vasoparesis' (Sheinker 1944; Langfitt et al. 1968;

Bruce et al. 1981). The result is an additional local or generalized brain swelling. This brain swelling compounds the effect of space-occupying haematoma, and increases brain shift—either from one side of the head to the other, or through the tentorial hiatus between the supratentorial compartment and the posterior fossa, or in posterior fossa clots, displacing cerebellum and brain stem up through the tentorial hiatus. The medulla and cerebellar tonsils may themselves be displaced down through the foramen magnum. Brain shift through the tentorial hiatus or foramen magnum produces the post-mortem appearance of 'coning' (Robbins et al. 1984). Coning leads to a rapid deterioration of conscious level, and death. Coning of the medulla through the foramen magnum is associated with acute respiratory failure and death, often with little prior warning.

The amount of energy required to fracture the skull and set in train these series of events is less than that required to produce unconsciousness (Gurdjian et al. 1950). In sport, therefore, a loss of consciousness associated with a head injury, of however brief a period, must be taken to indicate a head injury severe enough to lead to meningeal rupture, haematoma formation, brain swelling, and secondary deterioration, which may rapidly lead to death. In the classical head injury prototype, a lateral skull fracture tears middle meningeal vessels. An early recovery is made. The individual's conscious level improves, only to deteriorate later as brain swelling compounds growing space-occupying clots to produce raised intra-cranial pressure, cerebral distortion, brain-stem shift, and coning. Therefore, an individual who has been knocked out must be considered at risk until proved otherwise. One cannot determine at play or on the sports field whether or not such a fatal train of events has begun. The occurrence of unconsciousness has to be recognized and taken seriously. It requires at least careful observation in an establishment where the appropriate management can be provided immediately and effectively should secondary deterioration occur.

Acceleration

Acceleration is still poorly understood. Debate on its effects has raged since the Paris Academy of 1766. This confusion is compounded by the fact that acceleration exerts its effects by a series of further subsidiary mechanisms:

(1) bridging vessel disruption;

(2) shear;
(3) cavitation.

The brain floats like a gelatinous mushroom in the cerebrospinal fluid (CSF) within the skull. It is imperfectly anchored by arachnoidal ligaments, which traverse the subarachnoid space between arachnoid and pia mater. This anchoring is more marked at the skull base, and allows considerable freedom of movement both to the cerebral hemispheres and along its long axis, within the brain stem.

The injurious force available in any one situation reflects the general equation:

$$F = ma$$

In sport, mass is commonly the head itself and acceleration is the rate of change in velocity of the head—as in violent deceleration of the head on impact. Speed is less important than acceleration. Low speed, immediately halted by impact on a hard surface, will occasion more acceleration than progressive deceleration from high speed in an individual riding in a motor vehicle with a properly arranged safety harness and helmet.

Bridging vessel disruption

Aberrant vessels frequently run from the surface of the cerebral hemispheres to the overlying arachnoid and dura, bridging the subarachnoid and subdural spaces. These vessels may be arteries or veins. They are firmly anchored superficially to the dura, and fixed thereby to the inside of the skull. Their other end is on the surface of the brain. Sudden movement or acceleration of the head induces a differential motion between the skull and the mobile jelly-like brain within. A critical vector which may not cause unconsciousness can rupture such a vessel, usually at its dural end. Rapid bleeding from it causes a space-occupying clot (haematoma) between overlying dura and the brain, exploiting and spreading along the subdural space as a subdural haematoma. Its expansion is easy and rapid. Unlike extradural haematoma, which, to expand, has to strip the tough dura off the inside of the skull, a subdural haematoma can develop very rapidly, and may follow apparently trivial head injury. This injury is then followed by early rapid deterioration into coma and death. Subdural haematomas are more common in the elderly, but may occur at any age and are a plague of boxing. Their associated mortality is very high, owing to their rapid development which leaves little time for their surgical evacuation. The speed of development is compounded by local disturbance of cerebral blood flow and secondary brain swelling. In posterior fossa clots, hydrocephalus is a further hazard owing to obstruction of the circulation of the CSF by distortion of the aqueduct caused by upward displacement of the midbrain. This mortality is all the more regrettable, as the management of such haematoma is relatively simple. However, success depends upon prompt intervention before irreversible brain infarction has occurred. Such simple but rapid surgical intervention is rarely available, especially when the victim's attendants are lulled into a false sense of security by an early improvement in conscious level or the minimal disturbance caused by the initial injury.

Bridging vessel disruption may also be a problem in the brain stem. Under acceleration along its long axis, the brain stem acts like a column of gelatin. Head acceleration is transferred to the outside of the brain stem and its central core lags behind. Eventually the core is accelerated, and when the outer aspects of the stem are halted with the rest of the head, the centre continues to surge along the axis of acceleration producing the phenomenon of brain-stem 'sleeving' (Lindgren 1966). The effect is to pull the long perforating vessels of the brain stem and pons with arise from the basilar artery from their capillary beds in the floor of the fourth ventricle. Multiple punctuate brain-stem haemorrhages occur. These are not invariably fatal. They give rise to a great variety of subjective symptoms, sometimes with little by way of objective signs—a component of the 'post-traumatic syndrome'.

Shear

Shear is well described by Holbourn (1943) and Stritch (1956, 1961, 1969). As a gelatinous structure under acceleration, the brain's structural complexity induces differential movement, and thereby shear, within the brain itself. The shearing forces so induced disrupt both nerve cell axons (the cells' long processes running within and to and from brain and spinal cord), small blood vessels, and dendrites, the multitude of fine connections between adjacent nerve cells which bristle out from each nerve-cell body. The resulting disruption can have a catastrophic effect on brain function, with little apparent macroscopic (naked-eye) damage. This is a common finding in multiple repeated head injury—the 'punch-drunk' traumatic encephalopathy of boxing or the 'lame brain' jockey of former days, before the wearing of effective head protection (the British Standard Institution's BS 4472 specification) became mandatory under Jockey Club rules.

Cavitation

Under acceleration applied to the head, the brain lags behind the skull. It behaves much as coffee in a cup when the cup is struck against a wall. Like the skull, the cup comes to an abrupt halt, but the coffee flows on, and rising pressure subjacent to the impact site within the coffee causing it to rise up the side of the cup. The rising fluid reflects the increased pressure available under the impact point. At the other side of the cup the coffee level falls as the coffee flows away to the impact side. Oscillation to and fro then follows. In the intact head there is a sharp increase in local pressure under the impact point, producing a local percussion injury to the brain. This may just bruise (contuse), or actually disrupt, the brain substance. At the opposite side of the head, pressure falls acutely as the brain moves away. Pressure may fall below the tissue vapour pressure of gases in solution in the intracellular fluid in brain cells, in the extracellular space (between brain cells and their blood vessels), and within the blood vessels themselves. If the pressure becomes sufficiently low, bubble formation occurs, producing an explosive local decompressive lesion—the phenomenon of 'cavitation'.

As a result, in any one impact injury, acceleration can cause two severe injuries: one under the impact site (the French 'coup' = 'blow') and the other at the opposite side of the head (the 'contre-coup'). In practice a blow to the front of the head produces an impact, and percussion injury to the frontal poles of the brain and the tips of its temporal lobes. The fall in pressure at the back of the head is lessened by the ability of CSF to move up through the foramen magnum from the distensible subarachnoid space. The spinal dura covering the spinal cord is capable of expansion and contraction within the spinal canal, unlike the dura in the head which is firmly attached to the inner surface of the skull. Frontal impacts therefore produce frontal injury. Indeed, brain substance may be blown down the nose, to appear as white material at the nostrils. Conversely, occipital impact injury produces less of a percussion effect under the impact point, owing to the same ability of CSF to run out of the head through the foramen magnum, but the contre-coup cavitation effect on frontal and temporal poles may be devastating. Therefore both frontal and occipital impacts produce frontal devastation. Temporal blows—blows to the side of the head—not only involve the thinnest and most easily fractured part of the skull, with enhanced risk of haematoma formation from tearing of the underlying middle meningeal arteries, but also ensure both impact coup and cavitating contre-coup injury—injury to both sides of the brain in lateral impact. Any head injury may involve one, some, or all of these primary mechanisms in any combination.

Secondary complications

To these primary insults are added secondary complications. The first of these is the formation within the head of the space-occupying clots (haematomas) mentioned above. Bleeding may be extra-dural, subdural, or occur into bruised or cavitated and disrupted brain to form an intracerebral or intracerebellar haematoma. These haematomas may be above or below the tent—the latter in the posterior fossa. Initial injury is then secondarily complicated by the development of an intracranial space-occupying clot. This produces a generalized rise in intracranial pressure, as well as focal brain distortion and shift.

As if this is not enough, the normal auto-regulation of cerebral blood flow by terminal arterioles may be acutely abolished at impact or by brain compression or distortion. Auto-regulation, in normal brain, maintains a steady cerebral blood flow through each capillary bed, despite widely varying changes in systemic blood pressure. This mechanism, by controlling blood flow, controls cerebral blood volume and thereby the bulk of the brain. Teleologically it should be the most hardy of all physiological mechanisms. Unfortunately, one of the many fatal basic flaws in human design is that auto-regulation is easily abolished by any brain insult—including head injury. The resulting failure or loss of cerebral auto-regulation (vasoporesis) (Langfitt *et al.* 1968), is the cause of the brain swelling which complicates intracranial haematoma. More often it is a major post-traumatic complication in its own right.

Only one in three of those who die of head injuries have a space-occupying intracranial haematoma (Miller 1979). Many of the remainder die of raised intracranial pressure produced by the brain swelling, which itself is caused by vasoparesis—the loss of cerebrovascular auto-regulation. Brain swelling alone can produce a disastrous generalized rise in intracranial pressure, as well as brain shift by focal local brain swelling. In vasoparesis the loss of auto-regulation occurs at the terminal arterioles—the last arteries immediately before the capillary beds of the cerebral micro-circulation. It is a local mechanism, and therefore its failure does not necessarily involve the whole brain at one time. One or several parts of the brain may be rendered vasoparetic whilst others are still auto-regulating. This differential involvement produces irregular swelling, brain distortion, and shift. This brain swelling can be controlled, if caught early enough, by manipulating the other mechanisms which control cerebral blood flow—notably the carbon dioxide response. This requires ventilation—either immediately by mouth-to-mouth respiration, or subsequently by intubation and mechanical ventilation. While this is one purpose of an intensive care unit, the individual does not have to wait until he or she arrives at such a unit for cerebral blood flow (CBF) control to be instituted. CBF can be started immediately by mouth-to-mouth ventilation at the injury site. This in its turn means that effective cardiopulmonary

resuscitation should be available and practised at any sports site where head injury may occur. This may mean no more than basic training in resuscitation for coaches, linesmen, umpires, officials, etc, but such simple expertise should be available on any and every organized sporting occasion. The value of these precautions may be enhanced when immediate 'impact epilepsy' occurs, or an early post-traumatic seizure ensues. The latter can be fatal if the airway is not secured, but is self-limiting and recoverable if the airway is maintained.

Tertiary lesions

A further series of complications provide 'tertiary effects of head injury'. They may be early or late. They include acute hydrocephalus in posterior fossa lesions, epilepsy in cerebral contusion and haematoma, CSF leakage in basal skull fractures with later infection, meningitis, late post-traumatic hydrocephalus, and the phenomenon of post-traumatic encephalopathy.

Hydrocephalus

Acute hydrocephalus may complicate posterior fossa haematomata. The CSF circulation is obstructed at the level of the tent by distortion of the aqueduct within the brain stem. Expansion of the supratentorial, lateral, and third ventricles ensues, to add a symmetrical downward thrust through the tentorial hiatus to compound the local posterior fossa effects of brain-stem compression and enhance the likelihood of coning of medulla and cerebellar tonsils down through the foramen magnum (Robbins *et al.* 1984). Late post-traumatic hydrocephalus is outside the scope of this book, but is a cause of unexpected late deterioration in an individual already recovering from head injury, or of unexplained failure to recover. It should be considered in late failure to improve or late deterioration, once progressive recovery has been established.

Post-traumatic leakage of CSF from nose (CSF rhinorrhoea), ears (CSF otorrhoea), or through an open head wound carries with it the risk of bacterial contamination and infection of the central nervous system. Early post-traumatic management requires the re-establishment of the continuity of dura and scalp, to isolate the brain and limit the opportunity for post-traumatic infection. Immediate or early CSF rhinorrhoea commonly settles in ten days. If not, then neurosurgical closure is indicated. Later or recurrent leakage usually requires formal closure.

Post-traumatic epilepsy

Post-traumatic epilepsy may be considered as one of the following.

(i) 'Immediate' impact epilepsy: the immediate appearance of seizure-like movements on head impact. These do not carry with them a significant risk of later post-traumatic epilepsy.

(ii) 'Early' post-traumatic epilepsy—at any time immediately following impact or during the first week following injury. Such early epilepsy carries with it a 25 per cent chance of later post-traumatic epilepsy.

(iii) 'Late' post-traumatic epilepsy: epilepsy related to a head injury but occurring more than one week from insult. This is similar to late-onset epilepsy. It implies a risk of recurrence of further seizure of at least 16 per cent, and potentially an up to 65 per cent risk of a long-term epileptic problem. The risks of the occurrence of such late post-traumatic epilepsy are increased by several risk factors associated with the head injury itself.

1. Early epilepsy (25 per cent late epilepsy, as above).
2. Clinically significant intracranial haematoma (30 per cent).
3. Depressed skull fracture (4–64 per cent). The range of effects of depressed skull fracture are determined by the influence of further factors—the occurrence of early epilepsy, focal cerebral hemispheric signs, a demonstrated dural tear, and a post-traumatic amnesic interval of more than 24 hours (Jennett 1975).

Post-traumatic encephalopathy

The term 'post-traumatic encephalopathy' covers a number of states. Strictly, it is a post-mortem pathological diagnosis, and the result of multiple repeated head injuries with widespread shear damage. Clinically it is an alternative term to 'punch-drunkenness' in boxers and the 'lame brain' once seen in professional jockeys. It is also used to describe incomplete recovery from severe injury. Each case needs careful evaluation to exclude a remediable cause, of which post-traumatic hydrocephaly, due to the late CSF resorption block at the arachnoidal level or basal cistern occlusion, is amenable to CSF diversion or 'shunting'.

Prevention

This litany of potential disaster emphasizes the first law of head injury—'Prevention is better than cure'. All sports disciplines need to review their practice continuously, to define the present incidence and risk of head injury, and to develop their sports either to exclude or to minimize these risks. However, accidents may still happen despite every best endeavour.

The second law of head injury is 'If you can't prevent, protect'. The place of head protection should be carefully reviewed, and appropriate head protection worn at all times when the individual is at risk. A light-hearted attitude to head injury is inappropriate in today's world, where all have to live by their brains. Likewise, an irresponsible attitude to prevention and protection is likely to attract the attention of lawyers well versed in exacting punitive damages from those who ignore simple precautions.

Protection

Major strides are being made in head protection. Where a discipline is such that head injury remains a major hazard then full advantage should be taken of present progress—such as the wearing of protective helmets to the British Standards Institution's specifications (BSI 1986, 1988). No specifications are perfect, but they reflect the state of the art and are therefore the minimum acceptable in sporting disciplines. In sport no head injury is necessary; all head injury is potentially preventable, and therefore any head injury is unacceptable. To be effective, protective helmets have to form one unit with the head and skull at impact. Any relative motion between helmet and head may exacerbate injury and degrade the helmet's protective performance. Most helmets have an outer shape to give them aesthetic appeal—either 'hide' or 'silk'. Within this is a hard smooth shell to prevent skull penetration and deformation, and to assist the sliding of the head along surfaces so as to extend the period of deceleration. Within this 'shell' is an energy-burning or acceleration–attenuating lining—either an air gap, or some 'buffer' material which dissipates energy as it deforms. The air gap is a time-honoured solution to the requirement for energy dissipation, but it depends for its effectiveness on a very precise relationship between head and shell, with accurate separation of both by a critical margin. This must be checked every time that the hat is put on. Buffer materials act by absorbing energy in their own progressive deformation or destruction. They have made possible major improvements in helmet performance. But once deformed the buffer is destroyed, and the helmet has to be replaced as it will no longer protect if subjected to a further insult. Within the buffer or air-gap zone is the 'harness', 'cradle', or suspension, which provides the junction between head and helmet. It has to fit snugly, firmly, comfortably, and coolly, and to be retained in place under any acceleration and impact. It must not be displaced axially or in pitch, roll, or yaw. To maintain position under acceleration usually requires a four-point fixation system, with a chin-strap stabilized forwards and backwards in the sagittal plane by two points on either side of the head—four in all. A simple two-point chin-strap, even in complex 'full-face' helmets, may allow helmet loss or separation when the head is pitched forwards.

The basic requirements for helmet systems are that they should be:

(1) aesthetically attractive, so that all will want to wear them;
(2) mechanically and dynamically effective;
(3) comfortable and of light weight;
(4) easily, effectively, and conveniently secured, removed, and stored;
(5) not liable to exacerbate other injury, for instance to the cervical spine, or to introduce new hazards of their own (Firth 1985).

That these criteria can be met was demonstrated in the commercial introduction of motor cycle 'space helmets'. The success of this basic design as a fashion object can and should be emulated in other sporting disciplines where head protection is appropriate, particularly in horse-riding. Any protective device should comply with the appropriate British Standards Institution's specification to ensure minimum performance (BSI 1985, 1986, 1988).

Management strategies

The First Law is to PREVENT. If this fails: the Second Law is to PROTECT. If this also fails, the Third Law is to PREPARE: that is by PRUDENT PREPARATION, APPROPRIATE ASSESSMENT, and with SUFFICIENT SUSPICION of the potential for disaster posed by each head injury. Then careful management can minimize or exclude the secondary and later effects of the head injury.

In effect, the Third Law of head injury is 'Prepare for the worst'.

Having failed to prevent the head injury and to protect the brain, initial assessment is the basis for subsequent successful management. A problem is the infinite combination of mechanisms available in head injury—and therefore the variety of head injury presentation and development. Hippocrates noted the poor correlation between initial injury and outcome. A trivial injury can kill. A severe initial insult should not guarantee a poor outcome—given good management.

Head injury severity

Though head injury is very common, happily serious head injury is less so. A practical problem may exist immediately following a head injury in assessing its significance. 'Significance' is best considered as the transfer of sufficient energy from head to brain to occasion brain injury. A significant brain injury is indicated by any acute trauma-related neurological symptom or sign. A head injury must therefore be considered 'serious' if sufficient energy is transferred to the brain to render that individual unconscious, even if only momentarily. To be conscious requires the satisfactory function of all parts of the brain. An alteration in conscious level is the best indication of a significant disturbance of the brain. *An alteration of consciousness, however transient, has to be recognized as indicating serious brain insult.* That degree of insult is sufficient to cause auto-regulatory failure (vasoparesis) with brain swelling. Likewise the energy required to render an individual unconscious is less than that required to fracture the skull. The occurrence of unconsciousness carries with it the possibility of the subsequent development of an intracranial haematoma and all that that entails. The period of unconsciousness is accompanied by a longer period of amnesia—both before and after the injury (the pre- and post-traumatic amnesic intervals). The latter is considered to extend until the continuous return of memory, and may later be used to assess further the degree of brain insult. Pre-traumatic amnesia of up to ten minutes is commonplace. Longer than this probably indicates structural damage.

Basic assessment

Neck and spinal injury are commonly associated. Assessment is best made of the whole nervous system. As in all medicine, subsequent successful management depends on initial assessment—which in its turn is based on the following:

(1) history;
(2) signs.

In practice the *history* may have to be brief, and expanded later. However brief, one needs to determine the following:

(1) circumstance and detail of injury;
(2) potential for head penetration, deformation, and acceleration, together with that for an associated neck or spinal injury;
(3) unconsciousness, present or recovered from?
(4) occurrence of neurological symptoms or signs, including arms and legs.

The *immediate needs* are as follows.
(A) Airway—to get or keep it clear.
(B) Breathing—present and adequate; otherwise commence mouth-to-mouth ventilation.
(C) Circulation:
  (i)   lie flat with head/neck/spine moved in one and stabilized;
  (ii) stop bleeding points;
  (iii) external cardiac massage if adequate circulation is not demonstrated (with the patient flat cerebral circulation is likely to be adequate if there is a good carotid, radial, or femoral pulse, provided that venous outflow from the head is not obstructed).

Whilst achieving ABC one can define the VITAL SIGNS, which are the objective basis of the continuing assessment of the victim's progress.

Vital signs

The vital signs comprise the following.

I. *Conscious level*, assessed as response to conversation and pain, is the cardinal and most important sign of all (Fig. 2.1).

II. *'Hiatal signs'*—pupil equality, size, and reactivity; pulse and blood pressure; respiratory rate and rhythm; temperature. One or more of these signs changes with disturbance at the tentorial hiatus. This is the 'Piccadilly Circus' at the centre of the head. The first pupil to enlarge is usually on the same side as the clot large enough to cause a cone. Any major brain shift at the tentorial hiatus will be reflected in a change in one or more of these signs. Like conscious level, they are 'harbingers of mischief' within the head.

	Conversation	Pain
I	Normal	✓
II	Passive	✓
III	Shout	✓
IV	Nil	✓
V	Nil	Nil

FIG. 2.1 The indicators of conscious level.

III. *Long tract signs.* These are the ability of the individual to move hands, feet, arms, and legs, and his or her ability to appreciate light touch, pinprick, and joint-position sense throughout the body. These senses will be present or absent, and may change in both head and spinal injury. Like conscious level, their establishment is fundamental to the management of head and spinal injury. Motor power is best expressed in the MRC (Medical ·Research Council) scale (5 = normal, 4 = not normal but strong, 3 = can move against gravity, 2 = good movement but not strong enough to move against gravity, 1 = just detectable movement, 0 = no movement whatsoever) (Fig. 2.2). Neurological examination is also described in the chapter on spinal injury.

MRC Power Scale:

5. Normal

4. Strong, not normal

3. Against gravity

2. Good

1. Detectable

0. Nil.

FIG. 2.2 Motor signs in head injury: the MRC power scale.

Risk status

As head injury is so common, it is essential to assess, on the spot, the risk to an individual of later danger. This may or may not be obvious at this stage. At the very least, the patient should be carefully observed and managed as at risk if an alteration of consciousness has occurred or subjective symptoms or objective signs have been noted. *To continue to exercise after being knocked out is foolhardy.* It is the best way to swell a vasoparetic brain, and accelerate intracranial haemorrhage and haematoma formation.

If the head injury is not so serious as to warrant instant intervention, the medical attendant has to establish the risk of secondary complication in that individual. This will determine subsequent management. A period of observation is required. If conscious level is defined in terms of response to conversation and to pain, then a simple grading system can be constructed which can be used to demonstrate change, whether as improvement or as deterioration (Fig. 2.3). Under observation, every head injury falls into one of seven groups (Fig. 2.4).

Group 1 have not been knocked out.

Group II were unconscious, but make a rapid recovery, and are normal by the time that they are assessed on a second occasion.

Group III have impaired consciousness, but are undoubtedly improving at the time of that second assessment.

Response

Normal
    Passive
        Shout
            Pain
                Nil
CL

FIG. 2.3 A response scale against which to monitor changes in conscious level

RISK	STATUS	HEAD INJURY	SEEN	COMMENT
I	CL			Not knocked out
II				Knocked out but now well
III				Undoubted spontaneous progress
IV		At risk		Conscious level obscured or at risk
V		Static		No progress
VI				Deteriorating
VII		Resuscitate		

FIG. 2.4 Head injury groups in terms of changes in conscious level between two observations separated in time.

Groups II and III need observation to ensure that improvement is maintained and that subsequent, secondary deterioration does not occur.

Group IV require careful surveillance of neurological function, because assessment of neurological status is made difficult by other systemic injuries or epilepsy.

Group V remain static. They should be improving, which is the natural history of head injury. No improvement means intracranial clot formation, brain swelling, or both.

In *Group VI* undoubted deterioration, or initial improvement and then secondary deterioration, is occurring.

In *Group VII* the individual has had to be resuscitated following head injury. Generalized 'whole-brain' vasoparesis can be presumed.

Groups V–VII require the exclusion or removal of intracranial space-occupying haematomata, and the determined management of cerebral swelling—effectively neurosurgical management.

Of the more complex grading systems of conscious level assessment the Glasgow Coma Scale (Teasdale and Jennett 1974) is best known (Fig. 2.5). This depends on the assessment of eye opening, response to conversation, and best movement or motor function to provide a numerical score. Immediate scoring is very helpful for later assessment. After two or three days the Glasgow Coma Score gives a reasonable indication of later prognosis. However, an immediate score is no indication of improvement or deterioration. To establish a trend requires a second assessment after a period of time, though this can be short. In difficult circumstances, the simpler the assessment of conscious level the better, and that based on conversation and pain is commended, as it is easily established, readily recorded, and simply explained. Therefore conscious level should be established and recorded immediately following injury, and repeated at frequent intervals. Improvement or deterioration can then be clearly defined and provide the best basis for the individual's further management—whether to do no more than observe or to institute the full panoply of modern neurosurgical intensive care. If the Glasgow Coma Score can be recorded *together with* conscious level and vital signs, so much the better.

Associated injuries

Head and spinal injuries are commonly associated. Because the head is mounted on the neck, spinal injury must be presumed in all head injury until proved otherwise. The exclusion of spinal injury may be difficult, and requires careful clinical and radiological assessment in hospital. Spinal column injury is common in many sports. If disruption or distortion of the bony spine occurs, then injurious transfer of energy to the spinal cord can follow. The protection provided by the bony spine provides a high threshold for injury, which has to be exceeded to produce spinal cord injury. When that threshold is exceeded any excess can cause devastating spinal cord injury. The initial spinal cord injury may not be complete, but, once it has occurred, the cord is at risk in the destabilized spine. The spinal cord is unprotected from further spinal movement. One-third of spinal cord injuries are complete and irrecoverable from the moment of injury, but two-thirds are not and can recover if further damage is avoided. Therefore the greatest care has to be taken in moving, observing, and transporting head and spinal injuries because of the high probability of

	Eye opening (E)	Verbal response (V)	Best Motor Response (M)
1.	None	None	None
2.	To PAIN	Incomprehensible SOUNDS	EXTENSION
3.	To SPEECH	Inappropriate WORDS	Abnormal FLEXION
4.	Spontaneous	Confused CONVERSATION	Withdrawal
5.	-	Orientated	Localizes
6.	-	-	Obeys

FIG. 2.5 The Glasgow Coma Scale (Teasdale and Jennett 1974) for assessing conscious level.

causing further spinal cord insult by the injudicious or thoughtless distortion of the unstable neck or distal spine. In addition to the disturbance or abolition of motor and sensory function in limbs and trunk, spinal cord injury also affects the sympathetic nervous system at and below the level of injury. The sympathetic pathways maintain blood pressure by control of peripheral vascular resistance. Therefore cervical and dorsal spinal cord injury may deprive the individual of the ability to maintain the systemic blood pressure. A fall in blood pressure will be even more disastrous where the brain and/or spinal cord has been rendered vasoparetic by injury. The injured brain and spinal cord vasculature will not compensate for fluctuations in systemic blood pressure. Further cord insult is that much more likely if the blood pressure is allowed to fall, or the individual is sat up or stood up following head or spinal cord injury. Head and spinal injury are best managed with the patient horizontal, the airway clear, and breathing and circulation maintained.

Children are at particular risk from combined head and spinal complications. The anatomy of the paediatric cervical spine, its natural pliancy, and the carriage of a large head on a relatively small body, coupled with inexperience, poor balance, and, often, reckless enthusiasm mean that apparently minor injuries can occasion cord insult with no more than transient sensory symptoms in limbs and trunk. A child who complains of 'pins and needles' or other symptoms in arms, trunk, legs, or all three following injury should be considered as having sustained a spinal cord insult with established spinal cord vasoparesis. The child should be managed flat, with the neck stabilized until appropriate assessment can be made by a competent practitioner. In all cases of potential injury the child should be asked whether any sensory or motor disturbance, albeit transient, has occurred. *Presume cord injury until proved otherwise*

Head injury management

The first step is to maintain the brain's supply of oxygen and glucose by securing the airway, and ensuring ventilation and the circulation to the brain—ABC: Airway, Breathing, Circulation. If the patient is horizontal, if a central pulse (at groin or in the neck) is present, if the airway is clear, if spontaneous ventilation is maintained, and if the individual's tongue and mucous

membranes are pink, then all well and good. But if there is any doubt the airway must be secured by rolling the individual into the recovery position, with due caution for presumed neck injury, or by protruding the jaw to carry the tongue forward to maintain the airway. If ABC is inadequate then mouth-to-mouth ventilation and external cardiac massage should be instituted as necessary. Once these are secured, the rapid assessment of the individual's conscious level can follow. This is repeated as often as convenient, and should be recorded against time on a large label attached to the individual or written on skin or forehead. This is where the Glasgow Coma Score comes into its own—for the serial numerical recording of conscious level in time (Fig. 2.5).

Where a severe injury is present the ABC requirements are obvious, and the need for transport to hospital is mandatory. 'Minor' head injuries present their own difficulties. There may be uncertainty as to whether or not the conscious level was disturbed. A child or adult under stress may not complain of neurological symptoms or sensory or motor involvement of limbs and body unless asked specifically for them. Caution is the key, and a high index of suspicion is prudent. If the individual is obstreperous, uncooperative, anti-social and aggressive, this behaviour is itself a sign of frontal lobe injury—an additional reason for caution.

If the story of the accident or injury suggests that energy has been applied to head or spine, then significant injury should be presumed until proved otherwise. Recumbency in the recovery position is prudent, with continuous observation, serial recorded assessment, prompt transfer to a casualty department and preparedness to undertake the expeditious evacuation of intracranial haematomata.

When the individual appears well the situation may be even more difficult. If consciousness has been disturbed, then a risk of secondary neurological deterioration should be presumed until such a risk has been judged as remote by a properly qualified medical practitioner. An individual should not be allowed to risk further injury within a week of being knocked out—the period of early epilepsy. A month may be prudent. Though much of our sporting ethic is to 'press on regardless' in a heroic manner, this is foolhardy in head injury. The individual should be withdrawn from games or competition, and not allowed to return until assessed by a medical practitioner who is prepared to accept responsibility for the potential consequences. Once knocked out, even if well, the sportsman or sportswoman should remain in the care of a responsible adult and the general practitioner alerted.

If an epileptic fit occurs then the recovery position, with the same care for associated head and spinal injuries, should be adopted until the fit ends and a spontaneous recovery is made. Epilepsy complicating a head injury indicates sufficient focal cortical disturbance to cause the seizure, and warrants admission to hospital for observation and further management as indicated. It is a key prognostic indicator of further late post-traumatic epilepsy, and should be clearly recorded to guide later management.

Communications

Though immediate management is available at most accident and emergency departments, organizing the removal of intracra-nial clots and the relief of hydrocephalus takes time. In posterior fossa clots with pinpoint pupils and progressive deterioration a CT (computer-assisted tomographic) head scan may be the key to further successful management. Prior warning allows theatres to be made ready and scanners prepared. This may be possible over the ambulance radio network. However, sporting event organization should be prepared for the worst, and prior liaison well before an event is mandatory to establish lines of communication and an agreed plan of disaster management. Without these the opportunity to minimize head injury complication may be lost.

Ocular sports injuries

N. R. Galloway

The importance of ocular sports injuries has tended to be discounted in the past, perhaps because such injuries are not very common in ophthalmic practice and therefore are a rare event in general medical practice. To some extent the problem has been unmasked in recent years by the virtual abolition of perforating eye injuries following road traffic accidents. This has come about with the introduction of seat-belt law and public education concerning drinking and driving. By contrast, eye injuries in sport have been increasing, and to discount them is to ignore the sometimes devastating effect such an injury can have on an individual. Quite often, the severity of an eye injury is not apparent at first glance or without proper microscopic examination and delays in referral may occur as a result. The prompt treatment of a perforating injury can be sight-saving.

However, the treatment of severe eye injuries is not always satisfactory, even with the best of modern surgical techniques, and prevention is the best approach. Furthermore, in the case of sports injuries, prevention can often be achieved by relatively simple means.

The incidence of eye injuries

In the absence of a national reporting system for eye injuries sustained in sport, accurate statistics are not available in this country. Numerous attempts have been made to assess the problem in other ways, such as by the inspection of hospital records or through surveys conducted by means of questionnaires sent to practising ophthalmologists. A retrospective study of the records of those attending the Southampton Eye Hospital with various sports injuries in 1978–79 is of interest. In this study the number of playing sessions generating these injuries has been estimated by reference to the results of the 1977 General Household Survey published by Her Majesty's Stationery Office in 1979. The results indicate that squash produced the most injuries per playing session in the United Kingdom, as well as the greatest number of hospital admissions. The injury rate for squash was estimated at 5.2. per 100 000 playing sessions compared with 2.3 per 100 000 playing sessions for injuries from all causes (Barrell et al. 1981). There is some evidence, on the other hand, that squash does not produce the most long-term eye damage, since more severe though rarer injuries are seen in golf and football (Miller 1967; Burke et al. 1983). In Southeast Asia badminton seems to take a high toll. A series published from Malaysia indicates that badminton accounts for two-thirds of all ocular injuries, and 27 out of 63 patients suffered permanent visual impairment (Chandran 1974).

One source of information about sports injuries in the USA has been the National Electronic Surveillance System. This provides information on product-related injuries to consumers, and has been an important source of statistics for the National Society for the Prevention of Blindness. The data have been obtained from certain participating hospitals, but not from private ophthalmologists. Another source of sporting eye injury statistics in the USA is the National Athletic Injury/Illness Reporting System (NAIRS). This relies on information sent by active members of sports medicine teams. NAIRS also attempts to express frequency of injury as a rate. In order to obtain figures which can be compared from sport to sport and season to season it is necessary to know the 'althletic exposure', that is, the injury rate per hour of exposure to the given sport (Vinger 1981).

Hospital records can provide useful information concerning the more severe injuries. Table 2.1 shows the causes of traumatic bleeding into the anterior chamber ('hyphaema') seen at the Massachusetts Eye and Ear Infirmary from February to September 1980. It can be seen that 45 out of 90 cases were due to sports injuries and 'raquetball' accounted for the largest proportion of these. In an English series reporting sports injuries seen in hospital over a period of 18 months, 20 hyphaemata due to sports injuries were recorded, and the various sports causing these are shown in Table 2.2. Squash and badminton are the main offenders, but the number of injuries from Association Football is noteworthy (Gregory 1986).

Table 2.1. Causes of hyphaema, Massachusetts Eye and Ear Infirmary, USA, 1 February–30 September 1980 (Vinger 1981).

Injury	No. of patients
Traumatic	90
Sports	45
	(43 no eye protection)
Accidental	31
Mechanical/DIY	5
Alleged assault	9
Spontaneous, secondary to vitreous haemorrhage	2
Unknown	2
Total	94

Summary of sports injuries

Racquetball (ball)	10
Racquetball (bracket)	1
Tennis (ball)	9
Squash (ball)	2
Baseball (ball)	4
Baseball (bat)	1
Softball (ball)	4
Wiffleball (ball)	2
Hockeystick	3
Street hockey ball	1
Frisbee	2
Bicycle	1
Basketball	1
Volleyball	1
BB gun	1
Ball (unspecified)	2

Table 2.2. Sporting causes of hyphaema, Sussex Eye Hospital, England. October 1982–March 1984 (Gregory 1986)

Squash	3
Soccer	6
Badminton	7
Tennis	1
Rugby	1
Golf	1
Marbles	1
Total	20

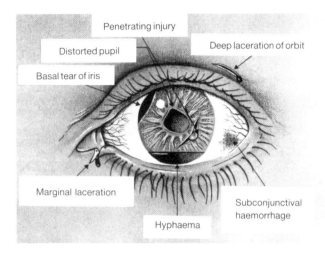

Fig. 2.6 Some typical ocular sports injuries.

A review of the incidence of the more severe types of injury has been achieved by analysing the reasons for surgical removal of eyes between 1960 and 1980. The percentage of eyes removed for injuries sustained in sport as against the percentage of eyes removed for other reasons appears at first sight to have increased considerably. This is likely to be because the total number of surgical enucleations has been reduced. Over the twenty-year period sports-related enucleations represented 3.04% of all surgical enucleations. It should be noted that about half of these were due to 'BB gun' (air pistol or air rifle) injuries, and these are probably less common in Great Britain, though just as dangerous (Portis *et al.* 1981). An analysis of all new cases attending the Bristol Eye Hospital Casualty department has shown that 2.5 per cent of all eye trauma cases are caused by sport (Vernon 1983). This might be compared with the claim that 23 per cent of all trauma *admissions* to the Massachusetts Eye and Ear Informary were due to sport (Elman 1986).

Of course, figures obtained from hospital files do not give a true incidence of the problem either among the general population or in the population at risk. For this reason one set is not comparable with another. Organized sport is in a position to provide better figures and this has been especially true of ice hockey. Here a high and increasing injury rate has been effectively reduced by preventive measures (Pashby 1985).

The incidence of eye injuries in boxing is worthy of special mention. The number of participants in this sport is relatively small, and reported statistics have not been as forthcoming as in ice hockey for example. It was reported in 1981 that retinal detachment is not a common occurrence in boxing (Whiteson 1981). This is contrary to the experience of individual ophthalmic surgeons, and indeed a questionnaire sent out to eye surgeons in the United Kingdom, which achieved a 50.35 per cent reply rate, gave a total of 38 cases of retinal detachment in boxers over the preceding five years (Elkington 1985). Even this figure, which is likely to be under-reported, suggests a higher incidence of retinal detachment than in the general population. In a different study, the routine examination of boxers with or without eye symptoms has revealed a surprisingly high incidence of signs of ocular contusion, and especially of lesions predisposing to retinal detachment (Giovinazzo *et al.* 1987).

Mechanisms of eye injury

Ocular contusion

The mechanical results of direct contusion depend to some extent on whether the eyelids were open or closed at the moment of impact, as well as on the size, speed, and weight of the missile. The squash ball, which measures 40 mm in diame-

ter, is an ideal size for causing compression of the globe whereas in the case of the larger tennis ball some of the force of impact is cushioned by the surrounding orbital margin. Unfortunately even a football may mould itself into the orbit and cause contusion of the globe, so that the larger size of the ball cannot always guarantee protection. A high-speed missile may contuse the globe through the closed lids but bruising of the eyelids can be an indication that the globe has been protected. A squash ball may be travelling at more than a hundred miles an hour, and can strike the eye before the blink reflex has had time to occur. In such cases the cornea tends to be abraded, causing severe sharp pain and photophobia. The more severe effects of such a contusion are due to distortion of the globe. The force of impact is usually upwards and inwards on the lower temporal quadrant. This causes stretching and tearing of the iris root, and may result in the rupture of tributaries of the major arterial circle of the iris. Typically, bleeding into the anterior chamber can occur with an associated iridodialysis or rip of the iris root (see Fig. 2.6). The blood forms a red fluid level, which is a sign that specialist advice should be sought immediately. This bleeding may recur more seriously after two or three days in 10 per cent or more of such patients (Wilson 1980). It is generally taken to be an indication for admission to hospital.

If the force of impact is centred more posteriorly, then the retina may be torn (retinal dialysis). Such tears may go unnoticed, until eventually the retina becomes detached, often after several weeks or months. These tears can be sealed by laser treatment or cryopexy immediately after the injury if spotted in time. The distortion of the globe can also cause splitting open of the angle of the anterior chamber, or 'angle recession'. This can affect the drainage of aqueous fluid, causing the intraocular pressure to rise, and, if untreated, pressure atrophy of the optic nerve head (secondary glaucoma). Sometimes the sudden stretching produces small tears in the iris sphincter at the inner margin of the pupil, and as a result the pupil may be fixed and dilated. This of course can cause great concern if a head injury is suspected, but the diagnosis can be clarified easily by proper ophthalmological examination. Contusion of the eye may also cause posterior subcapsular opacities in the lens, although these may take some days, or sometimes much longer, to develop. After some blows on the eye there appears to be a contracoup effect, in that most of the damage is found in the retina and choroid. Bruising of the retina is seen as grey patches with multiple haemorrhages; this may have a serious effect on the visual acuity if the fovea is involved. Distortion of the globe can cause ruptures of the choroid, seen as circumferential white crescents concentric with the optic disc. One final effect of contusion may be bleeding into the optic nerve sheath. After the impact the patient finds that he cannot see out of one eye. The physical signs may be minimal, apart from an afferent pupillary defect, in spite of the fact that the eye is completely blind and usually remains so. After a few weeks the optic disc becomes pale. Early decompression of the optic nerve may be helpful in these cases.

Effect on surrounding structures

It is perhaps surprising how often a contused globe is seen as an isolated injury but other injuries may mask the eye damage. Typically a larger 'missile', such as a knee or fist, may cause a 'blow-out fracture', in which the globe is forced posteriorly, causing fracture of the floor of the orbit and trapping of the inferior rectus muscle. The infraorbital nerve may be injured, causing anaesthesia of the cheek, along with the other typical signs such as enophthalmos (posterior displacement of the eye) and limitation of elevation of the eye, with diplopia on upward gaze. In the absence of a blow-out fracture, injury to the superior orbital margin may damage the pulley of the superior oblique muscle, thus causing diplopia by a different mechanism.

Ocular perforation

If the globe is severely contused by a blunt object scleral rupture may occur. More commonly, perforation of the globe is caused by a sharp object, and the site of perforation is in the anterior segment of the eye. If the cornea is perforated, aqueous fluid escapes, and the iris shoots forwards to plug the opening. A knuckle of iris may project through the wound, and on no account should this be mistaken for a foreign body by the first-aid attendant. Any perforating injury of the eye demands urgent surgical attention, because of the risk of infection and disruption of the intraocular structures. If the lens of the eye escapes damage then the visual outcome may be good, but once the lens is involved then a cataract inevitably forms. Cataract surgery may present technical difficulties after injuries, and even the best surgical result leaves the patient with no focusing power. This may be acceptable to the elderly patient with little focusing power before the injury, but may cause considerable handicap to the younger patient. If the perforation involves the sclera further posteriorly, then there is a high risk of retinal detachment. It can be seen that a perforating injury is a serious risk to the sight of the eye, and may result in the need for repeated operations and time off work. Most people have heard of sympathetic ophthalmia, and are aware that the uninjured eye may become inflamed after a perforating injury. Fortunately this is a very rare event indeed, and the risk is largely eliminated by careful reparative surgery.

Injuries related to particular sports

Racquet sports such as squash and racquetball are particularly likely to produce eye injuries, whereas eye damage is less common where the players are separated by a net, as in tennis and badminton. Hyphaema is the commonest injury from a squash ball. The ways in which a squash ball may damage the eye can be seen by inspection of Table 2.3. This series was

Table 2.3. Nature of eye injuries in squash players (Kennerley Bankes 1985)

Tissue	Injury	No. of injuries
Orbit	Fracture	3
Eyelids	Lacerations	50
	Bruising	40
Conjunctiva	Haemorrhage	18
	Lacerations	4
Cornea	Abrasions	54
	Perforations	2
Anterior Chamber	Hyphaema	147
	Angle recession	3
Iris	Iritis	30
	Mydriasis	8
	Dialysis	1
Lens	Subluxation	2
Vitreous	Posterior separation	4
	Haemorrhage	2
Sclera	Perforation	1
Retina	Haemorrhage/oedema	28
	Tear	3
	Detachment	2

obtained from a questionnaire completed by ophthalmologists (Kennerley Bankes 1985). The pattern of injury from ice hockey in Canada in 1972–73 showed 15 ruptured globes, 91 hyphaemata, and 13 orbital fractures. Out of the 287 injuries, 20 caused total blindness of the eye. Such a severe toll prompted vigorous protective measures, which have proved effective. In 1983–84 there were only 124 reported injuries, and none of these were in players wearing guards. The average age of injured players rose over this period, reflecting the more regular wearing of guards among younger players.

Some of the less common sporting eye injuries have their own peculiarities. Hurling can cause severe injuries; the solid 75 mm wooden ball is the commonest cause of sporting injury in the West of Ireland, where the game is played (Kelly and Nolan 1983). Golf balls nearly always cause devastating damage to the eye on impact (Miller 1967), as do airgun pellets and darts. Dart injuries are a serious problem in children either as a result of a direct perforation from the point of the dart or, curiously, in the shape of damage inflicted by the tail of the dart when it is pulled out of the board (Cole and Smerdon 1988). In spite of its size and hardness, the cricket ball can contuse the eye, and recent reports suggest that such injuries may be increasing (Coroneo 1985; Jones and Tullo 1986). Fishermen are not immune from eye injuries either, caused by penetration by fishhooks or by spears. The removal of a hook from an eye can pose a difficult surgical problem (Bartholomew and MacDonald 1980). Recently, a number of eye injuries have been reported by those participating in war games. The eye may be contused by pellets, and it is possible for dye to impregnate the conjunctiva. Such injuries are sustained because of inadequate protection by goggles (Acheson et al. 1989).

Economics and prevention of eye injuries

Canadian ice hockey provides a model for the study of prevention of sporting eye injuries. In the early 1970s eye injuries from this cause became a national problem, and public realization of this led to a change in ice hockey rules. Experimental work on masks led to the development of protective headgear. The Canadian Standards Association (CSA) published a standard for eye and tooth protection in 1977, and in 1981 the wearing of such CSA-certified masks was made compulsory for all Canadian minor league hockey players (Pashby 1985). This combination of measures—changes in the rules and the compulsory use of protective headgear—has resulted in a dramatic reduction of eye injuries, and a probable saving of several million dollars annually (Tolpin et al. 1981). It is worth noting that the less dangerous field hockey has recently seen rule changes which may increase the number of eye injuries. Whereas in ice hockey a 'high sticks' rule was introduced in 1975, preventing players from raising the stick above the shoulders, in field hockey this rule was relaxed in 1982 (Elliott and Jones 1984).

The history of preventive measures as applied to racquet sports is less encouraging. In 1980 an Eye Safety Committee of the American Society for Testing and Materials was formed, and by 1983 a performance standard for racquet sports eye protectors was published (Elman 1986). Spectacle wearers are at particular risk in racquet sports, and the wearing of open-type guards around the eye does not prevent a squash ball travelling at 50 miles an hour from causing a contusion (Feigelman et al. 1983). Eye guards with plano or prescription polycarbonate

plastic lenses appear to be the safest (Fig. 2.7). One of the problems concerning prevention in racquet sports is the reluctance of the individual to wear special protective guards (Genovese et al. 1990). It is often claimed that such items are cumbersome and impair the player's performance. It is important that all players are made to wear such guards in order to avoid increased vulnerability. The economic consequences of eye injuries resulting from sport are not easy to assess accurately, but one must consider the immediate cost of medical treatment and possible admission to hospital as being only a small part. The time lost from work must be included, and the greatest cost can arise from permanent handicap and possible unemployment.

First-aid management of sporting injuries

When a sporting injury involves the eyes, the first-aid attendant should make a simple assessment of the vision. If the vision is impaired and cannot be cleared by blinking, then immediate referral for specialist treatment is essential. The examiner can test the field by using finger movements in all four quadrants; if the examiner sees his own finger significantly before the injured athlete, then referral is indicated. A near vision test card can be a helpful item in such circumstances. A simple test of eye movements, in which the athlete is asked to follow the examiner's fingers, may reveal damage that needs expert attention. The majority of suspected eye injuries demand prompt referral, but the first-aid attendant may be able to assist with the removal of foreign bodies or the replacement of a dislodged contact lens. Many contact lens wearers can replace their own dislodged contact lenses if they have a small mirror, and such an item might be included in the first-aid kit, together with a pen-torch and sterile cotton swabs. A hard eye-shield is another useful item; this is taped over the injured eye to protect it. The first-aid kit should also include a sterile eye-irrigating solution. When a perforating injury of the eye is suspected no further attempt to examine the eye should be made. A protective shield should be applied, and the injured person should be given nothing to eat or drink in case an emergency anaesthetic is subsequently needed.

Preparticipation screening

It is possible to enjoy many sports with relatively poor eyesight, but certain eye conditions demand that careful consideration should be given before participating in high-risk sports. Highly myopic individuals are at risk of the development of retinal detachment, and such patients are usually advised to avoid sports where the head may be bumped. Heading a football or high diving are especially contraindicated. The one-eyed athlete is a special case who should certainly avoid such risks. Providing advice in an individual case is not always straightforward; the individual may earn his or her living from the sport, and many other factors may need to be taken into account.

Participation in sport should be avoided after any serious eye injury for a variable period of time, depending on the nature of the injury. Squash players are usually advised to refrain from playing squash for at least three months after an intraocular haemorrhage. After a retinal detachment participation in sport

FIG. 2.7 Eye guards with plano or prescription polycarbonate plastic lenses appear to be the safest. (Courtesy Thomas Bond and Partners, Nottingham Optometrist.)

may need to be curtailed for two or three months, although many surgeons now claim that the retina is likely to be more secure after successful surgery than it was prior to the injury. Patients with only one eye who wish to return to a sport should be strongly advised to wear suitable eye protection.

References

Acheson, J. F., Griffiths, M. F. P., and Cooling, R. J. (1989). Serious eye injuries due to war games. *Br. Med. J.*, **298**, 26.

Barrell, G. V., Cooper P. J., Elkington, A. R., MacFadyen, J. M., Powell, R. G., and Tormey, P. (1981). Squash ball to eyeball: the likelihood of squash players incurring an eye injury. *Br. Med. J.*, **283**, 893–5.

Bartholomew, R. S. and MacDonald, M. (1980). Fish hook injuries of the eye. *Br. J. Ophthalmol.*, **64**, 531–3.

Bruce, D. A., Alavi, A., Bilaniuk, L. *et al.* (1981). Diffuse cerebral swelling following head injuries in children. The syndrome of malignant brain oedema. *J. Neurosurg.*, **54**, 170–8.

(BSI) British Standards Institution. (1985). *BS6658. Protective helmets for vehicle users.* BSI, London.

(BSI) British Standards Institution. (1986). *BS 6473. Specification for protective hats for horse and pony riders.* BS1, London.

(BSI) British Standards Institution. (1988). *BS 4472. Specification for protective skull caps for jockeys.* BS1, London.

Burke, M. J., Sanitato, J. J., Vinger, P. F., Raymond, L. A., and Kulwin, D. R. (1983). Soccerball induced eye injuries. *J. Am. Med. Assoc.*, **249 (19)**, 2682–5.

Chandran S. (1974). Ocular hazards of playing badminton. *Br. J. Ophthalmol.*, **58**, 757–60.

Cole, M. D. and Smerdon D. (1988). Perforating eye injuries caused by darts. *Br. J. Ophthalmol*, **72**, 511–14.

Coroneo, M. T. (1985). An eye for cricket. *Med. J. Aust.*, **142**, 469–70

Elkington, A. R. (1985). Boxing and the eye: results of a questionnaire. *Trans. Ophthalmol. Soc. U.K.*, **104**, 898–902.

Elliott, A. J. and Jones, D. (1984). Major ocular trauma: a disturbing trend in field hockey, *Br. Med. J.*, **289**, 21-2.

Elman, M. J. (1986). Racket-sports ocular injuries. *Arch. Ophthalmol.*, **104**, 1453–4.

Feigelman, M. J., Sugar, J., Jednock, N., Read, J. S., and Johnson, P. L. (1983). Assessment of ocular protection for racquetball *J. Am. Med. Assoc.*, **250**(24), 3305–9.

Firth, J. L. (1985). Equestrian injuries. In *Sports injuries: mechanisms, prevention and treatment* (ed. R. C. Schneider, J. C. Kennedy, and M. L. Plant), pp. 431–49. Williams and Wilkins, Baltimore.

Genovese, M. T., Lenzo, N. P., Lim, Rik., Morkel, D. R., and Jamrozik, K. D. (1990). Eye injuries among pennant squash players and their attitudes to protective eyewear. *Med. J. Aust.*, **153**, 655–8.

Giovinazzo, V. J., Yannuzzi, L. A., Sorenson, J. A. Delrowe, D. J., Campbell, E. A. (1987). The ocular complications of boxing. *Ophthalmology*, **94** (6), 587–96.

Gregory, P. T. S. (1986). Sussex Eye Hospital sports injuries. *Br. J. Ophthalmol.*, **70**, 748–50.

Gurdjian, E. S., Webster, J. E., and Lissner, H. R. (1950). The mechanisms of skull fracture. *J. Neurosurg.*, **7**, 106–14.

'Hippocrates'. Cited in Knight, G. and Rains, T. J. H. (ed.) (1971). *Bailey and Love's short practice of surgery*, p. 376. H. K. Lewis, London.

Holbourn, A. H. S. (1943). Mechanics of head injury. *Lancet*, **2**, 438–41.

Jennett, W. B. (1975). *Epilepsy after non-missile head injuries* (2nd edn). Heinemann Medical, London.

Jones, N. P. and Tullo, A. B. (1986). Severe eye injuries in cricket. *Br. J. Sports Med.*, **20**, 178–9.

Kelly, S. and Nolan, J. (1983). Eye injuries in organised sports in a rural area. *Br. J. Ophthalmol.*, **67**, 837–39.

Kennerley Bankes, J. L. (1985). Squash rackets: a survey of eye injuries in England. *Br. Med. J.*, **291**, 1539.

Langfitt, T. W., Marshall, W. J. S., Kassell, N. F., and Schutta, H. S. (1968). The pathophysiology of brain swelling produced by mechanical trauma and hypertension. *Scand. J. Clin. Lab. Invest.*, **Suppl. 102 XIVB**.

Lindgren, S. O. (1966). Experimental studies on mechanical effects in head injury. *Acta Chir. Scand.*, **Suppl. 360.**

Millar, G. T., (1967). Golfing eye injuries. *Am. J. Ophthalmol.*, **64**, 741–2.

Miller, J. D., (1979). Intracranial mass lesions. In *Neural trauma* (ed. A. J. Popp *et al.*), pp. 173–80. Raven Press, New York.

Pashby, T. (1985). Eye injuries in Canadian amateur hockey. *Can. J. Ophthalmol.*, **20**(I), 2–4.

Portis, J. M., Vassalio, S.A., and Albert, D. A. (1981). Ocular sports injuries a review of cases on file at the Massachusetts Eye and Ear Infirmary Pathology Laboratory, *Int. Ophthalmol. Clin.*, **21** (4), 1–19.

Robbins, S. L., Contran, R. S., and Kumar V. (eds.) (1984). *Pathologic basis of disease* (3rd edn.), pp. 1374–7 Saunders, Philadelphia.

Sheinker, I. M. (1944) Vasoparalysis of the central nervous systems. A characteristic vascular syndrome. *Arch. Neurol. Psychol.*, **52**, 43 -56.

Strich, S. J. (1956). Diffuse degeneration of the cerebral white matter in severe dementia following head injury. *J. Neurol Psychiatr.*, **19**, 163–85.

Strich, S. J. (1961). Shearing of nerve fibres as a cause of brain damaged due to head injury. *Lancet*, **2**, 443–8.

Strich, S. J. (1969). Pathology of brain damage due to blunt head injury. In *Late effects of head injury* (ed. A. E. Walker, W. F. Covaness, and M.Critchley), pp. 501–26. Thomas, Springfield, Ill.

Teasdale, G. and Jennett, W. B. (1974) The Glasgow Come Scale. *Lancet*, **2**, 81–4.

Tolpin, H. G., Vinger, P. F., and Tolpin, D. L. (1988). Ocular sports injuries: *Int. Ophthalmol. Clin.*, **21** (4), 179–201.

Vernon, S. A. (1983). Analysis of all new cases seen in a busy regional centre ophthalmic casualty department during a 24 week period. *J. R. Soc. Med.*, **76**, 279–82.

Vinger, P. F. (1981). The incidence of eye injuries in sports. *Int. Ophthalmol. Clin.*, **21 (4)**, 1–45.

Whiteson, A. L. (1981). Injuries in professional boxing. Their treatment and prevention. *Practitioner*, **225**, 1053–7.

Wilson, F. M. (1980). Traumatic hyphaema. *Ophthalmology*, **87**, 910–19.

3 Injuries to the shoulder

W. A. WALLACE AND M. A. HUTSON

Basic anatomy and biomechanics

The shoulder is a complex anatomical area which allows the arm to be moved in a number of directions to position the hand for either everyday or sporting activities. The design is superb, and is arranged to allow the maximum amount of both power and fine control to the movements of the arm and hand. Unfortunately, because of its generous range of movement, it is potentially a very unstable joint, and this may lead to considerable problems when the soft tissues around the shoulder are injured.

There are four different 'joints' in the shoulder region, all of which contribute to arm movement: the glenohumeral or true shoulder joint, the acromioclavicular joint, the scapulothoracic joint, and—perhaps the most important joint—the subacromial joint. This last joint has only become appreciated in recent years, but is the one most likely to give rise to pain from the shoulder—particularly in athletes. Then there is the sternoclavicular joint, some distance from the shoulder, which anchors the shoulder girdle to the chest wall and may also sustain a number of sports-related injuries.

The *glenohumeral joint* (Fig. 3.1) is rather like a ball (the humeral head), sitting on a shallow saucer (the bony glenoid). The saucer is deepend by both the glenoid labrum—a fibrous structure in some ways very similar to the meniscus in the knee and the capsule of the shoulder joint, which provides some flexible restraint to the joint. Superiorly the humeral head is held down by the long head of biceps, which passes from its origin at the superior pole of the glenoid over the top of the humeral head and anteriorly downwards into the bicipital groove between the

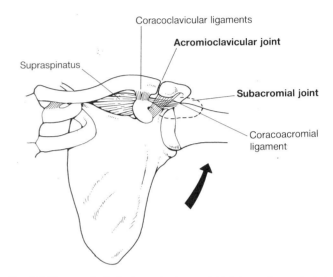

FIG. 3.2 The aromioclavicular and subacromial joints are demonstrated.

greater and lesser tuberosities of the humerus. Surrounding the humeral head and holding it in place is the rotator cuff, composed of four different muscles. Anteriorly is the subscapularis and superiorly is supraspinatus—both muscles becoming tendinous before reaching their insertions into the lesser and greater tuberosities of the humerus respectively. Posteriorly lies the infraspinatus, which is muscular right up to its insertion, and the teres minor, which is very thick indeed. The difference between a tendinous insertion and a muscular insertion is important with regard to both injury and treatment. Injury to the supraspinatus will behave more like an Achilles tendon injury, while the infraspinatus will react to injury in a similar way to a torn hamstring or gastrocnemius muscle.

The *acromioclavicular (A-C) joint* (Figs. 3.1 and 3.2) is unusual because its stability depends more on the coracoclavicular ligaments, which act as check reins, than on the local superior and inferior acromioclavicular ligaments. In fact if these superior and inferior ligaments are damaged there is little displacement of the joint. Within the A-C joint lies a meniscus, as in the knee, but this meniscus commonly becomes worn, and by the age of 30 is often only a peripheral tag. The A-C joint allows movement between the scapula and clavicle, which is required to allow the scapula its 60°–70° rotation on the chest wall during a full range of arm movement.

The *scapulothoracic joint* (Fig. 3.1) is important in sportsmen because it can be the site of inflammation, and later fibrosis, due to overuse. If this happens adhesions develop in the layer

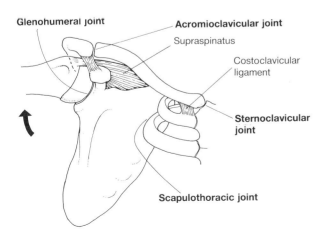

FIG. 3.1 The glenohumeral, acromioclavicular, scapulothoracic, and sternoclavicular joints are demonstrated.

Origin of middle fibres
of deltoid from acromion

FIG. 3.3 The mechanical effect of the deltoid acting
alone.

between the subscapularis and serratus anterior muscles and the chest wall. These adhesions cause abnormal soft tissue tethering, and result in a condition called 'snapping scapula'. This is normally painless, but occasionally can be a cause of pain and may result in limitation of further sporting activity—particularly in weight-lifters.

The *subacromial joint* (Fig. 3.2) has been ignored by anatomists for many years. It is formed by (1) a roof, the acromion posteriorly and the coracoacromial ligament and coracoid anteriorly, and (2) a floor, the supraspinatus tendon medially and the greater tuberosity of the humerus laterally. The joint cavity is formed by the subacromial bursa—a sac which contains only a thin film of fluid. The interesting feature of this subacromial area is that if a large force is transmitted across the subacromial joint then pain occurs due to local soft tissue injury. As a consequence *this joint is responsible for the majority of painful shoulders.*

The *sternoclavicular joint* (Fig. 3.1) lies outside the region of the shoulder, but it makes an important contribution to movements of the shoulder girdle, and if injured can result in limitation of shoulder movement. The joint is similar in some ways to the acromioclavicular joint. Although it does have joint ligaments passing from the sternum to the clavicle, the main stabilizing ligament of the joint is the costoclavicular ligament, which is attached to the clavicle lateral to the joint. The joint is divided into a medial and lateral compartment by an intra-articular meniscus, which also acts as a stabilizing ligament. This joint has no inherent mechanical stability, and is very dependent on these different ligamentous structures to hold the bones in place.

The biomechanics of the shoulder complex are difficult to grasp, but are perhaps best understood by concentrating first on the kinetics—the study of the actual movements of the joints—and second on the dynamics—the forces required to produce these movements.

The *kinetics* of the shoulder movement are as follows. When an arm is raised the movement is usually divided into two phases. The first 30° is described as the setting phase—during this there is a variable pattern of shoulder movement, but Poppen and Walker (1976) have noted that, for most shoulders, movement during this phase occurs at the glenohumeral joint while the scapula remains fairly static. From 30° onwards, however, there is a uniform pattern of movement, with 2° of glenohumeral movement for every 1° of scapular rotation. This means that if the arm is raised to 90° elevation, then 60° is glenohumeral while 30° is scapular; for 180° of elevation 120°

is glenohumeral and 60° is scapular. For the A-C joint, studies have shown that there is little movement of the A-C joint when the arm is raised to 90°, but movements increase from 90° upwards, with the maximum movement and the largest strain to the A-C joint occurring from 140° to 180° of arm elevation (Wallace and Johnson 1982).

The *dynamics* of shoulder movement highlight a delicately coordinated group of muscles, all of which are required for normal shoulder movement. If one considers the deltoid acting alone on the dependent arm trying to raise it (see Fig. 3.3) it can be seen that its action is to push the humeral head upwards, forcing it to impinge on the acromion and the coracoacromial arch through the subacromial joint. In order to prevent this the infraspinatus and teres minor posteriorly and the subscapularis anteriorly tend to apply traction to the shoulder through the greater and lesser tuberosities of the humerus respectively, pulling the head back down (see Fig. 3.4). This is further helped by the tendons of the supraspinatus and the long head of biceps which have a bowstring-type action which also pushes the humeral head down. An excellent study (van Linge and Mulder 1963) has demonstrated that if the supraspinatus and infraspinatus muscles are put out of action by a local anaesthetic block to the suprascapular nerve, then considerable weakness and loss of endurance of the strength of the shoulder for elevation occurs. This was highlighted by a reduced ability to lift a weight to shoulder height and keep it there, although in most cases the subjects were able to lift their arms up fully without

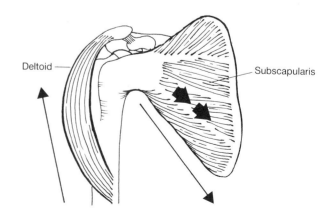

Deltoid

Subscapularis

FIG. 3.4 The mechanical effects of subscapularis, infraspinatus, teres minor, and supraspinatus.

FIG. 3.5 Previous rupture of the left pectoralis major due to water-skiing is demonstrated.

any weights. Howell *et al.* (1986) have confirmed this finding in their studies using isokinetic dynamometry.

An integrated system (the brain and spinal cord) controls these groups of muscles, and usually does this very well, but if the coordination of muscle contraction is not good then the humeral head will be driven up through the subacromial joint, which will result in shoulder pain.

Besides the deltoid (which flexes and extends the shoulder as well as acting as an abductor) other muscles also act as prime movers of the shoulder joint. The pectoralis major is a powerful adductor, and also medially rotates the arm. The latissimus dorsi extends, medially rotates, and depresses the shoulder. The deltoid is rarely injured, despite the fact that referred pain is commonly felt over its inferior attachment. Pectoralis major is occasionally ruptured (Scott *et al.*, 1992), for instance in weight-lifting or water-skiing (Fig. 3.5). Partial rupture of the latissimus dorsi has been observed (M.A.H.), although it is uncommon.

The relationship between neck pain and shoulder dysfunction is an interesting and ill-understood phenomenon. It is common for those with neck pain from disorders of the cervical spine to suffer secondary shoulder pain—particularly the subacromial impingement type of pain. In the authors' opinion this occurs as a consequence of pressure on the C5 and C6 nerve roots, causing incoordination of the C5 and C6 innervated muscles (supraspinatus, infraspinatus, deltoid, and biceps), and pain is produced as a result. The opposite also occurs—shoulder pain secondarily produces neck pain because with shoulder dysfunction there tends to be increased tone in the trapezius, levator scapulae, and rhomboid muscles as well as the sternomastoid, all of which may disturb the mechanics of the cervical spine and result in neck pain.

Dyscoordination of muscle action also occurs in shoulder instability—subluxation (which is a partial dislocation) and dislocation of the joint. In these situations muscle incoordination, either voluntary or subconscious (involuntary), may be the sole cause of the instability, and is perhaps the most common cause of multi-directional instability of the shoulder in teenagers. The forces required to produce normal shoulder movement are much larger than many realize. In a study carried out in Nottingham (Wallace 1984) the force required in either the supraspinatus or the infraspinatus to lift the arm was of the order of 30 to 40 kilograms, or 50 per cent of bodyweight.

Overuse syndromes of the shoulder

Problems with repetitive propulsive and explosive stress ('thrower's shoulder')

It may be seen from the foregoing account of the biomechanics of shoulder function that repetitive stress may give rise to a number of problems, of which attrition of the rotator cuff under the unyielding coracoacromial arch is a major one. The freely mobile glenohumeral joint is also at risk from the relative paucity of restraining capsular ligaments. A number of sports—for example, swimming, tennis, and those with a throwing component (for instance baseball, American football, and cricket)—involve repetitive propulsive, and sometimes explosive, activity in the overhead position (Fig. 3.6). The size of the problem may be gauged from the estimation of Richardson *et al.* (1980) that over 40 per cent of elite swimmers, particularly those using the crawl, the butterfly, and the back-strokes, complain at one time or another of shoulder pain. Perhaps this is not surprising when one appreciates that the competitive swimmer may perform up to ten thousand overhead strokes in any one week of training. In the game of cricket it is not unusual to find that at least one member of a team is unable to throw in a conventional overhead manner because of pain or the complaint of 'throwing the shoulder out'. A distinction should be made between throwing and bowling, as they have different biomechanical characteristics: a smoother action is required for bowling, which is less likely to cause injury. Pitchers in baseball and quarterbacks in American football also spend a considerable amount of time throwing during training as well as in matches. American sports physicians have developed a considerable insight into these problems, especially as they are advising a group of highly paid athletes. As a result of careful documentation of shoulder injuries, physicians have been instrumental in drawing up changes in the rules applied to baseball both in the junior 'Little Leagues' and in the senior games. Tennis, which is played more universally, imposes a considerable strain during the serve or overhead smash (see Fig. 1.4, p. 4). Although at first sight there may appear to be major differences between these various activities—for example, swimming as opposed to throwing—the following shoulder actions are common to all:

cocking (or recovery phase in swimming) involving abduction, external rotation, and extension;

acceleration (pull-through in swimming) involving forward flexion, internal rotation and adduction;

follow-through (deceleration).

Each phase with its attendant problems will be described separately.

Cocking

The muscles responsible are the posterior deltoid, infraspinatus, and teres minor. In addition there is biceps brachii activity to flex the elbow. In the fully externally rotated and abducted position the subscapularis is stretched across the anterior aspect of the joint, and is active during this restraining function. In this position the anterior capsule is stretched, and the shoulder is at risk from anterior subluxation. Such a risk applied to the underwater turn in backstroke swimming before the change of rules allowed a turn onto the front and the use of a tumble turn, as in

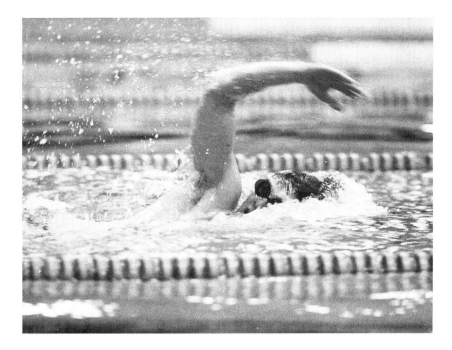

FIG. 3.6 A number of sports involve repetitive propulsive, and sometimes explosive, activity of the shoulder in the overhead position—crawl stroke swimming, baseball pitching, and cricket bowling.

front-crawl, on the approach to the wall. The main problems are thus related to anterior capsular strain and anterior instability, in addition to infraspinatus overactivity.

Acceleration

This is the main propulsive phase in throwing and racket overheads, and in company with follow-through accounts for the pull-through phase in swimming. The muscles involved are the anterior deltoid, pectoralis major, latissimus dorsi, subscapularis, and teres major. Attrition of the rotator cuff, principally the supraspinatus and the biceps brachii tendons, by *impingement* under the coracoacromial arch occurs in this situation, and probably accounts for the majority of those injuries that do not show much sign of early resolution. Other overuse conditions include stress fracture of the coracoid process, tendinitis of the conjoint tendon of the short head of biceps brachii and coracobrachialis, proximal epiphysitis of the humerus in youngsters, and stress fracture of the humerus. Tendinitis of the long head of the triceps, due to repeated elbow extension, occurs in swimmers and is also recognized in javelin throwers. Ringman's shoulder (insertional tendinitis of pectoralis major) is due to repeated maintenance of the iron-cross position in gymnastics. Andrews *et al.* (1985) have described superior labrum detachment in the region of the attachment of the long head of biceps. In throwers this is presumably related to overuse of the biceps (acting through the long head) during cocking and again in the deceleration phase. Ectopic calcification may be visible on radiographs in any of the above situations.

Follow-through

The restraining action of the infraspinatus and the further activity of biceps brachii in this phase may contribute towards shoulder soreness. Posterior shoulder strain is common and posterior subluxation (probably responsible for the arm being 'thrown out') may occur.

Impingement

Many factors may contribute to the development of impingement. A simple mechanical reason is a reduction in the sub-

acromial gap—narrowing the subacromial space that is available for the rotator cuff. This can occur due to encroachment by inferior osteophytes from the acromioclavicular joint (Petersson and Gentz 1983), and may result in thinning of the cuff due to degenerative processes in the mature athlete (Fig. 3.7; see Fig. 10.20(a), p. 179). It has already been established that the rotator cuff is subject to attrition. The postero-lateral aspect of the head of the humerus is particularly affected during the repeated combination of internal rotation, flexion, and adduction. 'Swimmer's impingement', for instance, typically occurs at the end of the recovery phase when the arm is brought into maximal internal rotation and forward elevation. Studies have shown that blanching of the cuff is a feature (Rathburn and McNab 1970), indicating that reduced vascularization plays a significant part, in combination with repeated microtrauma (Kennedy *et al.* 1978).

It is likely that a vicious circle develops: inflammatory swelling surrounding overused tendons provokes a friction effect underneath the coracoacromial arch, which gives rise to further microtrauma and further swelling. An inflammatory reaction occurs in the adjacent subacromial bursa, which is initially oedematous and invaded by inflammatory cells, and subsequently becomes fibrotic. Partial or full-thickness rotator cuff tears may develop as a result. Impingement of the humeral head occurs with a rotator cuff tear, as the head is allowed to rise up during abduction (Weiner and McNab 1970). Overuse tendinitis of the tendons of biceps brachii, subscapularis, supraspinatus, and infraspinatus may occur as a result of unaccustomed overhead exercise, giving rise to the painful arc syndrome as the affected tendon and the adjacent subacromial bursa are squeezed between the humeral head or greater tuberosity and the coracoacromial arch. Degenerative changes in the cuff may give rise to calcific deposits (Fig. 3.8), usually found in the supraspinatus tendon of the middle-aged. These contribute further to subacromial impingement.

Instability

Chronic instability usually manifests itself as recurrent bouts of subluxation which follow an initial dislocation episode. Beware the 'sprained shoulder', which is often the presentation of the first acute dislocation episode. These shoulders should be treated with a broad arm-sling under the clothes for four weeks to reduce the chance of recurrence. Recurrent anterior dislocation is particularly common in younger patients (aged 18 to 30). What is rarely appreciated is that if a dislocation occurs at this

age the chance of a normal shoulder later is only 20 per cent, with 60 per cent having recurrent dislocation episodes and 20 per cent recurrent subluxation symptoms (Simonet and Cofield 1984). A similar situation may apply to the less common posterior dislocation. Subsequent dislocations may be reduced by the patient; nevertheless he should be referred to an orthopaedic surgeon for consideration of surgical stabilization of the shoulder. The general rule is that patients are expected to 'earn' their operations, and most orthopaedic surgeons will only operate if there have been at least three dislocation episodes. Sometimes, however, the subsequent episodes take the form of subluxation rather than dislocation. These can be very disabling, and are often associated with a sudden click in the shoulder, a popping sensation, a 'dead arm', or a pain shooting down the arm or into the hand. These episodes are occasionally followed by a few days of shoulder dysfunction.

It is important to separate recurrent traumatic subluxation or dislocation, which is usually unidirectional, from recurrent

FIG. 3.7 Downward-pointing osteophytes from the A-C joint.

FIG. 3.8 Calcium (hydroxyapatite) deposits in the rotator cuff—usually the supraspinatus tendon. These may contribute to subacromial impingement.

atraumatic subluxation or dislocation, which is often multidirectional. Beware of the habitual dislocator who has no history of trauma, but is able to dislocate the shoulder either anteriorly or posteriorly at will. These patients are special cases. They should not be treated with surgery, and are best referred early to an orthopaedic surgeon with a special interest in shoulders, to have reassurance and rotator cuff-strengthening exercises.

Careful attention should be paid to the history, and in particular a detailed enquiry should be made into the position of the arm at the time of the initial dislocation and also the position of the arm during subsequent episodes of subluxation or dislocation.

Assessment

The history

Full details of the history should be obtained from every patient with a shoulder problem. As in the knee, approximately 50 per cent of patients can have a diagnosis made from the history alone.The pain from conditions in the subacromial region is often felt on the anterolateral aspect of the shoulder or close to the insertion of the deltoid, and frequently it radiates to the upper arm. In the condition of capsulitis, which enters into the differential diagnosis in patients aged 45 years or over, pain comes on gradually and may radiate down the arm as far as the wrist. However, pain may come on suddenly and, if associated with a fall on to the point of the shoulder, this is strongly suggestive of a rotator cuff tear, a fracture, an A-C joint injury (see p. 47), or occasionally a glenohumeral joint dislocation with spontaneous reduction. The pain may be accompanied by a click and be grossly disabling for a short while, suggesting instability. It may take the form of the typical overuse syndrome, in which the pain gradually becomes more severe and is felt earlier in the exercise programme, eventually totally preventing training or any exercise. Such a story is strongly suggestive of impingement. As with all cases of shoulder and arm pain, any associated or preceding neck pain should be noted. A history of paraesthesiae and numbness in a dermatomal pattern, suggesting true nerve-root irritation, should always be sought.

The examination

A logical pattern of examination of the shoulder is crucial:

LOOK *then* MOVE *then* FEEL *then* INVESTIGATE FURTHER.

(1) LOOK—*observation* might reveal muscle-wasting in the region of the deltoid or in the supraspinous or infraspinous fossa. Localized soft tissue swelling is sometimes observed over the humeral head, particularly in acute bursitis, but this is uncommon. The subacromial bursa is more commonly swollen in the presence of a full-thickness rotator cuff tear or in rheumatological conditions.

(2) Move—*active movements* are assessed first. Active abduction yields information on the presence of a painful arc (see later), and on any restriction of range of movement. Abnormal scapulo-humeral rhythm should be observed by standing behind the patient. One useful sign is to study the anterior bulge formed by the top part of the humeral head during the initiation of abduction or flexion. In the presence of a rotator cuff tear or weakness of the cuff the head will ride up at the start of movement. If the shoulder is normal, the head position does not change. Included at this stage are tests of serratus anterior function to identify winging of the scapula due to a long thoracic nerve palsy. This can occur from excessive stretching of the nerve from an indirect injury.

FIG. 3.9 Assessment of true glenohumeral abduction requires stabilization of the scapula.

Passive movements are assessed next. The full range of passive shoulder movements is performed with care, so that the examiner is clear in his own mind exactly which movements or combinations of movements are being tested. Initially the patient is examined in the standing position. True glenohumeral abduction is assessed by passive abduction of the arm, using one hand supporting the elbow for leverage and the thumb and index fingers of the other examining hand to stabilize the inferior angle of the scapula (Fig. 3.9). The degree of arm abduction from the vertical is measured to the point at which the scapula starts to rotate. External rotation (Fig. 3.10) should initially be performed with the arm dependent and the elbow held at a right angle. Functional internal rotation (Fig. 3.11) is compared with the normal side by determining the number of the spinous process reached by the *dorsum* of the subject's hand at the full range of movement. There is now increasing awareness that a tight posterior capsule can give rise to impingement. It is therefore important to check full passive internal rotation in patients with impingement. Passive adduction (Fig. 3.12) is tested by pushing the arm, held at shoulder level, across the front of the chest. In all these movements a note is made of any restriction in range and the degree of pain elicited.

Patterns to emerge

(a) *The capsular pattern.* The capsular pattern of the shoulder is greater restriction of passive external rotation than of abduction or internal rotation. At its earliest stage external rotation alone may be restricted; subsequently all movements are restricted, so that in its most severe form there is up to 20° of fixed internal

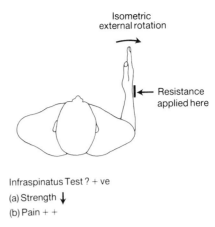

Isometric
external rotation

Resistance
applied here

Infraspinatus Test ? + ve
(a) Strength ↓
(b) Pain + +

FIG. 3.10 The elbow should be held by the examiner at a right angle prior to assessment of both the passive range of external rotation and the power of the external rotators (the infraspinatus test).

FIG. 3.11 Functional internal rotation (a) is compared with the normal side (b) by determining the number of the spinous process reached by the dorsum of the patient's hand.

(a)

(b)

FIG. 3.12 Passive adduction is tested by pushing the arm, held at shoulder level, across the front of the chest. (This is also used as the A-C joint stress test).

FIG. 3.13 The supraspinatus test is performed by resisting abduction with the arms in 20° abduction and 20° flexion.

rotation. These signs denote capsulitis, either post-traumatic or adhesive ('frozen shoulder').

(b) *The non-capsular pattern.* Chronic subacromial bursitis is one cause of a restriction of passive movements in a non-capsular pattern, although the possibility of more serious pathology (for instance, metastatic deposits) in the middle-aged and elderly should always be borne in mind. A typical pattern might be significant restriction of abduction and perhaps internal rotation, coupled with well-maintained external rotation. In acute bursitis, such as that which occurs in gout, all movements are grossly restricted. In this situation, the short history (hours or days), with no history of trauma, reduces the differential diagnosis to either gout or acute calcific tendinitis.

Assessing muscle balance

Apparent gross muscle weakness may be due to either pain inhibition or to neurological deficit, and should prompt regular examination over a few months. Winging of the scapula due to weakness of the serratus anterior may be a presenting feature of neuralgic amyotrophy—a disease which is still not clearly understood. Weakness of pectoralis major may be secondary to C7 nerve-root compression, but could also be due to direct injury (see Fig. 3.5). Occasionally minor tears of latissimus dorsi occur, giving rise to pain on resisted depression of the arm. Lesser degrees of muscle imbalance, possibly associated with loss

of flexibility, may not only indicate incomplete recovery, but may also be the precursors of a more substantial injury.

Assessment of the rotator cuff—the supraspinatus, infraspinatus, and subscapularis tests

The clinical assessment of the rotator cuff is an integral part of every examination of the shoulder. Rotator cuff injury in athletes and those participating in recreational sport is very common indeed. The muscles and their relationship to the subacromial bursa are examined as follows.

(a) *The supraspinatus test* (Fig. 3.13) is carried out with the patient standing. With the elbow straight the arm is placed in about 20° of both abduction and flexion, and the patient attempts to abduct the arm against resistance. The examiner assesses the strength of abduction, and the patient reports the amount of pain produced by this manoeuvre. The examiner then tests the opposite (normal) shoulder for comparison. If the test is painful, but there is no significant weakness, then this indicates supraspinatus tendinitis. Weakness on testing, however, indicates a rotator cuff tear. Unfortunately if there is a lot of pain during testing, weakness due to pain inhibition occurs, and the situation should be evaluated again after carrying out an impingement injection test.

(b) *The impingement injection test* (Neer 1983) allows the doctor to establish the exact site of the painful are syndrome. An injection of 5–10 ml of local anaesthetic (such as 0.25 per cent bupiva-caine or 1 per cent lignocaine) is given into the subacromial bursa in the region of the supraspinatus tendon. After ten minutes the patient is re-examined, and if the painful arc is improved or abol-ished, then the site of the pain has been established. After a supraspinatus test which is positive for pain an impingement test should be carried out to confirm the location of the pain, and then a further supraspinatus test should be carried out.

(c) *The infraspinatus test* (Fig. 3.10) is very similar to the supraspinatus test, and is a test of resisted (isometric) external rotation of the shoulder. The infraspinatus is the only efficient external rotator of the glenohumeral joint. Pain and weakness on testing are sought; pain denotes a tendinitis and weakness indi-cates a tear. Infraspinatus tears are particularly common in throw-ing athletes, but as the infraspinatus is almost totally muscular, tears usually heal, although they may have a protracted course.

(d) The *subscapularis* test (Fig. 3.14) is similar to but the oppo-site of the infraspinatus test—that is, resisted (isometric) *internal* rotation is assessed. Unfortunately this movement is produced by pectoralis major and latissimus dorsi, as well as subscapu-laris, and therefore this is not such a sensitive test.

(e) The *biceps* test (Fig. 3.15) is supposed to indicate biceps tendinitis. It is a test of resisted (isometric) elbow flexion, this being the activity which stresses particularly the long head of the biceps tendon. As biceps tendinitis is rare (despite comments made by other authors to the contrary), and a false-positive test

is common, particularly with subscapularis tendinitis, this test is unreliable. If the test is performed with a supinated forearm (instead of in neutral forearm rotation), an unstable biceps tendon may sublux from the bicipital groove.

(f) *Impingement signs* (Fig. 3.16) are produced by pushing the greater tuberosity upwards against the inferior aspect of the acromion—first when the arm is fully flexed, and secondly when the arm is internally rotated with 90° of forward flexion (Hawkins and Kennedy 1980; Gerber *et al.* 1985). The tests are positive when painful. Passive rotations of the shoulder are not significant restricted, although internal rotation is often painful—the non-capsular pattern emerges.

Other special tests to identify instability or specific joint pathologies are used at this stage. Which special tests are chosen depends on the differential diagnosis indicated by the previous history and examination. It is important not to carry out every special test on every patient, as this is both uncomfortable for the patient and time-consuming for the doctor. These special tests are described later.

(3) FEEL—*palpation* should be the final part of the examination because, again, where the examiner palpates depends on his likely diagnosis from the history and examination so far. Localized tenderness of the palpable portion of the subacromial bursa immediately inferior to the anterior margin of the acromion suggests subacromial bursitis. Tenderness of the inser-

FIG. 3.14 The subscapularis test is performed by resisting internal rotation.

FIG. 3.15 The biceps test is performed by resisting elbow flexion.

FIG. 3.16 The impingement signs: (a) full passive flexion; (b) 90° forward flexion combined with internal rotation.

(a)   (b)

tion of the supraspinatus tendon is most easily elicited when the arm is internally rotated behind the back, thus bringing the greater tuberosity to the fore.

Tenderness of the infraspinatus musculotendinous area should be detected with the patient prone, leaning on the elbow, and with the arm externally rotated 10°. Biceps tenderness (a non-specific sign) may be found in the bicipital groove. Subscapularis tenderness is felt more medially, over the anterior head of the humerus. Other anatomical sites—for instance, the coracoid process and the superior aspect of the A-C joint—may be palpated at this stage.

(4) FURTHER INVESTIGATIONS. Although most overuse syndromes of the shoulder are related to the soft tissues, radiographs can be helpful—particularly in excluding serious disorders (metabolic bone disorders and secondary tumours). Initially conventional AP and axial views are required. Two views of the shoulder are essential, and if it is not possible to abduct the arm sufficiently for a conventional axial view then a modified axial view as described by Wallace and Hellier (1983) should be taken. Ectopic calcification, resulting from degenerative change, may be seen in the region of the supraspinatus tendon (see Fig. 3.8). However, its presence is not necessary for the diagnosis of supraspinatus tendinitis; indeed it may be quite incidental, as demonstrated by one patient with clinical adhesive capsulitis who recovered fully following intra-articular steroid injections, but still had a large calcific deposit after treatment in a shoulder which was then painless. Nevertheless calcium may interfere mechanically with normal shoulder function. Not uncommonly, after a prolonged period lying 'dormant' within the cuff, an acute calcific tendinitis may develop suddenly. As the calcium liquefies an acute inflammatory response develops, causing the patient severe pain resulting in disturbance of sleep

and inability to move the arm. Degenerative changes within the A-C joint are common in middle-age, and again are usually of little significance. However, in weight-lifters and men doing heavy manual work the A-C joint occasionally develops a painful osteolysis, in which loss of bone, usually on the clavicular side of the joint, may be clearly seen on X-ray (Leyshon and Kessel 1982; Cahill 1982).

Further assessment and management of shoulder injuries

As highlighted in the previous section, the history is very important. In sportsmen and sportswomen the four common conditions which do not settle are:

(1) recurrent subluxation of the shoulder;
(2) chronic subacromial impingement syndrome (which may be secondary to recurrent subluxation);
(3) a rotator cuff tear;
(4) acromioclavicular disorders.

The assessment of the shoulder by an orthopaedic specialist will involve the following questions.

(a) What is your problem?
The problem will be pain, the giving way of the shoulder in certain positions, or inability to practise the sport to as high a standard as the athlete would wish. It should be remembered that it is not uncommon for a sportsman or sportswoman to fail to achieve a high standard and then to blame an injury for this, rather than to recognize that their failure of achievement is indeed due to a lack of skill.

(b) Where is the pain?

The pain will be identified either by the finger directed at the A-C joint area or by the palm of the hand directed to the front of the shoulder region or to the deltoid muscle.

(c) When does the pain occur—at rest? during activity? which activity?

Pain at rest normally indicates either early arthritis in the shoulder or a developing capsulitis ('frozen shoulder'), both of which are uncommon in the sportsman. Adhesive capsulitis may occur in the 45- to 60-year-old and, although not due to sport, nevertheless restricts activities, particularly racket sports. The capsular pattern of loss of movement is found on examination (Cyriax 1982). Management by intra-articular injection (see Fig. 12.9, p. 213), followed by stretching exercises (see Fig. 11.14, p. 198), has been found to be beneficial in most cases (Wallace and Echeverri 1987).

Pain on movement usually indicates a painful arc, and it is then necessary to identify which type of painful arc. There are four types: the subacromial painful arc, the A-C painful arc, the capsulitis painful arc, and the composite painful arc.

The *subacromial painful arc* (Fig. 3.17) typically produces a mid-arc pain during abduction (and less commonly during flexion) in the arc between 70° and 120° of elevation. It is accentuated by pronation of the forearm. This arc indicates pain arising from subacromial impingement. It will normally be improved or abolished by the impingement injection test.

The *A-C painful arc* (Fig. 3.18) is a painful arc at the extreme of flexion or abduction of the shoulder, occurring between 140° and 170° of elevation.

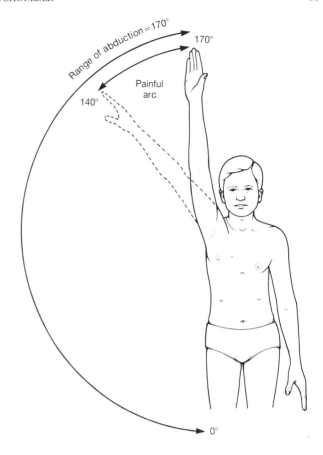

FIG. 3.18 A-C painful arc.

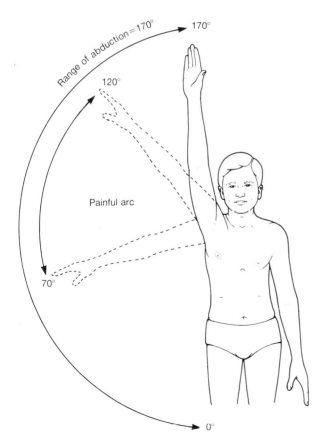

FIG. 3.17 Subacromial painful arc.

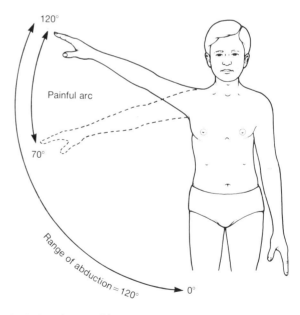

FIG. 3.19 Capsulitis painful arc.

The *capsulitis painful arc* (Fig. 3.19) is a terminal painful arc which occurs in a shoulder with a restricted range of movement—that is, elevation may be reduced to 120°, and the painful arc lies between 70° and 120°.

The *composite painful arc* (Fig. 3.20) is one where there is a near-normal range of shoulder elevation, but a painful arc from 70° to the top of the range. This is a fairly common situation. It

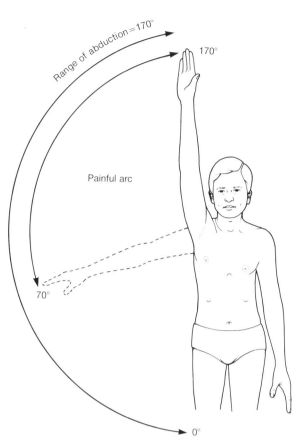

FIG. 3.20 Composite painful arc.

occurs in patients who have dual pathologies, such as A-C joint pain and a subacromial impingement, or subacromial impingement and an early capsulitis.

AN APPARENT SUBACROMIAL IMPINGEMENT SYNDROME IN A PATIENT UNDER THE AGE OF FORTY IS A TRAP FOR THE UNWARY—this is often a sign of shoulder instability, which produces secondary impingement.

(d) Is the shoulder unstable?
The patient will sometimes clearly say, 'I feel the shoulder jump out' or 'In some positions my shoulder seems to catch'. The patient is usually right, and it is important to explore the past history for a previous episode of possible traumatic dislocation. In a patient of under 30 years there is more than an 80 per cent likelihood of recurrent subluxation or recurrent dislocation following a reported past dislocation. A useful question to ask the patient is, 'Does your hand ever feel funny or develop pins and needles when your shoulder jumps?' If so, one can be confident that the problem is indeed an unstable shoulder.

Assessment of the shoulder for instability—anterior, posterior, and multidirectional

The doctor should assume that all patients with shoulder pain or a sensation of instability might have an unstable shoulder, and should carry out the following tests for instability, which have been well described by Gerber and Ganz (1984).

(a) Anterior apprehension test for anterior instability (Fig. 3.21)
The patient may be examined sitting though greater patient relaxation is usually achieved when supine. The problem shoul-

FIG. 3.21 Anterior apprehension test for instability.

der is passively abducted to 90° and is then passively externally rotated by the examiner into full external rotation. The arm is then pushed into the fully stressed position, while the patient's face is studied for apprehension and the anterior shoulder muscles are examined for muscle spasm. If pain is produced in an unstable shoulder, pressure backwards on the humeral neck may relieve it (the Jobe relocation test). The normal shoulder may then be stressed in the same way, and the two sides compared to detect loss of the passive range of movement. Finally on the problem side the arm is lifted higher under stressed external rotation, and then lowered through a range of 140° to 60° of abduction in order to identify any part of the abduction arc which produces apprehension. There is a risk during this test of provoking an anterior dislocation if the shoulder is grossly unstable; if this is suspected, extra care should be exercised.

(b) The sulcus sign (described by Neer and Foster 1980) for inferior subluxation (Fig. 3.22)
The patient is seated with both arms hanging downwards on either side of the chair and is asked to relax. The examiner applies a downward traction on the arm by holding the wrist and distracting the arm downwards firmly but not roughly. If the shoulder is inferiorly unstable, a sulcus will appear under the acromion—between the acromion and the humeral head—which will be both visible and palpable.

(c) Posterior stress test for posterior instability (Fig. 3.23)
The patient is examined lying supine on an examination couch. The arm is brought passively into 90° elevation in flexion. For examination of a right shoulder, the examiner's left hand is placed behind the glenohumeral joint—that is, under the shoulder blade. The humeral head is then pushed posteriorly by holding the elbow with the examiner's right hand and applying an axial loading to the humerus with the elbow at a right angle—that is, by pushing along the arm from the elbow, trying to push the humeral head backwards out of joint. If the joint is posteriorly unstable it will sublux posteriorly, and the examiner's left hand may feel this happening. However, it may not be picked up at this stage. The shoulder is next abducted in its 90° flexed position, with the shoulder axially loaded by the examiner's right hand—that is, the examiner continues to push hard along the length of the humerus, while *abducting* the shoulder. If the shoulder was posteriorly subluxed initially, as it is *abducted* it will jump back into joint and a clunk will be felt. Again, in the grossly unstable shoulder there is a definite risk of producing a complete posterior dislocation using this stress test.

These three tests are very valuable in the assessment of the problem shoulder. If one is positive the patient has a unidirectional instability, but if two or three tests are positive, then the instability is multidirectional and in general a very much more difficult condition to treat.

Further investigations for instability

All patients should have good quality radiographs—two AP views, one in external rotation and one in 60° internal rotation (Crawford Adams 1948). In addition a Stryker view is valuable

FIG. 3.22 The sulcus sign for inferior instability.

FIG. 3.23 Posterior stress test for instability.

in picking up the Hill-Sachs (Hill and Sachs 1940) or Broca (Broca and Hartman 1890) lesion, which is a bony dent in the humeral head. The other lesion typically found in 85 per cent of anterior dislocation patients (Rowe *et al.* 1978) is the Bankart lesion—an avulsion of the capsule and glenoid labrum from the anterior inferior portion of the glenoid rim. Usually this can be picked up only on an arthrogram (preferably a double-contrast CT arthrogram) or by arthroscopy; however, straight X-rays often show infraglenoid new bone formation (Hastings and Coughlin 1981). The indication for these further investigations is only when the diagnosis of instability is not definite or where there have been recurrent episodes of trouble with the shoulder and it has not been possible to make a diagnosis. Finally if the diagnosis is still in doubt it may be necessary to perform an examination under anaesthetic (EUA), which should be carried out by an orthopaedic surgeon with experience of shoulder instability.

Treatment for instability—anterior, posterior, and multidirectional

Anterior instability

If the shoulder is subluxing and not frankly dislocating, it is better to achieve stability, if possible, with rotator cuff-strengthening exercises. The supraspinatus will be built up with isometric and isokinetic abduction exercises, the infraspinatus with external rotation exercises with the arm by the side, and the subscapularis with internal rotation exercises. In general exercises should be restricted to below shoulder level, as subluxation is usually precipitated by elevation of the arm above shoulder level, and there is usually no problem with range of movement of the shoulder in these patients. The patient should be warned that some multi-gym activities do stress the shoulder and provoke rather than help anterior instability, and they should be given physiotherapy or medical guidance about which exercises are most appropriate for their instability.

  If anterior instability fails to respond to non-operative treatment for more than twelve months *and* the instability is unidirectional, then surgical stabilization of the shoulder should be considered. However, it is common after shoulder stabilization operations to lose at least 20° to 30° of elevation and external rotation, and in the cases of competitive athletes such as javelin

throwers, karate sportsmen, or cricket bowlers, this may end their sporting careers in these fields.

Posterior instability

This should also be treated with a conservative regime of strengthening exercise for a period of at least twelve months, again using rotator cuff-strengthening exercises, but concentrating on building up the infraspinatus and teres minor muscles posteriorly. Strengthening exercises appear to be more successful for posterior instability than for anterior instability.

  If posterior instability fails to settle with conservative treatment, then surgery may be considered. Although loss of range of movement is less of a problem with posterior stabilization operations, recurrence of the subluxation is not uncommon, and the patient should be warned before surgery that the surgeon cannot guarantee long-term success from this type of operation—perhaps a success rate of only 60 per cent.

Multidirectional instability

Patients who have instability in more than one direction provide a major treatment problem. Athletes—particularly swimmers and gymnasts—often have to retire early from their sporting careers if they develop this problem. Generalized joint laxity may exist, so that examination of the wrists, thumbs, elbows, and knees should be made to detect hyperextensibility (see Fig. 1.12, p. 11). The treatment is a conservative regime of strengthening of the rotator cuff muscles, with up to two years of physiotherapy and avoidance of activities which provoke the subluxation episodes. Sport may have to be discontinued during the treatment period. It has been felt by some shoulder surgeons that certain multi-gym exercises (particularly those which stretch the anterior shoulder capsule, as occurs with movements of 90° abduction with 90° external rotation) have been responsible for producing this kind of instability, and it is also more common in butterfly swimmers.

  If multidirectional instability continues for more than two years, and the patient wishes to accept a failure rate of 50 per cent, then surgery can be considered. Dr Neer in New York has devised an 'inferior capsular shift' operation for multidirectional instability, but, regrettably, recurrence of instability is fairly common after this procedure, and it is essential that the patient is warned about this before surgery.

Treatment for rotator cuff impingement and tears

Chronic rotator cuff impingement causes a recurrent subacromial painful arc syndrome. In the patient under 40 years of age the diagnosis of instability must first be excluded on clinical examination. Initial management is demonstrated in Fig. 12.10 (see p. 214), with an injection of the subacromial bursa (*not* the supraspinatus tendon) with a mixture of 5 ml of local anaesthetic (for instance, 1 per cent lignocaine or 0.25 per cent bupivacaine) and long-acting local steroid (for instance, 1 ml–20 mg of triamcinolone hexacetonide). Up to three injections (at intervals of four weeks between injections) may be necessary. If injection treatment fails, local physiotherapy, with ice-massage, ultrasound, pulsed electromagnetic field treatment (PEMF), interferential, and particularly deep transverse frictions (Cyriax 1984) directed to an individual cuff tendon, can be very successful.

Normally tendinitis and associated subacromial bursitis resolve following subacromial injections and the use of localized physiotherapeutic anti-inflammatory modalities. Occasionally insertional tendinitis (usually of the supraspinatus) proves to be refractory.

In this situation the insertion of the supraspinatus may be injected with low-dose steroid—such as 10 mg triamcinolone hexacetonide (M.A.H.) (see Fig. 12.11, p. 215). If symptomatic calcific tendinitis is present, 'dry' needling may be successful, though an additional injection of steroid and local anaesthetic for the associated inflammatory reaction is a more logical approach. Rarely, the insertions of infraspinatus and subscapularis into the greater and lesser tuberosities respectively require injection (see Figs. 12.12 and 12.13, p. 215 and 216). The infraspinatus lesion frequently lies at the musculotendinous junction, when it should be treated as a muscle tear. In all cases in which enthesopathies are injected it is particularly important to follow up with strengthening exercises. Biceps tendinitis is relatively uncommon; occasionally an injection around the tendon in the bicipital groove is helpful if physiotherapy is unsuccessful (see Fig. 12.14, p. 216).

Flexibility exercises

Aggressive stretching exercises must not be used in the inflammatory phase, as they may contribute to persistence of the condition. In the presence of painful restriction of shoulder movements the only flexibility exercises performed by the patient are Codman exercises (Fig. 3.24), which allow gravity to distract the glenohumeral joint. The therapist may utilize Maitland's passive exercises under gentle arm traction (Maitland 1986).

Once subacromial bursitis has resolved (or surgical stabilization has been achieved), graded stretching exercises with a stick or cane are encouraged on a home physiotherapy regimen (see Fig. 11.14, p. 198). Particular attention is paid to those movements which are relatively restricted: loss of passive external rotation, for instance, tends to occur in racket players and swimmers as a result of the overdevelopment of the medial rotators. Flexibility exercises should be considered later for prophylaxis.

Strengthening exercises

Isometric contraction within the painless range may be commenced as soon as there is sufficient healing of the cuff tendons to allow this to be performed painlessly. In due course exercises with surgical tubing or 'Cliniband' are instituted (Fig. 3.25), and followed if possible by isokinetic exercises. Attention is paid to the full complement of muscle groups responsible for internal

FIG. 3.24 The position of the patient is demonstrated for circumduction movements of the right shoulder under the effect of gravity (Codman exercises).

and external rotation, flexion, extension, abduction, and adduction. Once it has been determined that strength in all groups has improved to equal that of the normal side, isotonic contractions using hand-held weights and other available equipment may be started under the guidance of the therapist (Fig. 3.26). However, it is important that an inappropriate level of stress is not imposed on the shoulder too early in that position in which impingement or subluxation has been noted to occur.

Sports techniques

The mechanics of shoulder function, as applied to the specific sport, should be assessed to determine whether alterations of technique are possible to reduce stress. In swimming, impingement syndromes may be alleviated by measures such as raising the arm higher during the recovery phase, reducing extension of the arm by elevating the elbow at hand entry, and improving body-roll during the pull phase. Similar attention to biomechanical detail is often necessary in throwing and in racket sports, a sit-

(a)

(b)

(c)

(d)

(e)

Fɪɢ. 3.25 Strengthening exercises for the shoulder muscles may be performed with Cliniband (as shown) or surgical tubing: (a) abductors; (b) and (c) external rotators; (d) internal rotators; (e) extensors.

uation which demands close cooperation with the coach. Tennis servers, for instance, learn to rotate the side of the body towards the net as the racket arm is raised above the horizontal: failure to achieve correct body rotation forces the arm to be raised lateral to the functional arc of elevation, thereby risking a recurrence of symptoms. Adjustments may be made by baseball pitchers who learn to throw 'three-quarters side-arm' rather than full overhead.

Surgery

If the problem remains chronic and lasts for longer than nine months to one year, and temporary benefit has been achieved with injection treatment, then a subacromial decompression operation may be considered. The operation described by Neer in 1972 and shown in Fig. 3.27 is preferred to that described by Watson (1978), which in the experience of one of the present authors has less good results (W.A.W.). McShane *et al.* (1978) have shown that 40 per cent of patients have residual symptoms after this procedure, which are reduced if a powered burr is used for the surgery instead of an osteotome. Post-operative physiotherapy is important, and the athlete can expect to return to sport from twelve to sixteen weeks after surgery. An improvement can be expected in 80 per cent of patients treated sur-

gically, although only about 30 per cent will consider their shoulder completely cured. Since 1984 arthroscopic subacromial decompression operations, using a high-speed burr to remove the anterior and inferior acromion and coracoacromial ligament, have become increasingly popular in the USA (Ellman 1985). The recovery time using the arthroscopic technique is much quicker, and return to sport can be in as little as four to six weeks. However, this treatment has not yet been fully evaluated.

The most common cause of a chronic subacromial painful arc is a partial- or full-thickness rotator cuff tear. The diagnosis can often, but not always, be made with an arthrogram, but more recently arthroscopy of the shoulder has been found to be quite reliable in establishing the correct diagnosis (Bunker 1989). Full-thickness tears are categorized according to size, with small tears having a maximum dimension of 3 cm, medium tears 3 to 5 cm, and larger tears greater than 5 cm. In athletes chronic tears are much more common in the supraspinatus tendon, and it is rare to find a large tear. Fortunately both partial-thickness and full-thickness tears under 5 cm in maximum dimension can usually be satisfactorily repaired at the time of a subacromial decompression operation. Partial-thickness rotator cuff tears are best treated by opening the cuff fully and carrying out a formal

FIG. 3.26 Isotonic exercises using hand-held weights are demonstrated.

FIG. 3.27 Neer's anterior acromioplasty and decompression.

repair as for a full-thickness tear. The repair is carried out with interrupted non-absorbable sutures, with the repair technique varied according to the findings at operation. Again, post-operative physiotherapy is important, but recovery will take longer, with a return to sport delayed until sixteen to thirty weeks after surgery, depending on the size of the tear. Although the author (W.A.W.) has returned top-class sportsmen to their sport after surgical repair of rotator cuff tears, the outcome is not fully predictable and cannot be guaranteed.

The acromioclavicular joint

Assessment

Acute injury to the A-C joint usually results from a fall on to the point of the shoulder. It is particularly common in rugby football, and is often mistakenly diagnosed by the inexperienced traumatologist as a glenohumeral joint injury. A grade 1 injury involves a sprain of the superior A-C ligament. Further injury results in a subluxation (grade II) or a dislocation (Grade III), in which the coracoclavicular ligaments are torn. On inspection a

(a)

FIG. 3.28 A Grade III A-C joint injury: (a) Clinical—a step may be seen and palpated, (b) X-ray—confirms A-C joint dislocation.

step may be seen and palpated in grade III injuries (Fig. 3.28), but this may be missed during the first few days because of the local soft tissue swelling.

A-C joint pain is located at the point of the shoulder directly over the joint. It is aggravated by forced *adduction* of the shoulder

FIG. 3.29 Resisted adduction provokes A-C joint pain.

with the arm in 90° of flexion (Fig. 3.12). However, this test may also cause pain in a patient with a supraspinatus tendinitis. An additional useful test is resisted isometric *adduction* of the shoulder with the arm hanging close to the side (Fig. 3.29), which will aggravate pain in a patient who has pain arising from the A-C joint. In acute injuries a diagnosis of an A-C joint sprain, with subluxation or dislocation, should be explored with stress radiographs (Bannister *et al.* 1984). The site of the pain can be confirmed by a local anaesthetic diagnostic test—1 to 2 ml of local anaesthetic is injected into the A-C joint and 1 ml infiltrated into the superior A-C ligament (see Fig. 12.15, p. 217). If after five to ten minutes this improves or abolishes the pain on carrying out the above diagnostic tests, the diagnosis is established.

Treatment

The outcome from A-C joint injuries has been clearly highlighted by a randomized prospective study carried out by Bannister *et al.* (1984). In general a conservative expectant policy should be adopted, with early physiotherapy and muscle-strengthening exercises. Local pain will resolve over a period of six to eight weeks, and a return to sport may follow at around the same time. For recurrent chronic A-C joint pain, osteoarthritis of the A-C joint is the most likely cause. This is best treated with one to three injections of local steroid (10 mg triamcinolone hexacetonide) at two to three months intervals (see Fig. 12.15, p. 217). Local physiotherapy with ultrasound and 'mobilization' treatment of the joint can be very beneficial if injection treatment fails. Only a small proportion of patients fail to respond to such treatment, and if symptoms continue for longer than nine to twelve months, surgery (resection of the lateral 1 cm of the clavicle) can be considered. This is a very successful operation, with 90 per cent of patients satisfied (Taylor and Tooke 1977), but it often leaves the shoulder with a slight weakness for heavy manual tasks.

The scapulothoracic joint

Assessment

This joint is examined by positioning the patient erect and asking him to lift the arm, first in flexion and then in abduction, into full elevation. The scapula should slide smoothly over the posterior chest wall. If the scapula jerks, this indicates a disorder of the scapulothoracic joint, a glenohumeral joint disorder such as subluxation, or a subacromial joint disorder such as impingement or a supraspinatus tendinitis. If, in addition to jerking, the scapula makes a snapping sound, this indicates a problem in the scapulothoracic joint area. Crepitus may be palpated alongside the medial border of the scapula in the less severe case ('scapulothoracic bursitis'). If the snapping is pain free, it should be ignored completely and the patient should be reassured. If the snapping is painful, treatment should be considered.

Treatment

'Scapulothoracic bursitis' may be treated with local steroid injections and a short period of rest. However, a painful snapping scapula can be very disabling in an athlete, and can be responsible for prolonged disability. The first-line treatment is rest, and avoidance of aggravating the pain and snapping. This treatment is not popular with a sportsman, but should be carried on for at least four to six months. However, if the problem recurs on returning to sport and the athlete feels that the symptoms are excessively restrictive, then surgery may be offered. The results of surgical release of the plane between the subscapularis and serratus anterior and the chest wall (a subscapular mobilization) have been found to be promising (Foy and Wallace, personal communication).

The sternoclavicular joint

Assessment

The sternoclavicular joint can give rise to pain either from degenerative change (osteoarthritis) or from instability. The common situation is in the late teens when a girl athlete develops pain and an intermittent anterior displacement (or subluxation) of the medial end of the clavicle during elevation of the arm. The initial provoking injury is not usually a major one. A careful assessment of all joints is indicated because this condition may be associated with a generalized joint laxity. In particular it is vital to examine the other sternoclavicular joint very carefully, because usually it is also found to be abnormal. On examination the affected joint will be found to be slightly tender, and will displace obviously on full elevation of the arm (Fig. 3.30). The joint may also produce a palpable click on displacement. Radiographs are rarely helpful.

Fig. 3.30 An anterior sternoclavicular joint subluxation.

Treatment

For instability of the joint non-surgical local treatment with ultrasound or PEMF therapy may result in a reduction of the tenderness. Surgical treatment should only be considered as a last resort, as most patients with this problem do learn to live and cope with it (although that may involve giving up sport). Surgery to the sternoclavicular joint area is dangerous, and deaths have occurred even in the best surgical hands. The author (W.A.W.) has attempted to stabilize six joints surgically, with four relative successes; however, if the joint has been successfully stabilized there is usually a loss of up to 40° of arm elevation, and this may in itself limit the patients' capacity to carry out their chosen sport. Osteoarthritis of the sternoclavicular joint is uncommon, but when it occurs and causes persistent symptoms, surgical resection of the medial 1 cm of the clavicle can be very successful.

Don't forget the neck

The neck and the shoulder are closely related, and the relationship between neck pain and shoulder pain is complex. If smooth coordinated movements of the shoulder are lost owing to shoulder pathology, then an increased muscular strain is placed on the neck, particularly by the trapezius, sternomastoid, and levator scapulae muscles. This commonly causes secondary neck pain. A reduction of spasm with massage or relaxation therapy will help this. It is also worth trying cervical mobilization or traction, even when the problems are obviously primarily in the shoulder.

As indicated at the beginning of this chapter, the authors believe that one reason why shoulder pain is so common is because of primary C5 nerve root irritation resulting in secondary C5 muscle incoordination and weakness, and resulting pain in the subacromial joint. Therefore it is necessary to perform a full assessment of the cervical spine (see Chapter 5) and direct treatment, if indicated, to the neck as well as to the shoulder in patients with shoulder disability. It is also important to recognize the corollary—it is often possible to relieve neck pain, even if the neck is the primary problem, by treating a disordered shoulder.

Summary of examination procedures

(1) LOOK
Observation
- of deformity—dislocation of A-C or glenohumeral joints —fracture
- of swelling—acute bursitis
- of muscle wasting

(2) MOVE
(a) Active movements:
- flexion—range of movement/painful arc
- abduction—range of movement/painful arc

(b) Passive movements:
- flexion
- abduction—both combined and glenohumeral
- flexion and adduction
- rotation—internal and external

(3) FEEL

Palpation for tenderness	● A-C joint
	● subacromial
	● rotator cuff insertions

(4) SPECIAL TESTS

(a) Rotator cuff (resisted contraction)	● supraspinatus test = abduction
	● infraspinatus = external rotation
	● subscapularis test = internal rotation
	● biceps test = elbow flexion at 90°
(b) Impingement	● signs
	● injection test
(c) Instability	● anterior apprehension test
	● inferior—sulcus sign
	● posterior stress test

References

Andrews, J. R., Carson, W. G., and McLeod, W. D. (1985). Glenoid labrum tears related to the long head of biceps. *Am. J. Sports Med.*, **13**, 337–41.

Bannister, G. C., Stableforth, P. G., Wallace, W. A., and Hutson, M. A. (1984). A prospective study of the treatment of acromio-clavicular dislocation. *J. Bone Jt. Surg.*, **66B**, 279.

Broca, A. and Hartman, H. (1890). Contribution à l'étude des luxations de l'épaule. *Bull. Soc. Anat. Paris*, **5me Série, 4**, 312.

Bunker, T. (1989). Shoulder arthroscopy. *Ann. R. Coll. Surg.*, **71**, 213–17.

Cahill, B. R. (1982). Osteolysis of the distal part of the clavicle in male athletes. *J. Bone Jt. Surg.*, **64A**, 1053–8.

Crawford Adams, J. C. (1948). Recurrent dislocation of the shoulder. *J. Bone Jt. Surg.*, **30B**, 26–38.

Cyriax, J. (1982). *Textbook of orthopaedic medicine*, Vol. 1 (8th edn). Ballière Tindall, London.

Cyriax, J. and Russell, G. (1984). *Textbook of orthopaedic medicine*, Vol. 2 (11th edn). Baillière Tindall, London.

Ellman, H. (1985). Arthroscopic subacromial decompression: a preliminary report. *Orthop. Trans.*, **9** (1), 43.

Gerber, C. and Ganz, R. (1984). Clinical assessment of instability of the shoulder—with special reference to anterior and posterior drawer tests. *J. Bone Jt. Surg.*, **66B**, 551–6.

Gerber, C., Terrier, F., and Ganz, R. (1985). The role of the coracoid in the chronic impingement syndrome. *J. Bone Jt. Surg.*, **67B**, 703–8.

Hastings, D. E. and Coughlin, L. P. (1981). Recurrent subluxation of the glenohumeral joint. *Am. J. Sports Med.*, **9**, 352–5.

Hawkins, R. J. and Kennedy, J. C. (1980). Impingement syndrome in athletes. *Am. J. Sports Med.*, **8**, 151–8.

Hill, H. A. and Sachs, M. D. (1940). The grooved defect of the humeral head. A frequently unrecognised complication of dislocation of the shoulder joint. *Radiology*, **35**, 690–700.

Howell, S. M., Imobersteg, A. M., Seger, D. H., and Marone, P. J. (1986). Clarification of the role of the supraspinatus muscle in shoulder function. *J. Bone Jt. Surg.*, **68A**, 398–404.

Kennedy, J. C., Hawkins, R., and Krissof, W. B. (1978). Orthopaedic manifestations of swimming. *Am. J. Sports Med.*, **6**, 309–22.

Leyshon, A. and Kessel, L. (1982). Post-traumatic osteolysis of the distal clavicle. In *Shoulder surgery* (ed. I. Bayley and L. Kessel), pp. 183–7. Springer-Verlag, Berlin.

McShane, R. B., Leinberry, C. F., and Fenlin, J. M. (1978). Conservative open anterior acromioplasty. *Clin. Orthop.*, **223**, 137–44.

Maitland, G. D. (1986). *Vertebral manipulation* (5th edn). Butterworths, London.

Neer, C. S. (1972). Anterior acromioplasty for the chronic impingement syndrome in the shoulder. *J. Bone Jt. Surg.*, **54A**, 41–50.

Neer, C. S. (1983). Impingement lesions. *Clin. Orthop.*, **173**, 70–7.

Neer, C. S. and Foster, C. R. (1980). Inferior capsular shift for involuntary inferior and multi-directional instability of the shoulder. *J. Bone Jt. Surg.*, **62A**, 897–908.

Petersson, C. J. and Gentz, C. F. (1983). Ruptures of the supraspinatus tendon. The significance of distally pointing acromio-clavicular osteophytes. *Clin. Orthop.*, **174**, 143–8.

Poppen, N. K. and Walker, P. S. (1976). Normal and abnormal motion of the shoulder, *J. Bone Jt. Surg.*, **58A**, 195–201.

Rathbun, J. B. and MacNab, I. (1970). The microvascular pattern of the rotator cuff. *J. Bone Jt. Surg.*, **52B**, 540–53.

Richardson, A. B., Jobe, F. W., and Collins, H. R. (1980). The shoulder in competitive swimming. *Am. J. Sports Med.*, **8**, 159–63.

Rowe, C. R., Patel, D., and Southmayd, W. W. (1978). The Bankart procedure—a long-term end result study. *J. Bone Jt. Surg.*, **60A**, 1–16.

Scott B., Barton, M. A. J., and Wallace, W. A. (1992). Diagnosis and assessment of pectoralis major rupture by dynamometry. *J. Bone Jt. Surg.*, **74B**, 111–13.

Simonet, W. T. and Cofield, R.H. (1984). Prognosis in anterior shoulder dislocation. *Am. J. Sports Med.*, **12**, 19–24.

Taylor, G. M. and Tooke, M. (1977). Degenerative of the acromio-clavicular joint as a cause of shoulder pain. *J. Bone Jt. Surg.*, **59B**, 507.

van Linge, B. and Mulder, J. D. (1963). Function of the supraspinatus muscle and its relation to the supraspinatus syndrome. *J. Bone Jt. Surg.*, **45B**, 750–54.

Wallace, W. A. (1984). Evaluation of the forces, ICR and the neutral point during abduction of the shoulder. *Transactions of the 30th Annual Meeting of the Orthopaedic Research Society*, **9**, 5.

Wallace, W. A. and Echeverri, A. (1987). Intra-articular distension with local anaesthetic, steroid and air in the treatment of capsulitis of the shoulder. In *The Shoulder* (ed. N. Takagishi), pp. 204–8. Professional Postgraduate Services, Tokyo.

Wallace, W. A. and Hellier, M. (1983). Improving radiographs of the injured shoulder. *Radiography*, **49**, 229–33.

Wallace, W. A. and Johnson, F. (1982). A biochemical appraisal of the acromioclavicular joint. In *Shoulder surgery* (ed I. Bayley and L. Kessel), pp. 179–82. Springer-Verlag. Berlin.

Watson, M. (1978). The refractory painful arc syndrome. *J. Bone Jt. Surg.*, **60B**, 544–6.

Weiner, D. S. and McNab, I. (1970). Superior migration of the humeral head: a radiological aid in the diagnosis of tears of the rotator cuff. *J. Bone Jt. Surg.*, **52B**, 524–7.

4 Injuries to the upper limb

M. A. HUTSON AND N. J. BARTON

Overuse injuries

M. A. HUTSON

It is a natural consequence of most sports and recreational activities that loss of balance may result in a fall onto the outstretched hand and thus incur the risks of *trauma* to the elbow or wrist. An ensuing dislocation or fracture is of the same type as that sustained in most other circumstances, although any subsequent loss of flexibility (for example, loss of extension at the elbow) may result in grave problems for the athlete. For an understanding of the major joint injuries or fractures at and above the wrist, however, the reader should refer to suitable texts on orthopaedic surgery. The team doctor or general practitioner may be called upon to advise on hand injuries, for in certain sports such as cricket there is a commonly held view that 'getting on with the game', using strapping and early mobilization, is better than the enforced rest that otherwise may be prescribed upon the diagnosis of a fracture. To clarify this situation, hand and wrist injuries are included in the second part of this chapter, 'injuries to the hand and wrist'. *Overuse* injuries are common, especially in the forearm, and are covered in some depth. They arise particularly in racket sports and, in common with impingement problems at the shoulder, in those sports that involve throwing.

Applied anatomy/biomechanics

The function of the elbow is principally to allow the hand to be positioned for maximal efficiency; it is aided by the joints between radius and ulna. The *humero-ulnar* joint is inherently stable, being of the uniaxial hinge type. In extension there is a natural carrying angle of 10°–15° of valgus, greater in women than men. This is obliterated when the forearm is pronated or when the elbow is flexed. The *radiohumeral* joint is a shallow ball-and-socket joint, with the head of the radius being protected by the annular ligament; it is involved in the transmission of forces across the elbow, rather than in contributing towards stability. Since most stresses to the elbow are in the form of axial compression and medial tension, the medial ligament is strong. It has several components which produce tautness in both flexion and extension. Rotation of the forearm (into pronation and supination) is allowed at the superior and inferior *radio-ulnar joints*, which are pivotal in type. Injury to the distal radius may involve the inferior radio-ulnar joint and thus affect rotation. Displaced fractures of the distal third of the radial shaft are invariably associated with disruption of the inferior radio-ulnar joint (Galeazzi fracture-dislocation); although uncommon, they usually occur in the young adult. Angulated fractures of the proximal ulna are accompanied by a dislocation of the superior radio-ulnar joint (Monteggia fracture-dislocation). Thus it is important to examine (and X-ray) the elbow and wrist in the presence of a fracture of the radius or ulna, so that disruptions of the radio-ulnar joints may be diagnosed and treated.

The biceps brachii (Fig. 4.1) and triceps muscles are primarily responsible for flexion and extension at the elbow (as well as contributing towards flexion and extension at the shoulder). In addition, as a result of its distal attachment to the radius, the biceps is a powerful supinator of the forearm. Overall, supination is more powerful than pronation: hence the clockwise direction of the screwdriving mechanism. If greater power is required, the forearm may be locked and the rotator muscles of the shoulder recruited. Wrist and hand movements involved in the process of gripping are controlled by the extensors and radial deviators of the wrist arising from the lateral epicondyle of the humerus, and the flexors and ulnar deviators arising from the medial epi-

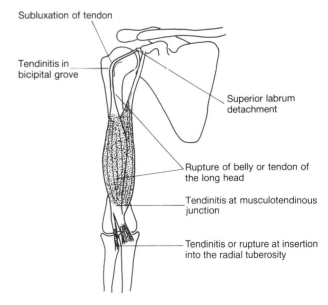

FIG. 4.1 Lesions of the biceps brachii are demonstrated.

condyle. The pronator teres also arises from the medial epicondyle—a fact which is of some significance in determining the cause of chronic medial elbow pain.

In throwing (see Chapter 3) the elbow is flexed to approximately 45° during the cocking phase, and forcibly extended towards the end of acceleration and in follow-through. The forearm is pronated, and the wrist flexed, in follow-through. Such propulsive efforts involving elbow extension may be seen in cricket, racket overheads and backhand, baseball pitching, swimming, discus and javelin throwing, and shot putting (Fig. 4.2). In these circumstances injury may occur as a result of the olecranon being forced into the olecranon fossa and the application of valgus stress during acceleration.

Acute injury to the elbow

Injuries to the elbow usually result from a fall onto the outstretched hand with the elbow locked into extension. Should the elbow be flexed, protection may be afforded by the shock absorption of the relevant muscle groups. In a child, epiphyseal fracture and avulsion fracture of the medial epicondyle may occur. In the adult, posterior dislocation of the elbow is a potentially serious injury; it may be complicated by vascular impairment, which, if it persists after reduction, needs very urgent surgical intervention. Subsequent loss of extension is likely. In children, the common supracondylar fracture also threatens the vascular supply and, if mismanaged, may give rise to Volkmann's ischaemic contracture. If involved in rehabilitation, the physician is advised to treat the elbow with the utmost respect, as any attempt to be aggressive

FIG. 4.2 Forceful elbow extension occurs in shot-putting.

towards the recovery of elbow extension may be counterproductive and lead to myositis ossificans. In the early stage, flexion exercises only should be countenanced.

In the child the elbow may be 'pulled out' when the head of the radius is avulsed from its restraining annular ligament: further advice should be sought. Fracture around the elbow should always be referred to an orthopaedic surgeon, as fixation may be required. However, the undisplaced olecranon fracture due to forced stretching of the contracting triceps may be managed by a few weeks in a sling. Similarly, a fracture of the radial head requires no more than support for a couple of weeks, though the period required to regain a full range of movement is often frustratingly prolonged.

A *haemarthrosis* may result from a relatively inconsequential undisplaced fracture. It may be recognised by the restriction in active and passive elbow movements in the capsular pattern (relatively greater restriction of flexion than extension) and by a boggy swelling which can be seen and felt either side of the olecranon process. X-rays usually show the 'fat pad' sign (Fig. 10.6, p. 172). Aspiration relieves pain—a posterolateral approach between the head of the radius and the humerus is desirable (Fig. 12.17, p. 218). Subsequently elbow extension tends to lag behind during recovery.

Overuse injury—elbow and forearm

Impingement syndromes

Repeated high-velocity elbow extension in throwers may provoke hypertrophy of the olecranon process as a result of impingement on the humerus in the olecranon fossa (Fig. 4.3). Symptoms include pain on throwing and impairment of throwing efficiency, as the capacity to extend the elbow fully is insidiously lost. Forced passive extension of the elbow is painful. Initially an appraisal of the throwing technique is necessary, and liaison with the patient's coach is desirable. In the established case, surgery is required to trim the posteromedial aspect of the olecranon (Wilson *et al.* 1983); recurrence of hypertrophic impingement may occur nevertheless. Stress fracture of the olecranon has been described from the same cause, and would be expected to resolve uneventfully following a suitable period of rest.

Medial distraction: avulsion of medial epicondyle

Contracture of common flexor origin

Chronic sprain/laxity of medial ligament

Posterior impingement of the olecranon in the olecranon fossa

Osteochondritis of capitellum: *lateral compression*

FIG. 4.3 'Thrower's elbow'. Repetitive throwing or pitching may give rise to elbow problems. These include posterior impingement of the olecranon in the olecranon fossa, valgus stress to the medial structures of the elbow joint, and compression injuries to the radiohumeral joint.

Medial joint injuries

Overload in throwing (for instance, discus throwing and baseball pitching) imposes repeated valgus stress upon the medial joint structures, principally the medial collateral ligament and common flexor origin, and compressive stress to the radio-humeral joint (Fig. 4.3). The medial collateral ligament undergoes repeated micro-tears, culminating in ectopic calcification and bony spur formation. Rupture may eventually occur. In the child and adolescent, 'Little Leaguer's elbow' (in baseball pitchers) is a descriptive label for recurrent medial joint pain, the causes of which include traction avulsion of the medial epicondyle. Baseball pitching is clearly a common source of elbow pain in the USA, and has been well documented (Slocum 1978); the combination of olecranon hypertrophy, chronic medial ligamentous strain, and contracture of the common flexors at their origin from the medial epicondyle leads to fixed flexion contracture in the elbows of 50 per cent of professional baseball pitchers (King *et al.* 1969). In the less established case, active and passive extension of the elbow are comfortable; the imposition of valgus stress with the elbow flexed to 30° provokes pain, and laxity may also be present. Isometric contractions are usually painless. Injections of small doses of steroid (for example, 10 mg triamcinolone hexacetonide) assist in the resolution of the symptoms, though recurrences are common unless biomechanical stress is reduced by an appropriate alteration of technique.

Medial epicondylitis (golfer's elbow)

Although less common than lateral epicondylitis, this is nevertheless a troublesome condition that is often difficult to eradicate. It is an enthesitis of the common flexor/pronator origin from the medial epicondyle. Localized discomfort that may radiate to the flexor aspect of the forearm is the principal complaint. Although isometric contraction of the wrist or finger flexors may be uncomfortable, it is predominantly the pronator teres that is affected, thus reflecting the aetiology of the condition. Over-pronation of the forearm, for instance, may be seen in a tennis player with a technically faulty topspin forehand, or in a golfer with an overdominant right hand. Short-term improvement may be gained by steroid injections and other anti-inflammatory measures. Correction of abnormal biomechanics is essential for a long-term cure.

Lateral epicondylitis (tennis elbow)

This is an extremely common condition, which arises from overload in industrial and domestic situations as well as in sport. The middle-aged male in particular is at risk from indulgence in occasional DIY activities, including repetitive screwdriving and bricklaying. In the sporting context, racket sports—for example, tennis, badminton, and squash—are the likely causes. Essentially it is an enthesitis, involving the common extensor origin from the lateral epicondyle, and is associated with repeated grasping. Pain or discomfort is felt over the lateral aspect of the elbow, frequently radiating either proximally or (more commonly) distally to the extensor aspect of the forearm. Grasping is painful—even simply holding a tea-cup. The aetiological factors include:

(1) overload—related to the sheer frequency of shots played;
(2) incorrect technique, particularly on the backhand;
(3) too small a racket handle;
(4) recent change of racket—for instance, from wood to graphite;
(5) too tight a grip between shots;
(6) muscle imbalance/loss of flexibility.

On examination, passive elbow movements are usually painless, though in the acute case extension is painful and may be slightly restricted. Passive stretching of the musculotendinous structures arising from the lateral epicondyle by the combination of elbow extension, pronation of the forearm, and palmar flexion of the wrist may be painful. The typical pattern on isometric contraction is pain on testing one or more of the wrist extensors, radial deviators, and finger extensors. Of these, the wrist extensors (extensors carpi radialis longus and brevis) are primarily affected. Tenderness is localized to the common extensor origin from the lateral epicondyle.

Initial management should be in the form of a short period of rest from sport, combined with ice and ultrasound. Subsequent treatment includes friction massage (for example, thrice a week for eight weeks) in addition to ice and ultrasound. This may be followed by Mills' manoeuvre, in which the examiner fully pronates the forearm, flexes the wrist, and then forcibly extends the affected elbow (Cyriax 1982). Regrettably, however, patients may develop a traumatic synovitis of the elbow joint if the procedure is over-vigorous. By far the most rapidly effective treatment is steroid injection. If accurately placed, one injection of 10 mg triamcinolone will suffice in 90 per cent of cases and two injections, ten days apart, in most of the remaining 10 per cent (Fig. 12.16, p. 218). However, it is necessary to identify any appropriate aetiological factors, often by referral to a coach. The player should be restrained from playing for several weeks, during which suitable stretching and strengthening exercises are considered. If imbalance is detected, the flexors may be strengthened. Regular stretching of the extensors is also logical. An epicondylitis clasp or medisplint may be prescribed in refractory cases.

Despite all this, recurrence is sufficiently common for the sufferer to be sceptical of a 'cure' being achieved. Once a recurrence has occurred, steroid injections tend to give relief for shorter periods, so that some cases appear refractory to all conservative methods. Cyriax has stated that, if left untreated, tennis elbow resolves spontaneously over a year or fifteen months, though few sportsmen have this patience. Alternatively, a muscle slide operation may be performed, although the results are by no means uniformly successful. At best, an attempt may be made at surgery to exclude nerve entrapment masquerading as tennis elbow. Entrapment of the dorsal branch of the radial nerve or the posterior interosseous nerve by the supinator or extensor carpi radialis brevis muscles has been described, though in the author's experience it is very uncommon. Tenderness is then usually felt over the anterior aspect of the radial head rather than over the common extensor origin from the humerus, and resisted extension of the middle finger with the elbow extended (thereby tightening the origin of extensor carpi radialis brevis) is stated to be invariably painful (Roles and Maudsley 1972).

Muscle lesions

Repetitive stress may give rise to minor tears occurring in muscle bellies around the elbow. Presenting as a variety of tennis elbow, the lesion occurs in one of the extensor muscle bellies some centimetres distal to the lateral epicondyle. Similarly, on the medial aspect of the antecubital fossa, the pronator teres may be tender 2–3 cm from the medial epicondyle, as a variety of golfer's elbow. Lesions of brachioradialis may occur, and insertional lesions of biceps brachii are perhaps slightly more common (Fig. 4.1). Occasionally, the distal biceps tendon is ruptured in the middle-aged. Early surgical reconstruction should be considered; otherwise, loss of power of supination as well as elbow flexion usually results in significant loss of function. Identification should be made by tissue tension tests (pain on resisted contraction of the respective muscles) and confirmed by palpation. Most minor muscle lesions respond to a course of deep friction massage.

Osteochondritis dissecans

In common with osteochondritis at the ankle and knee, the aetiology continues to be debated, though it seems logical that repeated impingement between the articular surfaces of the radial head and the capitellum is a likely cause. Thus it is common in those sports requiring throwing or pitching (Fig. 4.2; see also Fig. 3.6, pp. 34–5), in which forceful elbow extension is combined with lateral compression in valgus overload, such as baseball (Little Leaguer's elbow). Repeated weightbearing stress resulting in injury to the radiohumeral joint also occurs frequently in gymnasts (Fig. 4.4).

It is a lesion of the articular cartilage and subchondral bone, only occurring on convex articular surfaces, suggesting a traumatic aetiology. The lesion occurs most commonly in the capitellum in the 11–14-year old girl. It is probable that the condition is the same as that described by Panner (1929) and subsequently termed osteochondrosis (Singer and Roy 1984).

In the early case, discomfort is experienced on use, but rest may prevent the occurrence of fragmentation. In the established case loose bodies form, and give rise to temporary locking of the joint and repeated effusions. If an effusion occurs, both passive flexion and extension of the elbow are restricted; otherwise examination is essentially normal. X-rays reveal typical features. If ignored, the condition progresses to osteoarthritis in later life.

Osteoarthritis (OA) of the elbow

This may be the long-term result of a fracture, or possibly the result of a long period of stress—for instance, in baseball pitchers, weight-lifters, or gymnasts. In common with OA at other joints, the onset is often insidious, being recognized by the patient when a bout of pain reveals the accompanying restriction of movements in the capsular pattern. Whether due to a loose body or microfracture, pain is often accompanied by an effusion that may be expected to resolve gradually. As the condition progresses, however, pain may be anticipated when the elbow is stressed, a situation that is incompatible with sports which require a throwing or racket arm. The findings are restriction of movements in the capsular pattern, that is, in the proportion of 30° loss of flexion to 20° of extension. Tissue tension tests are negative. X-ray confirms the typical features of OA (Fig. 4.5). In the absence of degenerative changes in the elbow joint a restricted range of movements may be due to synovitis secondary to chondral damage.

Olecranon bursitis

A serous or haemorrhagic bursitis may develop as a result of repeated friction or contusion respectively. The initial complaints are of pain and swelling; tenderness and the presence of 'seedlings' within the bursa may be noted. If accompanied by redness there may be a significant acute inflammatory reaction which requires treatment by local anti-inflammatory measures. The presence of infection should be excluded, if necessary by microscopy and culture of the aspirate, and antibiotics prescribed if indicated. A localized steroid injection is indicated (in the non-infected case) if the acute reaction settles yet the swelling persists.

Tenosynovitis of the forearm

This condition is well recognized by the occupational medical officer and union official in a number of industries, where it is

FIG. 4.4 Repeated weightbearing stress resulting in injury to the radiohumeral joint occurs in gymnasts.

Fig. 4.5 Osteoarthritis of the elbow joint due to weight-lifting.

colloquially known as 'teno'. In the workplace, home, or sports arena it is an overuse injury to those tendons that pass through the forearm and cross the wrist to be inserted into the hand. As 'intersection syndrome' it presents as a crepitating swelling of the tendon sheaths of extensor pollicis brevis and abductor pollicis longus in the forearm some 4–6 cm proximal to the wrist where they cross over the tendons of the extensor carpi radialis. Often, however, these florid features are absent and the discomfort, unaccompanied by swelling, is to be found over the radial aspect of the wrist. At this anatomical level it was once known as 'styloiditis radii' but is now usually referred to as 'de Quervain's tenovaginitis' or 'tenosynovitis' (see Fig. 12.18, p. 219). Although common practice, it is fallacious to label all wrist and distal radius discomfort as tenosynovitis; in the absence of gross signs differentiation should be made from chronic dorsal wrist ligament sprain (in which localized tenderness of the relevant ligament should be sought). Stress injury to the distal radial epiphysis should be suspected in young gymnasts. In the industrial setting, many patients and unions regard 'teno' as an occupational injury, and commonly sue the employer. Thus it is particularly important not to diagnose a repetitive strain injury (RSI) without good evidence.

Any activity in which grasping is frequent or repeated may provoke RSI. It is more likely if acceleration or deceleration forces at the wrist are involved. Any of the dorsal wrist compartment tendons, including the finger extensors, may be affected as well as the thumb extensors/abductors. Rowers and weight-lifters are frequently affected by intersection syndrome. Golfers and racket sportsmen are prone to de Quervain's tenovaginitis. Dog-handlers are another vulnerable group. Whatever the cause, gripping and activities involving use of the forearm and thumb become excruciatingly painful.

On the volar aspect of the wrist overuse injury occurs in both the flexor carpi ulnaris and flexor carpi radialis tendons. Calcific deposits may form, when the condition presents as an acute inflammatory reaction with redness and swelling (Fig. 1.10, p. 9).

Identification is made by careful examination. Although there is usually a full range of active and passive movements in the forearm and wrist, passive ulnar deviation of the wrist with the thumb forcibly opposed across the palm is usually painful in de Quervain's disease (Finkelstein's test). Pain on resisted contraction of the respective contractile structures is to be expected. In the acute case crepitation, resulting from a synovial reaction in the sheath, may be felt. Pin-point tenderness must be elicited in the less florid case.

A short period of rest from sport is required while treatment using the normal anti-inflammatory options, including ice, ultrasound, and non-steroidal anti-inflammatory drugs (NSAIDs) is applied. Steroid injections are rapidly curative if there is tendon sheath swelling (Fig. 12.18, p. 219). Injections should be made into the sheath—that is, parallel to the tendon using the bent needle approach demonstrated in Fig. 12.24 (a) (p. 221), and in no circumstances should intratendinous injections be given. A critical analysis and, if appropriate, a subsequent adjustment of sporting technique may be undertaken. In discus throwing, for instance, de Quervain's disease may be due to overemphasis of the power snap at the wrist. A graded re-introduction into sporting activity is then required.

In·the hand, stenosing tenovaginitis of the flexor tendons may occur at the level of the metacarpophalangeal (MCP) joints, giving rise to a triggering effect—hence the term trigger finger (or thumb). A tender thickening is palpable on careful examination. Resolution may be expected after one steroid injection to the sheath; surgery is required in resistant cases.

Nerve entrapment

Direct trauma to a nerve causes paralysis. Compression (in a tunnel) of the median, ulnar, or radial nerves or their branches results in entrapment neuropathy, giving rise to pain and/or paraesthesiae in the forearm, hand, and digits.

The *median nerve* may be compressed occasionally in the proximal forearm by overactivity of the pronator teres. Since pronation is a component of the follow-through of a throw, repetitive throwing may cause nerve compression and give rise to forearm discomfort with or without sensory symptoms. Weight-lifters are also at risk, as a result of hypertrophy of the forearm muscles. Forceful isometric forearm pronation with the elbow at 90° may provoke discomfort during examination (Cabrera and McCue 1986). More commonly the median nerve is compressed at the wrist, giving rise to the *carpal tunnel syndrome*. In the sports context it is postulated (and disputed!) that this may be secondary to repeated wrist flexion and extension, or tight gripping, which clearly may be associated with any number of sports. In men, it may be due to an osteoarthritic wrist following old injury. Painful paraesthesiae in the radial three and a half digits, and discomfort in the wrist and forearm are features. Patients typically are woken at night, and obtain relief by moving or using the hand in some way. The condition should be suspected, and a provisional diagnosis made, on the symptomatology: in early cases objective sensory signs may not be detectable and motor weakness may not be evident. Only in late untreated cases will thenar atrophy and weakness of abduction and opposition of the thumb become obvious. Tinel's sign or Phalen's test may be positive. Diagnosis is confirmed by nerve conduction studies or by the therapeutic response to the injection of 5 mg (0.5 ml) triamcinolone and 0.5 ml lignocaine into the carpal tunnel (Fig. 4.6 (a); see also Fig. 12.19, p. 219). When the compression is due to sport surgical decompression is rarely necessary.

The *ulnar nerve* may also be compressed at the elbow or wrist. In its canal posterior to the medial epicondyle it is superficially positioned, and at risk from direct trauma; more insidiously it may be compressed by osteophytic encroachment. Deadness in the ulnar one and a half fingers, with additional extension to the dorsal aspect of the ulnar border of the hand (distinguishing it from distal compression) are noted. If nerve compression is unremitting, decompressive or transposition surgery should be carried out *before* motor weakness becomes evident. Should a patient present at a later stage, weakness of the small muscles of the hand supplied by the ulnar nerve—for instance, the

Fig. 4.6 (a) The ulnar nerve is at risk, for instance in cyclists, in the canal of Guyon. 'Handlebar neuropathy' may ensue. The site of injection of the carpal tunnel for median nerve entrapment is also demonstrated. (b) Various handlebar grip positions are shown by these cyclists. Padded gloves help prevent 'handlebar neuropathy'; the use of upright or aero bars may also be helpful.

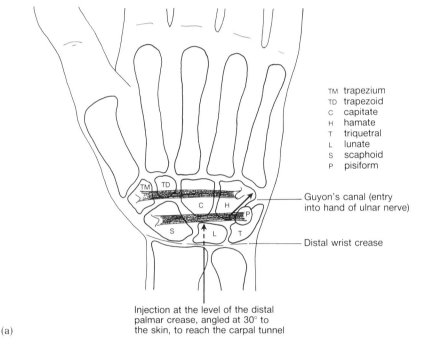

TM trapezium
TD trapezoid
C   capitate
H   hamate
T   triquetral
L   lunate
S   scaphoid
P   pisiform

Guyon's canal (entry into hand of ulnar nerve)

Distal wrist crease

Injection at the level of the distal palmar crease, angled at 30° to the skin, to reach the carpal tunnel

(a)

(b)

thumb adductor, the interossei, and the hypothenar muscles—may be detected. At the wrist the nerve is at risk in the canal of Guyon between the pisiform and hamate bones (Fig. 4.6). Direct trauma may result in contusion, though in the case of cyclists repeated pressure from handlebars is the cause ('handlebar neuropathy'). A similar situation may arise in golf and racket sports. A sensory branch is given off in this region: entrapment syndromes may be motor and/or sensory, depending upon the exact site of compression. In the case of chronic compression suitable padding may eliminate the symptoms. Gradual resolution is usually to be expected in distal entrapment neuropathy if the source of external compression is identified and remedied.

The *radial nerve* may be injured by fractures of the humerus or, very rarely, by repeated contraction of the forearm muscles, notably the supinator. Compression of one of its branches may be a cause of extensor forearm pain and, if so, it must be differentiated from tennis elbow. Forceful maintained isometric contraction of the elbow supinators in elbow extension is stated to provoke pain.

Other neuropathies have been described (Cabrera and McCue 1986). Compression of the anterior interosseous nerve in the forearm gives rise to weakness of 'pinch' between the tips of the thumb and the index finger. Repetitive digital compression may cause paresthesiae and numbness—for example, compression injury of the ulnar digital nerve of the thumb in ten-pin bowlers.

FIG. 4.7 Stress fracture of the distal radial epiphysis, due to compression loading during rotation, occurs in gymnasts. In this patient the injury resulted from incorrect water entry in high diving.

Capitate

Lunate

Epiphyseal
stress fracture

Overuse injury—the wrist

Stress fracture of the distal radial epiphysis

This occurs principally in gymnasts, and is considered by Read (1981) to result from compression loading during rotation, for instance in the Tsukahara vault. The complaint is usually of dorsal wrist pain. Examination reveals localized tenderness and slight swelling, but no articular or tissue tension signs. Radiographic changes (Fig. 4.7) include widening of the distal radial epiphysis, cystic changes, beaking of the distal or proximal aspect of the epiphysis, and haziness within the growth plate area (Roy *et al.* 1985). Stress changes at the epiphysis due to incorrect water entry when diving have been noted by the author in adolescents who complain of dorsal wrist pain while high diving. Abstinence from provocative stress for up to three months is normally sufficient for symptoms to resolve.

Ganglia

These occur over the dorsal aspect of wrists and feet, and occasionally elsewhere—for instance, over the flexor aspect of the wrist. If asymptomatic, which is often the case, they should be left. If painful during activity—for example, during racket sports or golf—aspiration with a 20 G needle (anything less is ineffective) may release the typically viscous fluid. If recurrent, surgical referral is indicated. It should not be assumed that any wrist pain is due to the ganglion, and other causes should be considered and excluded.

Chronic ligament sprains of the wrist

These occasionally occur, and should be differentiated from tenosynovitis by the pattern of discomfort felt on passively stretching the ligament (for example, the dorsal wrist ligament or ulnar collateral ligament) and the absence of pain on isometric contraction. Transverse friction massage is usually curative once the relevant ligament has been located by fingertip palpation.

Degenerative conditions

Osteoarthritis of the wrist is usually secondary to an old injury, such as an ununited scaphoid fracture. It causes a chronic ache that is aggravated by exercise. A restricted range of palmarflexion and dorsiflexion is found. Disturbance of the inferior radio-ulnar joint (for example, following a Colles' fracture) may give rise to permanent loss of rotation. A chronic sprain of the ulnar collateral ligament (which may also result from Colles' fracture) should respond to friction massage or steroid injection. Disruption of the triangular cartilage that forms the ulnar border of the proximal articular surface of the wrist joint results in recurrent pain and clicking on repeated wrist movements. There are few signs on examination: an arthrogram of the wrist reveals dispersal of dye into the proximal radio-ulnar space (Fig. 4.8).

Summary of examination procedures

For elbow, forearm, and wrist

| Inspection | Malalignment or deformity—for instance, cubitus valgus |
| | Effusion of elbow joint |

(a)

(b)

FIG. 4.8 (a) and (b) An arthrogram of the wrist joint reveals leakage of dye through a disrupted triangular cartilage. The additional presence of loose bodies in this patient gave rise to considerable disability.

	Swelling—for instance, olecranon bursitis, ganglia Muscle wasting—for example, thenar eminence
Active movements	Elbow flexion and extension Forearm pronation and supination Wrist flexion and dorsiflexion
Passive movements	Elbow flexion and extension (note 'end-feel') Forearm pronation and supination Wrist palmarflexion, dorsiflexion, ulnar deviation, and radial deviation
Stress tests	Valgus/varus stress to the elbow in 30° flexion Finkelstein's test: thumb opposition with ulnar deviation of wrist
Resisted movements (tissue tension tests)	Resisted elbow flexion in neutral, then in supination (to differentiate biceps from brachioradialis) Resisted elbow extension Resisted pronation and supination Resisted wrist palmarflexion and dorsiflexion, ulnar deviation, and radial deviation Resisted thumb movements—abduction, adduction, flexion, extension, opposition

	Resisted finger movements—flexion and extension (plus adduction and abduction if neuropathy suspected) Functional tests–pinch and grip
Additional tests	Tinel's sign (reproduction of paraesthesiae on tapping over a nerve, such as the median nerve in the carpal tunnel, plus sensory examination if required) Phalen's test (reproduction of the sensory symptoms of median nerve compression by maintaining full palmarflexion of the wrist—usually performed by pushing the dorsal surfaces of the hands together—for one minute)
Palpation	Localized tenderness Crepitus (tenosynovitis) Nodules (rheumatoid, stenosing tenovaginitis) Warmth (bursitis)

For thumb and digital examination procedures add:
active and passive flexion, extension, abduction and adduction at MCP, PIP, and DIP joints,
abduction/adduction stress tests at MCP and IP joints in 30° flexion
resisted flexion/extension at IP joints
specific 'fingertip' tenderness

Injuries to the hand and wrist

N. J. BARTON

Almost any type of hand injury could occur during sport—for example the hand might be pierced by a flying javelin or crushed by the collapse of a heavy stand, but in practice sports injuries to the hand and wrist are almost always closed injuries, usually to bone or joint. Therefore the rest of this chapter will be restricted to these kinds of injury, which, of course, are by no means unique to sport but are part of the common coinage of hand injuries.

These injuries are often minor, but sometimes not as minor as they may seem at first sight. What is required is the ability to make an accurate diagnosis, and to detect those which need serious treatment.

Causes of injury

A ball

The commonest cause is that the hand is struck by a ball which is either hard, like a cricket or hockey ball (Belliappa and Barton 1991), or heavy, like a football (Curtin and Kay 1976).

In most cases the ball knocks the finger or hand back into extension, breaking a bone or dislocating a joint, but more damage is done when the ball strikes the end of the finger, compressing it longitudinally so that the concave base of one bone is split upon the convex anvil of its proximal partner and the joint surface is disrupted.

In games in which the ball is hit with an implement, it may strike the player's hand instead as he holds the implement. There is then an element of crushing, with skin damage, but this is usually not serious and fractures tend to be comminuted but undisplaced and stable. Occasionally this mechanism may produce the damaging end-on blow to the fingertip.

The ground

In those games where players run around, they may fall onto their outstretched hand and sustain any of the injuries which this can produce, from a fractured finger to a dislocated shoulder. Such injuries are, of course, especially common when the nature of the sport is to move on a slippery surface, as in skating or skiing. They are likely to be worse if the sportsman is travelling at speed (for example, in skiing and cycle, motorcycle, or car racing) or falls from a height, as in jumping sports, gymnastics, riding (especially over jumps), mountaineering, or—the extreme cases—hang-gliding or flying.

The boundary of the playing area

In games such as squash or fives, which are played in small courts surrounded by a wall, the players sometimes run into the wall. This can result in injuries similar to those caused by falling on the outstretched hand, but the impact may be on the back of the hand or wrist, causing a contusion or a forcible flexion injury. In games played on a large field the player may run into a fence surrounding the ground, and, since his finger or hand may go in between the rails or wires, this can produce more complicated injuries.

An opponent

Clearly this is most likely to occur in sports whose aim is to injure the opponent, especially boxing; the fracture of the neck of the fifth metacarpal is sometimes known as 'the boxer's fracture'. Bennett's fracture–subluxation of the base of the first metacarpal has also been described as 'an injury which owes its origin to the disparity between an individual's pugnacity and his pugilistic technique' (Blum 1941). Unfortunately it is not unknown for similar blows to be exchanged in anger between players of other games, or in the semi-secrecy of the rugby football scrum. In the latter situation, the finger may also be pulled, wrenched, or twisted backwards or sideways to detach it from the ball, and similar injuries may occur in wrestling.

A special type of injury occurs in rugby football, where a player trying to tackle another succeeds only in catching his grasping fingers in the opponent's clothing, and the opposing extension force can rupture the tendon of the flexor digitorum profundus, usually to the ring finger.

A sporting implement

The player may be hit accidentally (or on purpose) by an opponent's racquet, stick, club, bat, etc. However, the damage may be done by his own implement, especially if it suddenly strikes a hard object in mid-swing, as when a golfer's club hits the ground. The upper end of the handle is driven forcibly against the front of the wrist, and this is actually the commonest cause of a rare but important injury—fracture of the hook of the hamate.

Sporting guns may, of course, also cause hand injuries, though it is more common for the victim to shoot himself in the foot while climbing over a fence.

Assessment of acute injuries to the hand and wrist

The first step in this process is to obtain a detailed history, as the mechanism of the damage often suggests the precise nature of the injury.

Clinical examination follows the usual pattern for orthopaedic assessment of an acute injury in which a fracture is a possibility: look, feel, move. Bruising, swelling, and deformity are looked for. In sportsmen seen immediately after the accident, bruising and swelling may not yet have appeared, but careful palpation with the tip of one finger to localize tenderness as precisely as possible is a most valuable—often *the* most valuable—part of the examination.

In palpating the wrist, it is particularly important that care is taken in the region of the anatomical snuff box. It is *normal* to be tender there because of pressure on the terminal sensory part of the radial nerve. Therefore, tenderness must always be assessed by comparison with the opposite wrist. Additionally, although the scaphoid is the most common carpal bone to be fractured, it is not the only one: any of the carpal bones may be fractured, and all are palpable clinically except the trapezoid. Moreover, the injury may be a fracture of the distal end of the radius or ulna, or the base of a metacarpal. Therefore palpation should start with the distal radius, and progress around the wrist at that level. Subsequent levels of examination are the proximal row of the carpus, the distal row of the carpus, and the bases of the metacarpals. It should not be forgotten that the injury may be to a joint, not a bone: this is especially important because if that is the case it will probably not be revealed on the X-ray, and the localization of the tenderness may be the only positive finding. As palpation proceeds along the metacarpals to the digits it is equally important that tenderness is precisely localized.

The patient is asked to put the part through a full active range of movement. If he can manage a *full* range there is probably no serious joint injury. If one is suspected, it is necessary to examine for abnormal movements (for example, sideways laxity of finger-joints), but it is probably wise, and certainly kind, to defer this until after an X-ray in case there is a fracture.

X-rays are usually necessary, but they are no substitute for clinical examination. X-rays may not reveal a joint injury, and will not reveal a fracture unless they are taken at the correct projection and angles to show that particular type of fracture. If X-rays of the wrist are requested, ordinary postero-anterior (PA) and lateral views are taken, which often do not reveal a scaphoid fracture, for which scaphoid views are needed. In the same way, fractures of the hook of the hamate will be visible only on special views taken for that purpose. *Therefore, clinical examination is necessary, not only in its own right* because of the information which only it can yield, *but to enable the examiner to order the appropriate X-ray views* without which the diagnosis will not be made.

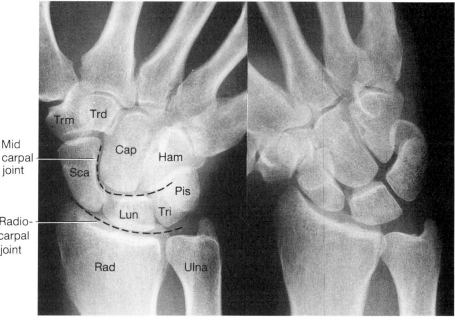

Fig. 4.9 PA views of the wrist in ulnar (left) and radial (right) deviation. In radial deviation, the scaphoid flexes and is therefore seen more end-on: a better view is obtained in ulnar deviation. Therefore, if 'scaphoid views' are requested, they will be taken with the wrist in this position. The shallow bowl of the radiocarpal joint and the deeper cup of the mid-carpal joint are seen in both positions.

Fig. 4.10 The smooth C-shape of the mid-carpal joint is not present, indicating a dislocation: in this case a dislocation of the lunate, which instead of being four-sided, looks five-sided. There is not always a gap between the dislocated lunate and the scaphoid; if present, it indicates an injury to the scapholunate ligament which may be isolated (see Fig. 4.16) or part of a dislocation.

It is necessary to study the X-rays carefully—something which does not always happen, as the examining doctor may not be familiar with the anatomy seen from certain angles, for example the lateral view. For this reason important injuries such as dislocation of the lunate or of the carpo-metacarpal joints are more often overlooked than diagnosed.

On the PA view of the wrist, one must look at each bone in turn: radius, ulna, scaphoid, lunate, triquetrum, pisiform, trapezium ('articulates with the thumb'), trapezoid, capitate, hamate, and each of the five metacarpals. In addition one should always and specifically look for the C-shape of the mid-carpal joint (Fig. 4.9); if it is not there, or is discontinuous, then something is badly wrong with the wrist (Fig. 4.10). The radiocarpal joint forms a second but shallower C.

On the lateral view of the wrist (Fig. 4.11), one can identify the radius with the proximal pole of the lunate fitting into it (a third C), the capitate fitting into the distal pole of the lunate (a fourth), and the superimposed second to fifth metacarpals, which should be in line with the capitate. At an angle of about 45° to these, one can also see the scaphoid, with its proximal pole overlapping the lunate and its distal pole and tuberosity projecting anteriorly, overlapping the pisiform. Figure 4.12 shows an abnormal lateral view.

In the fingers, one must not diagnose as a fracture the nutrient artery, the overlapping skin edge of the web between the fingers, an epiphyseal line, or the pseudo-epiphysis sometimes seen at the distal end of the first metacarpal.

Having studied the X-rays, it is usually wise to examine the patient again. Any doubtful features on the X-ray will be assessed in relation to the clinical findings: if it is not tender, it is probably not a recent injury. If there are no fractures, then the joints should be tested for lateral stability to detect injury to the collateral ligaments. It is especially important to do this after reducing a dislocation.

Fractures around the wrist

Fractures of the distal radius and ulna

Colles' fractures, though most common in elderly people, also occur in athletes, in whom they are more serious. The athlete will make greater demands upon the wrist and therefore expect a higher standard of result; in addition the bone is stronger, requiring a more violent force to break it, so that the injury is inherently worse. Treatment will be along orthodox lines (Charnley 1961; Burke 1988) but with a greater readiness, if the fracture slips, to remanipulate or resort to other methods such as external fixation.

Smith's fractures, in which the distal end of the radius displaces forwards instead of backwards, are often unstable and frequently require internal fixation. (Smith was Colles' pupil and successor, and it was he who carried out the post-mortem examination on Colles' body.)

Fractures of the scaphoid

Almost everything that is taught about scaphoid fractures rests upon sand rather than rock. Texts are full of dogmatic statements which are passed on to medical students, but the truth is that it is not really known what the answers are to any of the

FIG. 4.11 Lateral view of normal wrist: the proximal convex curve of the lunate ('moon-shaped') fits into the concavity of the distal radius and the convex head of the capitate fits into the distal concavity of the lunate: two more Cs. These three bones should be in line with each other and with the bases of the finger metacarpals.

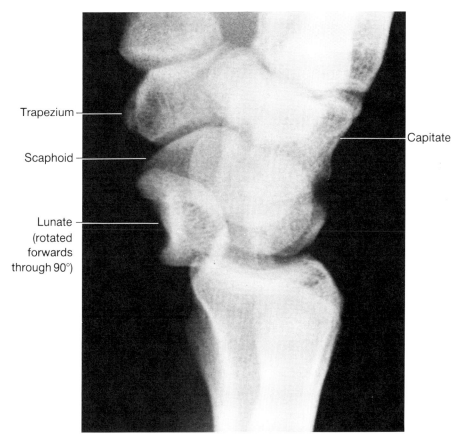

Trapezium

Scaphoid

Lunate
(rotated
forwards
through 90°)

Capitate

Fig. 4.12 Abnormal lateral view: anterior dislocation of the lunate which is rotated through 90°. Its proximal convex curve is not contained within the radius and its distal concavity does not contain the head of the capitate.

Capitate

Scaphoid

Lunate

Fig. 4.13 Fracture of the waist of the scaphoid. Often the fracture is less obvious than this.

important questions, such as how to diagnose them, how to treat them, and how to tell whether they are united (Barton 1992).

What is known is that they are fairly common, that they usually result from a dorsiflexion injury, that they are often missed, and that they are subject to non-union, especially if they are not treated.

Clinical signs, apart from tenderness and some pain on movement, are conspicuous by their absence, and indeed the triviality of the symptoms is the reason why many patients dismiss the injury as a sprain, and do not seek medical advice at all—only to turn up some time later with an un-united fracture of the scaphoid.

X-rays are essential (Fig. 4.13). A sprained wrist should never be diagnosed unless at least one set of adequate X-ray films has been taken. One of the myths is that fractures of the scaphoid often 'do not show up' on the original films, and only become visible a few weeks later after resorption of the bone ends adjoining the fracture. In fact, Leslie and Dickson (1981) found that the fracture was visible on the first X-rays in 98 per cent of cases. In 75 per cent it could be seen on the PA film, and in 77 per cent on the semi-pronated view; in only six out of 222 patients was it not visible on one of these two films taken at the first attendance.

Nevertheless, it remains the usual practice for a patient with a suspected scaphoid fracture to be treated in plaster for two weeks and then have further X-rays out of plaster, despite the fact that this hardly ever results in a fractured scaphoid being discovered later. The main reason for this practice is fear of medico-legal problems and of being considered negligent; but it seems reasonable as a symptomatic method of treatment, even if, at the end of the day, no fracture is shown and the retrospective diagnosis of a sprain is made.

The variety of methods of conservative treatment is amazing, varying both in the extent of the plaster and the position of immobilization. The traditional method in Britain, now sanctified by description as a 'scaphoid plaster', is in a below-elbow plaster extending to the interphalangeal joint of the thumb, with the wrist slightly extended. There is no convincing evidence that this is any better than the type of cast used for Colles' fractures, in which the thumb is left free; it has been shown to make no difference (Clay *et al.* 1991).

The real difficulty, though this is not mentioned in any of the textbooks or even in most of the papers in specialist journals, is in deciding for how long the plaster should be kept on or, to put it another way, when the fracture is united. The bone is too short for test by angular stress, as one would in the tibia. Tenderness is very subjective. The assumption is that the decision can be made on radiological grounds, despite the fact that on X-rays taken after eight or even twelve weeks of immobilization it is often—even usually—very difficult to decide whether the fracture is united or not. Dias *et al.* (1988) have shown that a group of eight consultants (four orthopaedic surgeons and four radiologists) frequently disagreed with each other as to whether the fracture was united, and, more significantly still, when they were shown the same films again some time later, often disagreed with what they themselves had said the first time! Thus all the papers which say that such-and-such a treatment led to union in X weeks must be taken with a large pinch of salt.

The author's current practice is to immobilize all fractures of the waist of scaphoid in a Colles' plaster for eight weeks and then assess them clinically and radiologically. If union is doubtful on either ground, they are given a further month in plaster; at the end of that time no further films are taken, as they will be left free of the plaster anyway. Most will progress to union. Those who develop non-union but have no symptoms do not need an operation. Those who have symptomatic non-union need a bone-grafting operation, though even this is not invariably successful (Green 1985; Warren-Smith and Barton 1988).

Thus the need to diagnose and treat these fractures in the first place is emphasized. Even if the sportsman has an important contest pending, it is not worth taking a chance by failing to immobilize a scaphoid waist fracture adequately and for long enough; the risk of lasting disability from non-union is too high.

In contrast, fractures of the scaphoid tuberosity are seldom a problem, and need only four weeks in plaster.

UP

DOWN

FIG. 4.14 Carpal tunnel view of the wrist of an international cricketer showing, on the right, pisiform and fractured hook of hamate and, on the left, first metacarpal, trapezium, and scaphoid tuberosity. The trough in the centre is the carpal tunnel.

Other carpal fractures

The most common is a flake of bone pulled off the back of the triquetrum by the distal attachment of the capsule of the wrist joint. It is visible only on a lateral X-ray, where it may look as though it has come from the lunate. This is essentially a ligamentous injury, and four weeks in plaster is adequate treatment.

Uncommon, but interesting because it is almost exclusively a sports injury, is the *fracture of the hook of the hamate*. Occasionally this may be due to a fall or a crushing injury, but as a sports injury it occurs when a golf club, tennis raquet, cricket bat, or similar implement hits something in mid-swing and the force is transmitted through the end of the handle to the base of the palm over the hook of the hamate. This lies about 1 cm distal and radial to the pisiform, where it can be felt by deep palpation. Stark *et al.* (1977) reported twenty patients (four tennis players, seven golfers, and nine baseball players) all with old un-united fractures of the hook of the hamate. If a golf club hits the ground instead of the ball, the impact is particularly severe and such an injury is more likely. It was always the upper hand which was injured. The correct diagnosis had been made in only two cases; the others had been treated by rest, physiotherapy, and steroid injections—without benefit.

There are two reasons why this injury is usually overlooked. The first is that doctors are not aware of it. A history such as that above, with tenderness localized to the hook of the hamate, suggests the diagnosis. Pain on flexing the ring or little fingers (whose flexor tendons pass alongside the hook) or paraesthesiae in those fingers (whose sensory nerves pass over the hook) strengthen the suspicion. The second reason is that ordinary X-rays of the wrist are unlikely to show the fracture. As previously explained, the history and examination enable one to order the correct X-rays to demonstrate the fracture. In the patient whose X-ray is shown as Fig. 4.14, only two films were requested: this view through the carpal tunnel, and an oblique view, which also showed the fracture. If pain prevents the patient from dorsiflexing the wrist enough to obtain a satisfactory carpal tunnel view showing all the hook, it can be demonstrated by CT scan.

Non-union is treated by excision of the hook of the hamate. Care is required, as it is quite deep, and there are sensory nerves superficial, a motor nerve distal, and tendons radial to the hook. The results are excellent, and professional sportsmen can quickly return to full activity. These fractures are so rarely diagnosed as fresh injuries that there is no guidance in the literature on treatment. It would appear that the attachment of the flexor retinaculum to the hook would tend to separate it, and that it might not heal even after a period in plaster. In the cricketer shown in Fig.4.14 the fractured hook was excised by the author, following which the patient resumed first-class cricket in six weeks.

Joint injuries of the wrist

A variety of *dislocations and fracture-dislocations* can occur involving the carpus. All are rare; the least uncommon are the following.

(a) An anterior dislocation of the lunate (Figs. 4.10 and 4.12) which, since it has displaced into the carpal tunnel, may cause acute compression of the median nerve although, surprisingly, dislocation of the lunate is hardly ever followed by avascular necrosis of that bone (Kienböck's disease).

(b) Perilunar dislocation (Fig. 4.15), where the lunate remains in its proper relationship with the radius, but everything distal to and around it is dislocated dorsally. It is thought that this is the first stage of the injury described above, after which the carpus moves anteriorly again, pushing the lunate forwards out of place.

(c) Trans-scaphoid perilunar dislocation, which is similar, except that the scaphoid fractures across its waist and its distal pole displaces with the rest of the carpus, while the proximal pole and lunate remain in the correct position. The dislocation is usually dorsal.

These are serious injuries. If PA and lateral X-rays are taken and studied carefully they should not be missed, but it still happens. An experienced orthopaedic surgeon should carry out the reduction as soon as possible. Even if a trans-scaphoid perilunar dislocation is reduced satisfactorily, the scaphoid fracture should be treated by open reduction and internal fixation: the former because there may be torn ligament interposed between the two halves of the scaphoid (Wilton 1987), which would prevent union, and the latter because this is an unstable injury and this too means that there is a strong chance of non-union.

One would also expect carpal instability after these dislocations, which must involve considerable ligamentous damage, but in practice the wrist usually becomes rather stiff instead (Panting *et al.* 1984).

Helal (1978) has described a condition that he calls *racquet player's pisiform*. The pathology is of chondromalacia of the articular cartilage between the pisiform and triquetral bones. He wrote that 'the probable mechanism is a torsional stress upon the capsule of the piso-triquetral joint by the sharp and powerful pronation-supination movements at the wrist which occur when wielding a racquet, the racquet acting as an additional lever upon the wrist. I believe that it is only those sports in which stroke play is mainly from the wrist which give rise to the syndrome: although in tennis a heavier racquet is used, the stroke is made from the shoulder'. Three squash players and one badminton player were cured by excision of the pisiform. A similar condition is said to have been seen in a golfer.

Moving distally, *dislocations and fracture-dislocations of the carpometacarpal joints* are missed far too often (Henderson and Arafa 1987). Clinically, the displacement is obscured by the soft tissue swelling. Radiologically it is discernible, provided that lateral views are taken and that the observer checks that the distal row of the carpus and the superimposed second to fifth metacarpals are in line.

Carpal instability

It is now clear that it is possible to tear ligaments around the carpus in such a way that, although the bones do not actually dislocate on each other, their relationship is altered. The most common pattern is that the lunate tilts so that its distal surface is pointing somewhat dorsally (dorsal intercalated segment instability); this extension of the lunate is accompanied by flexion of the scaphoid. The opposite pattern (volar intercalated segment instability), in which the lunate tilts in a palmar or volar direction, is less common. In extreme cases, the ligaments between the scaphoid and lunate are completely disrupted, so that a gap appears between these bones, a radiological finding known as the Terry-Thomas sign from its resemblance to the gap between that actor's front teeth (Fig. 4.16). Since the instability may not be present all the time, X-rays may fail to demonstrate it. A series of films with the wrists in various positions is recommended; alternatively the wrist may be screened whilst the patient attempts the movement that provoked pain or click-

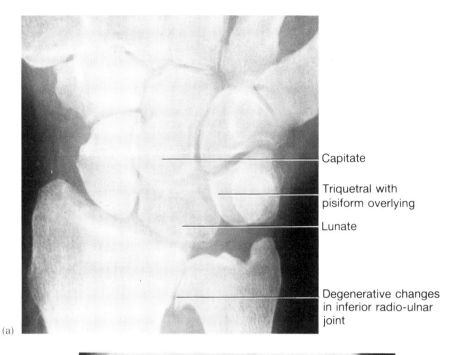

(a)

Capitate

Triquetral with
pisiform overlying

Lunate

Degenerative changes
in inferior radio-ulnar
joint

FIG. 4.15 (a) PA and (b) lateral
views of perilunar dislocation of
wrist. Note the loss of smooth
curve of mid-carpal joint on PA;
adjoining surfaces of lunate and
capitate are not parallel. The
patient also has a dorsal radial
fracture and degenerative changes
in the inferior radio-ulnar joint.)

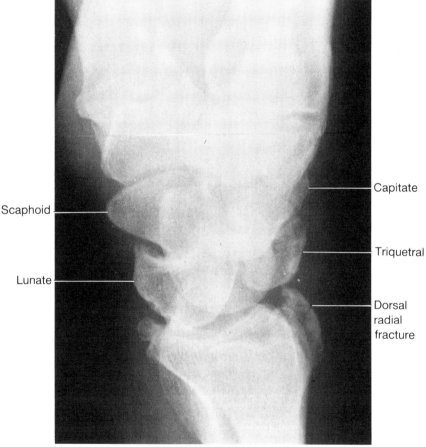

(b)

Scaphoid

Lunate

Capitate

Triquetral

Dorsal
radial
fracture

ing. Both the radiologist and the physician or surgeon should be
present. It is very helpful if the examination is recorded on
videotape so that it can be studied repeatedly.

Jones (1988), in an important paper entitled 'Beware the
sprained wrist', reviewed the findings in a consecutive series of

100 wrist injuries in which, in addition to the conventional X-
rays, an extra AP view was taken with the patient clenching his
fist tightly (Fig. 4.16); this is one of the views most likely to
demonstrate carpal instability. Only those patients with obvious
fractures of the distal radius were excluded; all others had this

Trapezium

Scaphoid
(flexed with ring sign)

Triquetral

Lunate

FIG. 4.16 AP film with the patient gripping. This is the film most likely to show, as it does here, a gap between the scaphoid and lunate bones (Terry-Thomas sign). The other wrist must always be X-rayed for comparison. A unilateral gap indicates a ligamentous injury. The scaphoid moves into a flexed position in which the cortical outline of its tuberosity appears as a ring.

extra view taken. In 76 patients, the films were considered normal: four had fractures of the scaphoid, three of the trapezium, and fourteen of the distal radius. However, the most important finding was that nineteen patients had a gap of more than 2 mm between the scaphoid and lunate; of these, it was found that in fourteen this finding was bilateral, and therefore presumably not caused by the injury, leaving five (that is, 5 per cent) thought to have had a significant injury to the scapholunate ligament complex, with clinical and radiographic evidence of instability. Clearly, this type of injury is not uncommon if one looks for it properly.

The treatment of these instability patterns in the carpus is still being determined; on the whole, ligamentous reconstructions have not proved to be very successful, and current opinion favours a limited or partial arthrodesis, for example, between the scaphoid, trapezium, and trapezoid. For further information on this complex subject, the reader is referred to the paper by Taleisnik (1988) and the book edited by Lichtman (1988).

What is clear, however, is that there are patients complaining of pain in the wrist in whom ordinary examination and X-rays reveal no abnormality, but who have a genuine if intermittent instability. This is comparable to the knee, where twenty years ago the instability patterns were not understood, and the

patients were either dismissed as hypochondriacs or just had to put up with it (or had their menisci removed). Unfortunately, even effective treatment of wrist instability may not succeed in allowing the patient to resume top-class sport.

Lastly on the topic of ligamentous injuries to the carpus, it must be admitted that probably a wrist sprain can occur, and this may be the pathology in those patients in whom a fracture of the scaphoid is suspected but never confirmed. The old adage 'sprained wrist does not exist' is not quite true, but it remains true that this is a diagnosis which can be made only after thorough clinical and radiological investigation and only in retrospect, by which time treatment is unnecessary as a true (acute) sprain settles quickly with rest. Persisting symptoms indicate the possibility of a more serious injury, perhaps one of the forms of carpal instability mentioned above.

Fractures of the hand

These are exceedingly common, and sport is a common cause. It is probably the *most* common cause of the end-on blows which result in severe damage to joints.

The essential principles of treatment of hand fractures are the same as for anywhere in the body, and comprise the three Rs of fracture treatment: reduction, retention, and rehabilitation. In the hand, however, the principles are applied in a rather different way (Barton 1984). The first step, of course, is to define the nature of the fracture; this requires an X-ray. In the femur, a subcapital fracture is not treated in the same way as a shaft fracture, and in the phalanges there are many different types of fracture, each needing different management.

Reduction

Frequently the fracture is undisplaced or minimally displaced: this does not need to be reduced. However, a displaced fracture of the shaft of the proximal phalanx will leave a step in the floor of the tunnel in which the flexor tendon runs, and this is not acceptable. Rotational deformity *must* be corrected, and therefore the finger must be examined specifically to look for this; the fingers of both hands should be studied end-on (Fig. 4.17). Usually, despite the fracture, the patient can be persuaded to flex the finger to some extent, which renders the deformity more obvious (Fig. 4.18); unless corrected, the finger will remain rotated permanently, making it almost useless. Spiral fractures, caused by a rotational force, are particularly likely to have rotational deformity.

Retention

Experience is required to determine which fractures are unstable and therefore need external or internal splintage. Figure 4.19 and 4.20, modified from London's book, give some guidance. Stable fractures should be treated by strapping the injured finger to an intact neighbour, giving some support and protection while allowing movement, with the normal finger acting as a dynamic splint (Fig. 4.21). The strapping must be applied in such a way as to *permit*, not prevent, movement. Any fracture which needs reduction also needs retention to ensure that reduction is maintained; this may be by external splintage or by internal fixation.

The hand tends to stiffen with the metacarpophalangeal (MCP) joints extended and the interphalangeal (IP) joints flexed. Therefore it must always be immobilized in the opposite position, with the MCP joints flexed and the IP joints extended (Fig. 4.22). This is often called the Edinburgh position because it was popularized by Professor J.I.P. James of Edinburgh (James 1970); he calls it the safe position. Whatever its name, nothing is more important in the treatment of hand injuries, whether minor or major, than to ensure that the hand is immobilized correctly to minimize the chance of permanent loss of movement. There are virtually no circumstances in which the interphalangeal joints should be immobilized in a flexed position.

External splintage of a single fractured finger may be achieved satisfactorily by a padded aluminium splint, such as one made by Zimmer; this must be put on correctly (Fig. 4.23), so that the finger is immobilized in the safe position and the fingertip can be inspected end-on to check that there is no malrotation. If more than one finger is fractured, anterior and posterior plaster slabs in the safe position provide the most effective immobilization. A fractured thumb which requires immobilization may be treated in a plaster cast extending almost to the tip of the thumb but leaving the fingers free.

Many fractures of the hand do not need to be immobilized, though clearly the digit should, if possible, be protected from further injury until the fracture has healed. This is determined *clinically*. Radiological union takes a long time, and one does not need to wait for it; in fact, once the position of the fracture is satisfactory, it is seldom necessary to take any more X-rays.

A very small proportion of hand fractures, not more than 5 per cent, need operative treatment. The *indications* are as follows:

(1) fractures of the shafts of the phalanges in which good reduction cannot be achieved by closed means;
(2) fractures involving joints in which there is either a large fragment carrying a lot of the joint surface or a small fragment associated with subluxation of the joint;
(3) multiple fractures within the hand.

The important early management decision is to identify the minority that must be treated by splintage or surgery from the majority, where simple strapping to a neighbouring finger is adequate treatment. Failure to do this is likely to result in per-

FIG. 4.17 Looking at fingers end-on to detect rotational deformity. The ring finger is pronated in relation to the other fingers. This is best seen by looking at the line of the finger-nail.

(a)

(b)

FIG. 4.18 (a)In extension, finger looks fairly normal; (b) in flexion, rotation deformity becomes obvious.

I   II–V   V

Fig. 4.19 Stable fractures, which do not need immobilization.

Fig. 4.20 Unstable fractures, needing either splintage or internal fixation.

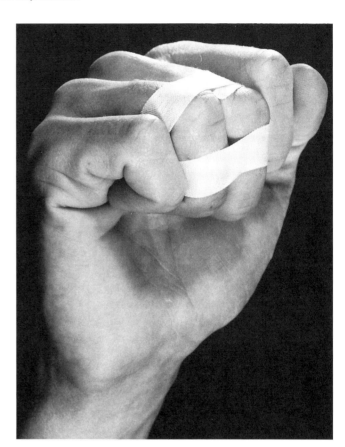

FIG. 4.21 The injured finger has been strapped to a neighbouring intact one in such a way as to allow full movement.

FIG. 4.22 The safe position, which should always be used when the hand has to be immobilized. It is not meant as a permanent position, but is the one from which it is easiest to regain a full range of movements.

FIG. 4.23 Finger splinted in the safe position on an aluminium splint. The splint is bent to 90° at the transverse palmar creases, which overlie the MCP joint (not the crease at the base of the finger, which is halfway down the proximal phalanx). The splint should not cross the wrist joint.

manent disability; little delay can be tolerated, as the fracture will begin to unite in the wrong position within a few days.

Rehabilitation

This is the most important part of treatment. In other parts of the body it must wait until the fracture has united, but in the hand it should start straightaway. In sportsmen, this is usually no problem; on the contrary, the difficulty is to persuade patients with more serious fractures that it is in their interest as sportsmen to accept a period of immobilization in order to achieve a satisfactory long-term result.

In stable fractures, active mobilization within the protective strapping is encouraged. The point when sport can safely be resumed is when tenderness has diminished to an acceptable level. Fractures which have been splinted or operated on may need physiotherapy to help the patient regain a full range of movement. Active exercises should be practised *with the hand empty:* squeezing a ball or bit of putty should be forbidden (though some well-meaning person will probably suggest it), because this promotes redisplacement of the fracture and prevents full flexion. What is required is a full range of movement, so that the finger does not stick out and become injured again; once a full range is regained, power quickly follows.

A detailed account of the management of each type of fracture of the metacarpal and phalanx is given elsewhere (Barton 1982), and so only brief comments follow on the most common or important types.

Fractures of the phalanges

Fingertip fractures

If the skin has burst or the nail is broken, the fracture is compound and must be treated as such. After careful cleansing, the nail may be replaced as a dressing (Henderson 1984). If the fracture is closed and there is a subungual haematoma, it should be released to relieve pain and speed resolution. A paper-clip may be opened up so that one end can be heated until it is red-hot and applied to the nail to burn a hole through; this is less painful than trephining and is also sterile.

The fracture itself is unimportant; it is the soft tissues which need treating.

Fractures involving joints

The most common are tiny flake fractures, avulsed by a ligament or capsule. There is no evidence that immobilization improves the outcome and so, provided that the joint is stable, activities can be resumed as soon as pain permits, with the protection afforded by strapping the finger to its neighbour.

However, if the joint is subluxed (Fig. 4.24), a very different situation exists. This is a major injury to the joint, requiring serious treatment. It occurs quite often in fielders in cricket and in Australian rules football. McElfresh *et al.* (1972) have described an ingenious extension block splint which allows flexion but prevents extension (which is the unstable position). The author prefers to use percutaneous Kirschner wire fixation to maintain the reduction for three weeks, and then an extension block splint for a further three weeks. In some cases, the small fragment may also need fixation.

(a)

(b)

FIG. 4.24 (a) Fracture-subluxation of PIP joint in a professional cricketer injured while fielding. The fact that the base of the middle phalanx is no longer congruous with the head of the proximal phalanx is more important than the small fracture. (b) Subluxation reduced and just held in correct alignment by transfixing Kirschner wire.

Fractures of the base of a phalanx without subluxation usually do surprisingly well without immobilization (Steel 1988). Fractures of the head of a phalanx nearly always need internal fixation (McCue *et al.* 1970).

Epiphyseal fractures

In boys, the epiphyses in the hand remain open until the age of 15 or later, and fractures in or near the growth plate are common in injuries sustained in games. A great deal of correction is to be anticipated from the processes of remodelling with growth, but it is important to correct lateral angulation near the interphalangeal joints and malrotation anywhere, because these do not correct themselves.

Fractures of shafts of phalanges

The front of the phalanx is the floor of the tunnel in which the flexor tendon glides up and down. If this is not restored to a smooth bony surface, one cannot expect the finger to work properly. The angulation, which is into extension, must be corrected, together with any displacement. A skilled manipulation can often achieve the desired perfect reduction. This is performed with the MCP joint flexed to stabilize the proximal fragment: the MCP joint is retained in the flexed position with the IP joints extended while the finger is immobilized. If perfect reduction cannot be achieved then, in the proximal phalanx at any rate, operation is indicated.

Comminuted fractures

These usually result from some sort of crushing injury, and the combination of many fracture lines with skin damage means that operation is often contraindicated. The periosteal envelope is usually intact, so that the fracture is stable and heals surprisingly well with early mobilization. Again, any rotational deformity must be corrected.

Fractures of the metacarpals

On the whole, these cause fewer problems than fractures of the phalanges. Metacarpal fractures usually angulate into *flexion* and so, if there is any permanent loss of movement, it is loss of extension, which is less likely to result in disability. Malrotation can occur, and, when it does, is serious because there is a greater length of digit distal to the fracture and greater deformity results; however, in most cases the deep transverse metacarpal ligaments and the interossei which connect adjoining metacarpals limit displacement of a single metacarpal fracture.

When one makes a fist and hits somebody, the impact is taken on the distal end of the metacarpal and commonly causes a fracture at that level, though the force may be transmitted down the shaft to the base of the metacarpal.

Fractures of the metacarpal heads

These are most often seen in the index and middle fingers, usually due to fighting. On the whole, they do surprisingly well, but again one cannot lump them all together. McElfresh and Dobyns (1983) have described ten different types of fracture of the metacarpal head.

Fractures of the neck of the metacarpals

These are usually the result of fist fighting, though not in a formal manner: unhappily this is increasingly common during sporting contests which are not intended to include fighting.

Considerable flexion deformity of this particular fracture is acceptable and compatible with normal function afterwards for the following reasons.

(a) Since the fracture is distal, an angulation of, say, 30° produces much less forward displacement of the metacarpal head than would the same angulation in the mid-shaft (Fig. 4.25).

(b) The joint between the hamate and the base of the metacarpal of the little finger (fifth carpo-metacarpal joint) normally allows about 30° flexion and extension, as may be observed by clenching one's fist tightly when the fifth metacarpal head moves forward.

Thus any flexion deformity at the neck of the fifth metacarpal can be compensated for by extending the joint at the base of the metacarpal. This applies less in the fourth metacarpal, whose basal joint has only about 15° of movement, and not at all in the middle and index fingers, whose basal joints have virtually no movement and therefore cannot compensate for more distal deformity.

Therefore the common fracture of the fifth metacarpal should not be overtreated. The author's practice is to treat it by a crepe bandage and early movements. The bandage reminds the patient and others that there is an injury. Often it takes some weeks to regain full active extension at the MCP joint, but hardly ever is there any permanent disability even in poorly

FIG. 4.25 Angulation at the neck of the metacarpal causes less deformity than angulation in the mid-shaft.

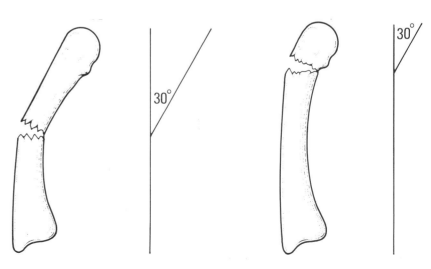

motivated patients (Ford *et al.* 1989). The old practice of strapping the finger in flexion has been rightly abandoned: it is true that in this position one can reduce the fracture by pressure along the proximal phalanx, but it is also true that immobilization with the proximal interphalangeal (PIP) joint flexed, even for a short period, can produce a permanent flexion contracture at that joint, which is worse than the effect of the original injury.

It is said that very severe angulation (e.g. 60° or more) in fifth metacarpal neck fractures requires operation: however in the author's experience surgical intervention seldom improves the result, and is occasionally very harmful.

Fractures of the shaft of the metacarpals

Often there is little or no displacement, and simple immobilization for three weeks is adequate treatment. However, it is important to make sure that there is no rotational deformity of the attached finger. Displaced or rotated fractures should be referred at once for orthopaedic assessment.

Fractures at or near the base of the first metacarpal

The most common type is a transverse fracture of the first metacarpal about 1 cm distal to the joint; the metacarpal is angulated into flexion. Since the first metacarpal normally lies in a rotated position compared with the other metacarpals, the injury results in the thumb becoming flexed across the palm—that is, extension of the thumb is restricted, and the span between the thumb and the index finger is reduced. Therefore, it is important to reduce these fractures, but they are usually easy to reduce and to hold corrected in plaster provided that the extension force is applied to the distal end of the metacarpal and

Fig. 4.26 Bennett's fracture-subluxation. The small piece broken off the base of the first metacarpal remains in place while the rest of the metacarpal, carrying most of the articular surface, subluxes laterally.

not to the phalanges of the thumb, which may merely hyperextend the MCP joint.

Bennett's fracture-dislocation of the first carpo-metacarpal joint (Fig. 4.26) is a rare injury, although much has been written about it. A surprisingly good functional result may occur despite poor treatment (Cannon *et al.* 1986), but as it involves an important joint, it seems right that such an injury should be managed by an orthopaedic surgeon. It may be treated conservatively provided that a very special and careful technique of plaster application is used (Charnley 1961), but frequently percutaneous fixation with a Kirschner wire is needed (Wagner 1959). Either way, the immobilization should be maintained for six weeks; the usual three weeks is not enough, and if the joint is left free at that stage it may redisplace.

Joint injuries to the digits

Fractures into the joints have already been considered; the following account is of soft tissue injuries.

Carpo-metacarpal joints

At the bases of the second and third metacarpals 'sprain-impaction problems are seen after flexion stress injuries resulting in volar impaction and dorsal stretch. A common example occurs when ice-hockey players crash into the wall or fend off an opponent. Compression-impaction is a serious problem in the professional boxer, whose repetitive stress to the stable longitudinal arch eventually results in cartilage damage, osteochondral fractures, and a chronically painful arthrosis.' (Dobyns 1988)

Metacarpophalangeal joints

As the *thumb* protrudes laterally from the hand at the level of the MCP joint, this joint is often injured. This is particularly common in skiing. If the ulnar collateral ligament of the MCP joint is torn (Fig. 4.27) it displaces superficial to the adductor aponeurosis (Stener 1962). It cannot heal with this aponeurosis interposed between the two ends of the ligament, and operative treatment is required. Therefore these patients must be referred to a surgeon for operation within a few days of injury. The diagnosis should be made upon the detection of bruising, the absence of fracture on X-ray, and the presence of ligamentous laxity (comparison should be made with the normal thumb). The radial collateral ligament is less often torn, but can be surprisingly troublesome. The anatomy is different on that side of the thumb, with little risk of soft tissue interposition, and conservative treatment in a plaster cast is satisfactory except in the more severe cases.

The acute injury (skier's thumb) should be distinguished from chronic instability due to an old injury and from gamekeeper's thumb, a condition confined to gamekeepers, which is not due to a single injury but to gradual attenuation of the ligament over many years while breaking the necks of rabbits (Campbell 1955).

The MCP joints of the *fingers* are less often injured. If injury does occur it usually takes the form of a dislocation of the second or fifth MCP joint. This is either easy or impossible to reduce by manipulation. One try is permissible. If it will not reduce, the torn volar plate is probably interposed between the joint surfaces, and this must be dealt with by open operation (Kaplan 1957). Repeated and increasingly forceful attempts to reduce the dislocation can only do harm.

FIG. 4.27 Mechanism of torn ulnar collateral ligament of the MCP joint of the thumb: (1) normal anatomy; (2) radial abduction injury to thumb tears distal end of collateral ligament; (3) when the thumb returns to its normal position the adductor aponeurosis comes to lie deep to the torn ligament or even (4) is folded back. Operative replacement and repair are needed.

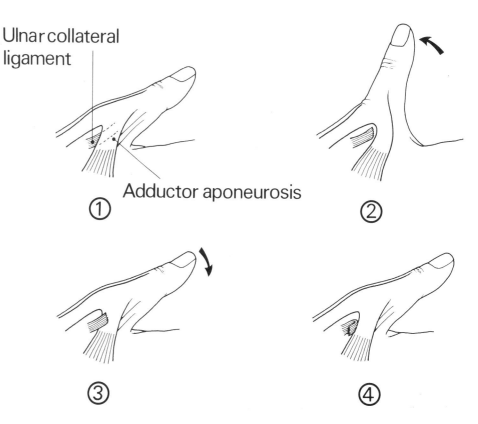

Proximal interphalangeal joints

Dislocation is easy to diagnose clinically and often easy to reduce, but it is always wise to have it X-rayed because an accompanying fracture makes it a much more serious injury, requiring expert treatment (see above). The usual dorsal dislocation (that is with the distal part of the finger displaced dorsally) is easily

FIG. 4.28 Stress views show abnormal lateral angulation due to torn collateral ligament of PIP joint. The patient, a famous Antipodean fast bowler, was treated by simple strapping, and regained full stability (perhaps to the regret of the English batsmen, as later that summer he took many England wickets).

reduced. The collateral ligaments are often intact, the base of the middle phalanx having swung round on them like a trapeze artist on his arms, but, after reduction, one must always test the collateral ligaments by applying first radial and then ulnar angulation to the extended finger. If the ligaments are intact, it is not necessary to immobilize the finger, though it may be wise to do so as some authorities believe that complete immobilization for ten days in a splint or in plaster will allow the finger to make a complete recovery more quickly (Eaton 1971).

If a collateral ligament is not intact, then the injury passes into the next category.

Tears of the collateral ligament of the PIP joint result from sideways force—for example, trying to catch a ball or falling onto the finger. With a complete tear, the instability is usually obvious; in cases of doubt, the finger may easily be anaesthetized by digital block, and stress X-rays performed (Fig. 4.28). Opinions differ as to whether operative repair is required. Provided that the X-ray shows the joint surfaces to be exactly parallel (that is, the torn ligament is not displaced into the joint), the author's practice has been to strap the finger to an intact neighbour to prevent further lateral stress but allow flexion and extension; the results have appeared satisfactory.

Sprains are partial tears of the collateral ligament, in which lateral stress causes pain but no abnormal lateral angulation. These would appear to be the least serious joint injuries in the fingers, but in practice they are often the most troublesome. Pain may continue for six months, and swelling for a year or even more. No treatment seems to make any difference, but eventually they make a full recovery and all the patients need is reassurance.

The *boutonnière injury* (known in France as 'le button-hole') is caused by a flexion force which tears the central slip of the extensor mechanism over the back of the PIP joint (Fig. 4.29). This injury is easily overlooked because at first the patient is

FIG. 4.29 The boutonnière injury: (a) clinical appearance; (b) pathology.

Lateral bands

Central slip

(A) Normal (B) Boutonniere injury (C) Boutonniere deformity (b)

FIG. 4.30 Mallet finger injury: (a) clinical appearance; (b) pathology.

(a)

Flexion force against extended finger

Rupture of tendon by shredding of the central fibres

Retinacular ligament usually remains intact

(b)

Fig. 4.31 Stack splint for mallet finger.

able to extend the PIP joint using the lateral bands of the extensor mechanism. However, there will be tenderness and pain on extension against resistance. Treatment is by immobilization in extension for four weeks, followed by a lively splint for another two weeks. If the injury is not diagnosed and treated, then over the next week or two the lateral bands slip forwards down the side of the joint until they can no longer extend it (Fig. 4.29(c)). A flexion contracture quickly develops, with the joint coming through between the lateral bands like a button through its hole. This is now the boutonniere deformity and is much more difficult to treat, though lively splintage is sometimes effective. Surgery is not recommended.

Distal interphalangeal (DIP) joint

Dislocation and collateral ligament injuries at this level are uncommon, because there is such a short length of finger distal to the joint.

However, *mallet fingers* are very common, owing to forcible passive flexion of the DIP joint when the extensor apparatus is contracting. The result is an injury to the extensor tendon rather like a rupture of the Achilles tendon: it is not a transverse tear with the ends apart, but an internal shredding, with the torn ends overlapping but in a lengthened position. The result is a lag in active extension, but full active flexion (Fig. 4.30). An X-ray should be taken, as the presence of a fracture may mean that different treatment is required. If there is no fracture, a decision must be made as to whether to treat the injury or not. A minor lag (e.g. 30°) may be taken up by the extensor mechanism, and an almost normal finger results; but a more severe one will, if untreated, be permanent: however, this causes no disability. Treatment consists of continuous immobilization of the DIP joint in extension for *eight weeks*. Any splint will do, *provided it is kept on all the time and not removed for any reason, even briefly.* Stack's moulded polypropylene splint (Fig. 4.31), which comes in various sizes and is available from Pryor & Howard Ltd, Manufacturers of Orthopaedic and Surgical Appliances, Willow Lane, Mitcham, CR44US, is probably the most satisfactory (Warren *et al.* 1988). It should be trimmed with a scalpel if the edge is pressing on the tender dorsum of the DIP joint. If the patient is not prepared to persevere with this treatment, there is no point in starting it, and he must understand that he will have to accept the minor deformity; however, function will be no problem. There is no need for surgical treatment of the acute injury, and very few indications for later surgery either.

Forcible extension of the finger can produce a corresponding, but much rarer, injury: *rupture of the flexor digitorum profundus (FDP) tendon* on the front of the finger. This is classically seen in rugby football players failing to make a tackle; they clutch despairingly at the trouser-band of the other player, whose determined departure pulls the distal end of the FDP tendon, sometimes with a fragment of bone, from the distal phalanx. It is nearly always the ring finger which is injured. This is often a more severe injury than an open cut of the flexor tendon, because the force of flexion pulls the tendon right down into the palm, ripping the vincula and filling the empty tendon sheath with blood, which will, if allowed, turn into restrictive fibrous tissue. A surgeon specializing in the hand should be given the opportunity to carry out primary repair within a day or two. If this chance has been lost, active flexion of the DIP joint can only be restored by a tendon graft—never a very predictable procedure. Provided that the patient has full active flexion of the PIP joint (by the intact flexor digitorum superficialis), it may be wiser to do nothing, as lack of flexion at the distal joint seldom causes much difficulty in using the hand. If it does, a tenodesis or arthrodesis of the DIP joint in slight flexion can be offered.

Conclusion

Many, but not all, sports injuries to the hand and wrist are minor and need little treatment or time off sport. Some, which may at first sight appear to be minor injuries, will cause permanent disability if not treated energetically. All must be assessed with great care including X-rays in most cases, to ensure recognition of the more serious injuries, so that they may be referred to an expert. The average casualty officer is not an expert, and the doctor in charge of the patient may be wise to arrange an urgent referral to a hand surgeon or an orthopaedic surgeon, which should take place within two or three days.

References

Barton, N. J. (1982). Fractures and joint injuries of the hand. In Watson-Jones' *Fractures and joint injuries* (ed. J.N. Wilson), Vol. 2, pp. 739–88. Churchill-Livingstone, Edinburgh.

Barton, N. J. (1984). Fractures of the hand. *J. Bone Jt. Surg.*, **66B**, 159–67.

Barton, N. J. (1992). Twenty questions about scaphoid fractures. *J. Hand Surg.*, **17B**, 289–310.

Belliappa, P. P. and Barton, N.J. (1991). Hand injuries in cricketers. *J. Hand Surg.*, **16B**, 212–14.

Blum, L. (1941). The treatment of Bennett's fracture-dislocation of the first metacarpal bone. *J. Bone Jt. Surg.*, **23**, 578–80.

Burke, F. D. (1988). Colles' fractures: conservative treatment. In *Fractures of the hand and wrist* (ed. N. J. Barton), pp. 267–75. Churchill-Livingstone, Edinburgh.

Cabrera, J. M. and McCue, F. C. (1986). Nonosseous athletic injuries of the elbow, forearm, and hand. *Clin. Sports Med.*, **5**, 681–700.

Campbell, C. S. (1955). Gamekeeper's thumb. *J. Bone Jt. Surg.*, **37B**, 148–9.

Cannon, S. R., Dowd, G. S. E., Williams, D. H., and Scott, J. M. (1986). A long-term study following Bennett's fracture. *J. Hand Surg.*, **11B**, 426–31.

Charnley, J. (1961). *The closed treatment of common fractures* (3rd edn). Churchill-Livingstone, Edinburgh.

Clay, N. R., Dias, J. J., Costigan, P. S., Gregg, P. J. and Barton, N. J. (1991). Need the thumb be immobilized in scaphoid fractures? A randomized prospective trial. *J. Bone Jt. Surg.*, **73B**, 828–32.

Curtin, J. and Kay, N. M. R. (1976). Hand injuries due to soccer. *Hand*, **8**, 93–5.

Cyriax, J. (1982). *Textbook of orthopaedic medicine*, Vol. 1 (8th edn). Baillière Tindall, London.

Dias, J. J., Taylor, M., Thompson, J., Brenkel, I. J., and Gregg, P. J. (1988). Radiographic signs of union of scaphoid fractures. *J. Bone Jt. Surg.*, **70B**, 299–301.

Dobyns, J. H. (1988). Fractures and dislocations at the base of the metacarpals. In *Fractures of the hand and wrist* (ed. N.J. Barton), pp. 120–33. Churchill-Livingstone, Edinburgh.

Eaton, R. G. (1971). *Joint injuries of the hand.* Thomas, Springfield, Ill. USA.

Ford, D. J., Ali, M. S., and Steel, W. M. (1989). Fractures of the fifth metacarpal neck:is reduction or immobilization necessary? *J. Hand Surg.*, **14B**, 165–7.

Green, D. P. (1985). The effect of avascular necrosis on Russe bone grafting for scaphoid non-union *J. Hand Surg.*, **10A**, 597–605.

Helal, B. (1978). Racquet player's pisiform. *Hand*, **10**, 87–90.

Henderson, H. P. (1984). The best dressing for a nail bed is the nail itself. *J. Hand Surg.*, **9B**, 197–8.

Henderson, J. J. and Arafa, M. A. M. (1987). Carpometacarpal dislocation. An easily missed diagnosis. *J. Bone Jt. Surg.*, **69B**, 212–14.

James, J. I. P. (1970). The assessment and management of the injured hand. *Hand*, **2**, 97–105.

Jones, W. A. (1988). Beware the sprained wrist. The incidence and diagnosis of scapho-lunate instability. *J. Bone Jt. Surg.*, **70B**, 293–7.

Kaplan, E. B. (1957). Dorsal dislocation of metacarpo-phalangeal joint of the index finger. *J. Bone Jt. Surg.*, **39A**, 1081–6.

King, J. W., Brelsford, H. J., and Tullos H.S. (1969). Analysis of the pitching arm of the professional baseball pitcher. *Clin. Orthop.*, **67**, 116–23.

Leslie, I. J. and Dickson, R. A. (1981). The fractured carpal scaphoid. Natural history and factors influencing outcome. *J. Bone Jt. Surg.*, **63B**, 225–30.

Lichtman, D. M. (1988). *The wrist and its disorders.* W. B. Saunders, Philladelphia.

London, P. S. (1967). *A practical guide to the care of the injured.* Livingstone, Edinburgh.

McCue, F. C., Honner, R., Johnson, M. C., and Giech, J. H. (1970). Athletic injuries of the proximal interphalangeal joint requiring surgical treatment, *J. Bone Jt. Surg.*, **52A**, 937–56.

McElfresh, E. C. and Dobyns, J. H. (1983). Intra-articular metacarpal head fractures. *J. Hand Surg.*, **8**, 383–93.

McElfresh, E. C., Dobyns, J. H., and O'Brien, E. T. (1972). Management of fracture-dislocation of the proximal interphalangeal joint by extension splinting. *J. Bone Jt. Surg.*, **54A**, 1705–11.

Panner, H. J. (1929). A peculiar affection of the capitellum humeri resembling Calve-Perthes disease of the hip. *Acta Radiol.*, **10**, 234.

Panting, A. L., Lamb, D. W., Noble, J., and Haw, C. S. (1984). Dislocations of the lunate with and without fracture of the scaphoid. *J. Bone Jt. Surg.* 391–5.

Read, M. T. F. (1981). Stress fractures of the distal radius in adolescent gymnasts. *Br. J. Sports Med.*, **15**, 272–6.

Roles, N. C. and Maudsley, R.H. (1972). Radial tunnel syndrome. *J. Bone Surg.*, **54B**, 499–508.

Roy, S., Caine, D., and Singer, K. M. (1985). Stress changes of the distal radial epiphysis in young gymnasts. *Am. J. Sports Med.*, **13**, 301–8.

Singer, K. M. and Roy, S. P. (1984). Osteochondrosis of the humeral capitellum. *Am. J. Sports Med.*, **12**, 351–60.

Slocum, D. B. (1978). Classification of elbow injuries from baseball players. *Am. J. Sports Med.*, **6**, 62–7.

Stark, J. J., Hobe, F. W., Boyes, J. H., and Ashworth, C. R. (1977). Fracture of the hook of the hamate in athletes. *J. Bone Jt. Surg.*, **59A**, 575–82.

Steel, W. M. (1988). Articular fractures. In *Fractures of the hand and wrist* (ed. N. J. Barton), pp. 55–73. Churchill-Livingstone, Edinburgh.

Stener, B. (1962). Displacement of the ruptured ulnar collateral ligament of the metacarpo-phalangeal joint of the thumb. *J. Bone Jt. Surg.*, **44B**, 869–79.

Taleisnik, J. (1988). Carpal instability. *J. Bone Jt. Surg.*, **70A**, 1262–8.

Wagner, C. J. (1950). Method of treatment of Bennett's fracture-dislocation. *Am. J. Surg.*, **80**, 230–31.

Warren, R. A., Norris, S. H., and Ferguson, D. D. (1988). Mallet finger: a trial of two splints. *J. Hand Surg.*, **13B**, 151–3.

Warren-Smith, C. D. and Barton, N. J. (1988). Non-union of the scaphoid: Russe graft vs Herbert Screw. *J. Hand Surg.*, **13B**, 82–5.

Wilson, F. D., Andrews, J. R., Blackburn, T. A., and McCluskey, G. (1983). Valgus extension overload in the pitching elbow. *Am. J. Sports Med.*, **11**, 83–8.

Wilton, T. J. (1987). Soft-tissue interposition as a possible cause of scaphoid non-union. *J. Hand Surg.*, **12B**, 50–51.

5 Spinal injuries

M. A. HUTSON AND F. R. I. MIDDLETON

Soft tissue injuries

M. A. HUTSON

Biomechanics/applied anatomy

The spine has a number of functions that reflect man's upright stance, his capacity to bend and lift, and his desire to indulge in sport and recreation, which demand both stability and flexibility. It may be considered to be constructed in two columns, anterior and posterior. The *anterior* column is composed of vertebral bodies, their superior and inferior margins (the end plates) and the intervening discs. Each disc has a fibrocartilaginous annulus and a gelatinous nucleus pulposus. The anterior column resists axial compression loading of the spine. Associated with this shock-absorbing function of the disc is a little intervertebral movement in all directions (Bogduk and Twomey 1987). The *posterior* column is derived from the neural arches: movement occurs at the zygo-apophyseal (facet) joints, which are diarthrodial—that is, synovial in type.

In the cervical spine nodding movements and side flexion occur at the atlanto-occipital joints. At C1/2 (the atlanto-axial joint) approximately 50° of rotation is allowed around the odontoid peg. At the other facet joints in the neck side flexion, rotation, and flexion/extension occur. The greatest degree of flexion/extension occurs at C5/6. Intervertebral discs are present at all levels other than C0/1 and C1/2. The intervertebral foramina are reduced to their smallest diameter on ipsilateral side flexion, rotation, and extension—a fact of clinical significance when examining for evidence of nerve root entrapment.

The thoracic spine is inherently stable because of its kyphosis and its rib attachments. A limited range of movements (flexion, extension, rotations, and side flexions) occur at the facet joints. Most rotation/side flexion takes place between T10 and T12 and at the thoracolumbar junction. As a result these distal joints are vulnerable to injury. The ribs articulate with the vertebral bodies at the costovertebral joints and between T1 and T10 at the costotransverse joints; both these sets of joints are synovial. Further joints are found between the ribs and the costal cartilages (costochondral joints), between ribs 1 to 7 and the sternum (sternocostal joints), and between ribs and adjacent costal cartilages (ribs 5 to 9). The 'false' ribs 8, 9, and 10 join only with the costocartilage of the ribs above, and 'floating' ribs 11 and 12 do not have a distal articulation.

In the lumbar spine the facet joints are orientated to resist torsional and shear strain: rotation is minimal. Flexion/extension occurs maximally at the lumbosacral junction, thereby constituting a physiological pivot between trunk and legs. Trunk flexion is a combination of pelvic rotation (around the transverse axes of the hip joints) and lumbar flexion (essentially a reversal of lumbar lordosis). The smooth simultaneous movement at these different levels constitutes the dynamic *lumbar-pelvic rhythm* (Cailliet 1981). The extensor muscles of the spine are divided into three distinct groups. The erectores spinae (sacrospinales) are the longest and most superficial group, extending from the lumbosacral spines and the iliac crest inferiorly to the ribs and thoracic transverse processes superiorly. Lying underneath the erectores spinae are a second group of muscles (semispinalis, multifidus, and rotatores) which span three segments only. The third group of muscles in the lumbar spine (only) connect the spinous processes and transverse processes of adjacent vertebrae.

Intradiscal pressure studies (Nachemson and Elfstrom 1970) have identified the increased loading of the L3 disc in different postures and during different lifting techniques: both sitting and lifting with straight legs increase intradiscal pressure considerably. Farfan (1973) emphasizes the importance of torsional overload that results in injury to the facet joints and annulus. Cailliet (1981) identifies faulty posture as a major cause of 'static' back pain, and advises strengthening exercises for the abdominals and gluteals to reduce the lumbosacral angle (Fig. 5.1). Exercise-related (kinetic) problems are due to poor training and technique, inadequate flexibility, muscle imbalance, and fatigue caused by overload. In contrast, muscle-strengthening and spinal flexibility exercises improve the dissipation of forces arising from compression loads in particular, and reduce the incidence of injury.

On bending forwards and lifting, the powerful hip extensor muscles (the gluteals and to a lesser extent the hamstrings) may allow a dead lift of over three times bodyweight. In the lumbar spine the strain is then taken by the combination of contraction of the trunk musculature (powerful, though not as powerful as the hip extensors) and the ligamentous system. The paraspinal muscles create a compressive effect on the disc and some degree of shearing force. The ligaments comprise the spinal ligaments (supraspinous, interspinous, ligamentum flavae, posterior and

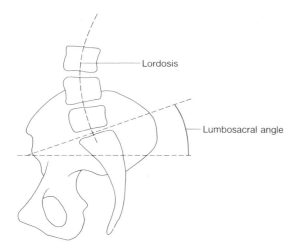

FIG. 5.1 The lumbosacral angle is made between the plane of the upper border of the sacrum and the horizontal in the standing position: it is affected by posture, and may be reduced by corrective exercises (using the abdominal and gluteal muscles).

anterior longitudinal ligaments, and facet capsules) and the lumbodorsal (or 'dorsilumbar') fascia. The abdominal muscles create extra tension in the lumbodorsal fascia, and are thus essential in the balance of external loads applied to the spine. An important function of the ligaments is to minimize the compressive and shear forces applied to the intervertebral joints.

Two important points may be emphasized. The first is the importance of a satisfactory range of extension at the hip joints. If this is absent, and fixed hip flexion develops as a result of degenerative disease, excessive extension strain occurs at the low lumbar joints during walking and lifting. This explains the increased risk

of low back problems in association with hip disorders. The second is the importance of strong abdominal musculature, which is understood by weight-lifters who often employ a tight abdominal/lumbar belt during lifting (Fig. 5.2). The abdominal muscles help increase tension within the abdominal cavity, and thus assist with transmission of lifting stress through arms, shoulders, thorax, abdomen, and pelvis. They also help to reduce shear forces posteriorly and reinforce ligamentous function as described.

With the exception of spondylolysis, which is almost exclusively caused by repetitive hyperextension, for example during back walkovers in gymnastics, the patho-anatomical changes in evidence when an athlete injures his back are the same as in the general population. In the latter group, however, inadequate musculature, particularly in the abdomen and thighs, and poor working positions are often aetiological factors. In sport the usual causes are simply excessive loads applied repetitively to the spine. Inadequate or imbalanced muscle function may be seen under occasional circumstances—for example, inadequate strength in the neck muscles in adolescent rugby players or in the lumbar and abdominal muscles in the middle-aged who do not maintain regular physical conditioning. A correct technique is thus crucial when recurrent loading of any type is applied to the spine in sport. This is particularly important in weight training (as well as weight lifting), the more so as this type of training is now used in a multitude of different sports. The maintenance of the correct degree of lumbar lordosis and pelvic angle during heavy lifts requires adequate coaching. Fatigue is more of a problem in circuit training, particularly with barbells, so that the athlete may not be aware of the tendency towards hyperextension that may accompany upper body work. Faulty technique in almost all (if not all) sports may allow overload to create structural problems of any of the pathoanatomical types subsequently described.

Pain transmission has been researched, though it continues to be debated. The articular nerves supplying the facet joints are branches of the posterior primary rami. Although the

FIG. 5.2 Strong abdominal musculature is necessary for weight-lifters, who often use a tight abdominal belt (courtesy of Supersport).

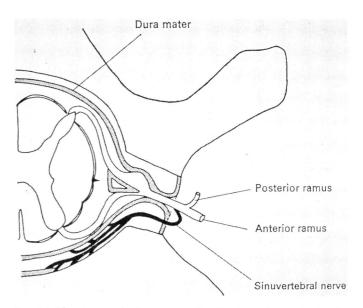

FIG. 5.3 The sinuvertebral nerve supplies the dura, the contents of epidural space, and the posterior margin of the annulus of the disc articular nerves to the posterior apophyseal joints are branches of posterior primary rami

intervertebral discs were thought at one time to contain no sensory nerve endings, it is now apparent that the sinuvertebral nerves (small branches from the common spinal nerve) supply the posterior annular margins (Fig. 5.3). The sinuvertebral nerves also supply the dura and contents of the epidural space. It is probable that dural compression and irritation are responsible for the pain caused primarily by disc herniation.

A comment about 'spondylosis' is necessary: this radiological entity, present in the cervical and lumbar spines as a response to stress at the vertebral margins above and below the disc, does not cause pain, has no relationship to painful syndromes, and is not referred to again in the text.

Cervical Injury

Patho-anatomy and Epidemiology

In addition to fractures and fracture-dislocations, injuries to the soft tissues are naturally most common in those sports in which physical contact is part of the game. Rugby football, American football, and wrestling are three of the sports associated with a relatively high incidence of cervical injury. In common with the other areas of the spine, facet strains and disc injury also occur in the absence of a history of direct trauma.

The injury that is typically found in American football and wrestling is the 'burner' or 'stinger'. This takes the form of a temporary painful loss of function in the affected arm immediately following a blow to or angulation of the neck. There are two types of causation. In one, the neck is laterally flexed away from the site of injury whilst the ipsilateral shoulder is depressed, thus stretching the brachial plexus. In the other, the neck is extended and rotated/side-flexed towards the injured side: it is likely that this mechanism irritates the nerve root by diminishing the size of the intervertebral foramen. The feeling of electric shocks in the arm (from shoulder to fingers) is followed by numbness and partial paralysis lasting for several minutes. Complete subjective and objective recovery is often made within a few minutes, though neurological deficit occasionally persists for longer.

Neurological deficit in the arm may result also from a cervical disc prolapse, though the onset is not so acute. Radicular pain, paraesthesiae, and numbness are usually preceded by a short history of stiffness and discomfort felt in the neck. Occasionally, particularly in C7 root palsy, the pain may be felt largely in the pectoral region and axilla. Dermatomal identification is made by recording the distribution of paraesthesiae/numbness (confirmed by subsequent neurological examination). The most common sites of prolapse are at C5/6 and particularly C6/7. The root that emerges inferior to the vertebral body is traumatized, commonly C6 (tingling in the thumb and index finger) or C7 (tingling in index, long, and ring finger). If the C5 root is involved (due to C4/5 disc prolapse) the radicular pain is usually unaccompanied by sensory symptoms.

Facet syndromes are particularly common. Theories abound as to the exact nature of facet dysfunction: the author envisages structural pathological changes, though proof is lacking in the acute (clinically reversible) lesion. The osteopathic concept is one of neurophysiological (functional rather than structural) disturbance. Undoubtedly degenerative changes occur in the older age groups, though *per se* these are unlikely to be the cause of bouts of pain. Relatively minor trauma, often involving axial compression or torsional stress, may be recorded in acute facet dysfunction. The complaint is of pain in the neck and radiation of discomfort (referred pain) to almost anywhere in the head and shoulders, depending upon the level of dysfunction. Reference of pain from both facet syndromes and disc prolapses in the distal cervical spine to the base of the neck and the region just medial to the superomedial border of the scapula is particularly common. Tenderness may also be elicited, either in the skin and subcutaneous tissues (positive skin rolling) or within the underlying muscle (known as a 'trigger point'). Facet injury also occurs in whiplash, when sudden hyperextension of the neck stresses both facets and connecting ligaments, and in more severe cases the intervertebral disc and ligamentum flavum. This

FIG. 5.4 CT scan at C4/5 revealing a disc prolapse on the left. Compression of the emerging C5 nerve root affected the anterior deltoid, supraspinatus, and infraspinatus muscles, resulting in inability to actively abduct the arm beyond 30°.

most commonly occurs in car accidents, when a stationary vehicle is hit from the rear.

Examination

In the standing position active movements, followed by passive movements, are performed in the six directions: flexion, extension, rotations (right and left), side flexions (right and left). Pain and restriction of movement are noted; end-feel is determined at the extremes of passive movements. Neurological assessment in the upper limbs is most usefully made by examination of the motor system to detect muscle weakness due to nerve root compression:

Shoulder shrug	C4
Shoulder abduction	C5
Shoulder external rotation	C5
Elbow flexion	C5, 6
Wrist extension	C6
Elbow extension	C7
Shoulder adduction	C7
Wrist flexion	C7
Wrist ulnar deviation	C8
Thumb abduction/extension	C8
Fingers 4/5 approximation	TI

Wasting of some muscle groups—for example, pectorals in C7 root entrapment—may also be observed.

In the presence of arm pain a neural tension test may be used: the C5 and C6 roots are stretched when the neck is contralaterally flexed, the ipsilateral shoulder is abducted, extended, and depressed, the forearm is supinated, the elbow is extended, and the wrist is dorsiflexed. Exacerbation of arm pain indicates the presence of a root (or brachial plexus) lesion.

The patient should then lie in the supine position on the examination couch, with his head cradled in the examiner's hands. Accessory passive movements known as joint play are performed (Fig. 12.6(a), p. 210):

anteroposterior glide;
lateral glide;
side bending.

These tests yield further information on the mobility at each cervical segment. Palpation of the facets for localized tenderness and muscle spasm assists in localization. Maitland's segmental vibratory techniques may also be used (Maitland 1986). Assessment of function of the neck muscles by isometric contraction may be performed at this stage, although it is unlikely to be helpful as a diagnostic procedure (as intrinsic muscle lesions are very uncommon). X-rays should be taken when there is root involvement: although of limited value, they help to exclude bony pathology, and to identify the capacity of the intervertebral foramina. Occasionally CT scans and MRI are helpful (Fig. 5.4).

Interpretation and Management

The capsular pattern in the neck is limitation of all movements other than flexion. This is seen in (painless) osteoarthritis in the elderly, and ankylosing spondylitis in the young. When spondylitis is present in the neck, the lumbar spine is 'flat' on examination, and the sacroiliac joints are sclerotic on X-ray (see Fig. 6.9, p. 108).

All the soft tissue lesions subsequently described give rise to a partial articular (non-capsular) pattern, in which some movements of the neck are painful and restricted, and others are not. The only exception to this pattern occurs in the acute stage of an injury such as whiplash, burner, or torticollis owing to acute disc protrusion, when all movements may be uncomfortable and appear to be restricted. The partial articular pattern emerges before long even so.

The presence of persisting radicular pain in the arm, particularly when radiating below the elbow and when associated with paraesthesiae/numbness, strongly suggests *disc prolapse*. The nerve root is affected, and the radicular pain is usually provoked by a combination of passive neck extension and ipsilateral rotation. Additionally the neural tension test may be positive. The presence of motor palsy should be sought: it has some prognostic significance. If absent, cervical traction is likely to be successful. It is not unreasonable for an experienced therapist to initiate treatment using gentle mobilization techniques to the affected segment. If the affected nerve root is irritated rather than severely compressed, it seems probable that the accompanying oedema may be improved by passive motion (Elvey 1986). In the author's experience traction is normally required nevertheless. If motor weakness is present there is little prospect of improvement of symptoms by repeated distraction force, although nerve blocks may produce dramatic relief of pain. However, the patient may be reassured that spontaneous resolution is to be expected within three months: since nocturnal pain is troublesome the patient may gain relief by sleeping with the ipsilateral hand placed behind the neck.

In *facet dysfunction* a partial articular pattern is also found, though the restriction in mobility is not gross. Usually rotation towards the painful side is restricted. Joint play signs are particularly useful; when combined with palpation for tenderness they localize the level and give a guide to the type of mobilization or manipulation that is required (Fig. 12.6(b), p. 210). Mennell suggests that manipulation is merely an extension of the examining technique (Mennell 1960). Cyriax insisted on manipulation being carried out during manual traction (Cyriax and Russell 1984). Stoddard's techniques are also commended (Stoddard 1980). In general, 'mobilization' is the use of passive stretching without thrust. 'Manipulation' uses thrust at the extreme of range. A few sessions of treatment, using a technique with which the physician or therapist has become familiar, at intervals of two or three days is a reasonable regime. 'Muscle energy' techniques may also be helpful: passive stretching is facilitated by a preceding isometric contraction of the relevant muscle groups. In recovery from neck injury and for prophylaxis in those sports requiring strong neck musculature, for instance in forward play in rugby football, neck-strengthening exercises should be prescribed.

Thoracic Injury

Patho-anatomy and epidemiology

As a result of rotation strains, injuries occur to spinal joints, intercostal muscles, and costochondral joints. In addition, a form of osteochondritis known as Scheuermann's disease affects the distal thoracic and proximal lumbar spine in adolescents. Although the aetiology of this growth disorder is unproven, it is possible that repeated trauma is responsible for the vertebral

(a)   (b)

FIG. 5.5 The typical radiological appearances of Scheuermann's disease: (a) irregularity of the antero-
inferior epiphyseal ring and adjacent sclerosis at D9; (b) anterior erosions at L1/2 and L2/3

end-plate degeneration, with subsequent propulsion of nucleus pulposus into adjacent vertebral bodies and anterior wedging (Fig. 5.5). Occurring in 14–18-year-olds, it may be a painless condition, though it often gives rise to discomfort on or after exercise. An exaggerated thoracic kyphosis may be observed. If symptomatic, exercise restriction needs to be applied for some months. At least one authority (Stoddard 1980) considers that there is an association between Scheuermann's disease and the incidence of low back pain in later life. More recently, Sward *et al.* (1991) have confirmed the correlation between disc degeneration and the presence of Schmorl's nodes in the thoracolumbar spine in an MRI study of elite gymnasts. Reduction in thoracic mobility and premature degenerative changes in the thoracic spine in the third and fourth decades may also restrict the capacity for certain types of exercise, such as rowing.

The exact nature of the patho-anatomical process involved in posterior thoracic 'strains' is unknown. Disc prolapses occasionally occur, though they are relatively uncommon. It is more likely that the facet joints or costovertebral joints are the source of problems which are clinically of two types. An acute sprain occurs as a result of rotational stress combined with either flexion or extension; pain is felt to one side of the thoracic spine, particularly in the D5-D8 range. Spontaneous resolution may be expected inside a week. A more chronic lesion presents as discomfort in a similar area, commonly with radiation unilaterally around the chest as far as the sternum, and occasionally presenting as anterior chest pain alone (thereby mimicking cardiac

pain). Lesions at the thoracolumbar junction are not uncommon in the 30-45 year age-group: pain is often referred to the iliac fossa and iliac crest. Discomfort in thoracic joint lesions is predominantly felt after exercise.

Pain that is felt unilaterally around the chest and related to exercise may either be referred from the spinal joints or be a manifestation of more local pathology, such as intercostal muscle strain. The latter condition is seen typically in fast bowlers (cricket). In other sports, such as rowing and sculling, unilateral thoracic pain may be due to a stress fracture of a rib. Holden and Jackson (1985) consider that stress during weight training and serratus anterior overload are the aetiological factors. Resolution is to be expected with modification of activity. Mechanical derangement may occur at a costochondral junction in the form of a 'sprung rib'. Sudden well-localized pain is felt, and may be accompanied by clicking and swelling, which reflect repeated subluxation.

On the question of scoliosis, there may be a primary (structural) deformity in which there is a marked rotational element, or it may arise as a consequence of intense muscle spasm ('sciatic scoliosis') or a short leg. Although a mild degree of structural scoliosis of the thoracolumbar spine (such as idiopathic adolescent scoliosis) is relatively common, it has little or no relationship to sports injuries of any kind. The underlying cause for a secondary scoliosis must be determined: in the absence of back pain or sciatica, leg-length inequality may be detected. Of particular relevance is its association with overuse injury in the lower limbs.

Examination

The natural primary curvature of the thoracic spine may be exaggerated in the form of a kyphosis or, when acutely angulated, for instance when due to wedge fractures, in the form of a kyphus. Neck flexion is initially performed in the standing position: when pain is felt in the thorax this indicates dural irritation—for example, by disc protrusion. Active posterior approximation of the scapulae by the patient tests the upper thoracic joints by traction on the dural sheath of the T1 and T2 nerve roots. Active movements, followed by passive movements, of the thoracic spine then follow:

flexion;
extension;
rotations (right and left);
side flexions (right and left).

During flexion a mild primary scoliosis may be detected by the presence of a 'rib hump' that is indicative of the rotational element of the deformity. A scoliosis that is present on standing, though absent on sitting, is probably due to leg-length inequality.

It is often easier to determine the passive range of rotation with the patient sitting with his fingers interlocked behind his neck. In the sitting position isometric contraction may be tested; it is of more relevance in the thoracic region than elsewhere in the spine, as muscle injury may occur in the supporting (intercostal) muscles. Segmental (extension) pressure and skin rolling are best performed in the prone position to identify the affected level. Tests for the stability of the thoracic cage include rib springing (both AP and bilateral), pain on deep inspiration, and localized tenderness or swelling (indicating the possibility of rib callus or a sprung costochondral joint).

Interpretation and Management

The partial articular pattern in which two, three, or four active and passive movements hurt, though not all are restricted, denotes *thoracic joint dysfunction*. Usually at least one rotatory movement is affected. Resisted contraction is painless, and localizing signs are positive (localized segmental pressure and skin rolling). Treatment is by manipulation, which should be successful over two or three sessions (see Fig. 12.7, p. 211). Recurrent dysfunction may require management by sclerosant injections to the interspinous and (facet) capsular ligaments. The uncommon thoracic disc protrusion is characterized by pain on neck flexion and substantial restriction of forward flexion of the thoracic spine. Any suspicion of cord compression (symptoms or signs of an upper motor neurone lesion in the legs) should stimulate further investigation for the presence of disc prolapse or spinal tumour.

Although an *intercostal muscle strain* will also give rise to discomfort on certain thoracic movements (by stretching the affected muscles), there is likely in addition to be pain on coughing and deep breathing, and localized tenderness. Although it is difficult to resist the temptation to prescribe localized treatment, the muscle tear will nevertheless take two to three weeks to heal. The important aspect of management is the initial restriction of rotational stress, followed during rehabilitation by graded passive rotational stretching exercises in order to prevent recurrence.

A *sprung rib*, indicating at least a sprain, and more probably instability of the affected costochondral joint, may be a difficult problem to resolve. In the presence of swelling and clicking intra-articular steroid injections may be tried: occasionally surgical excision is required.

FIG. 5.6 Nerve root compression due to HNP in the lumbar spine. L5 root entrapment results from L4/5 disc prolapse. S1 root entrapment results from L5/S1 disc prolapse.

Lumbar and Sacroiliac Injury

Patho-anatomy and Epidemiology

Acute Injury

An acute strain occurring at a motion segment (the intervertebral disc and its accompanying facet joints) often reflects pre-existing patho-anatomical changes in both the anterior and posterior columns. Thus radial tears in the disc and ligamentous laxity in the facetal supporting structures are probably coexistent in the majority of cases. However, on a clinical basis, specific syndromes are identifiable, which may be localized to the individual parts of a motion segment and demand a variety of therapeutic approaches.

As a result of a crack in the annulus of the disc, prolapse of nuclear material may take place (herniation of nucleus pulposus (HNP)). Initially, mild lumbar discomfort may be experienced, worsening overnight to give rise to the typical appearance of lumbago the following morning: low lumbar pain and stiffness accompanied by restricted flexion, and possibly by a 'pelvic tilt'. Such a protrusion is *central*—that is, posterior—and gives rise to severe low back pain (LBP), with some radiation to the thighs. Commonly the protrusion moves *posterolaterally*, and compression of the nerve root ensues (Fig. 5.6). Sometimes HNP may be primarily posterolateral, in which case sciatica is not preceded by LBP. Paraesthesiae and numbness may be experienced in the dermatomal pattern: the most commonly involved of the dermatomes are L5 and S1, giving rise to posterolateral and posteriorly distributed symptoms respectively. L4 root symptoms are felt anterolaterally in the leg, and account for approximately 5–10 per cent of cases. Disc prolapse is not confined to middle age: patients in their twenties and thirties are commonly affected. Porter and colleagues (1978) have stressed the relationship between symptomatic disc disease and the diameter of the spinal canal: patients with narrow canals are at considerable risk.

The nature of acute LBP, often felt unilaterally without sciatic referral and with less pronounced articular signs, is subject to much debate. Although devotees of the Cyriax approach consider that a common cause would be a displaced tag of annular fibrocartilage (Cyriax 1982), the author's opinion is that *facet dysfunction* is responsible—even so, the structural changes which occur in an acute bout of pain are conjectural. Stress tests for the facet joints may be performed, and are often found to be positive. Rotational stress in flexion is an important aetiological factor. Repetitive hyperextension may also be incriminated. Thus backache in oarsmen has been considered to be facetal in origin (Stallard 1980). Cricket bowling may cause a number of different types of back injury, of which facet dysfunction is common. A technically correct golf swing is less likely to be associated with facet dysfunction unless overload is extreme: youngsters, in attempting to achieve extra distance on their drives, may sustain back strain by exaggerating the arched and rotated position on the backswing or follow through.

Pain felt over the sacroiliac joint is a common symptom, and commonly ascribed (wrongly) to a lesion at this joint. It is often *referred* from a lumbar segment. However, despite the fact that normal sacroiliac joint mobility is apparently minimal (a few millimetres only on clinical measurement, by Colachis *et al.* 1963, of the inter-PSIS distance in different postures such as sitting and lying) mechanical problems do arise. Hypermobility is the underlying cause of *sacroiliac dysfunction*: pain may radiate from the sacroiliac region into the groin and posteriorly down the thigh as far as the heel.

A stress fracture of the pars interarticularis (*spondylolysis*) (Fig. 5.7) has a relatively more subacute onset. Although it was thought at one time to be present as a congenital abnormality, studies have shown that the lytic defect develops principally during childhood and adolescence (Fredrikson *et al.* 1984). The overall incidence of spondylolysis in the population is of the order of 2–6 per cent, becoming rather higher in selected groups such as female gymnasts (eleven per cent in a group of average age 14 years studied by Jackson *et al.* 1976, Jackson *et al.* 1981). Little (or no) backache may have been recalled on retrospective enquiry amongst such groups. Spondylolysis that develops in the teenager may give rise to exercise dependent backache, either unilateral or bilateral. It is particularly common in children who indulge in repetitive hyperextension and rotation, as in gymnastics, circuit training, field athletics and cricket bowling (Fig. 5.8; see also Fig. 11.5(a), p. 188). Apprentice soccer players are also at risk if they are trained too vigorously. Although the author has seen an acute spondylolysis (confirmed by bone scan) in a 26-year-old it is most uncommon after the late teens (Elliott *et al.* 1988). The identical biomechanical stresses may give rise to facet strain in an older age group.

Chronic or Relapsing Injury

As degenerative changes progressively take place in the facet joints and are associated with disc degeneration and narrowing, the likelihood of *lumbar instability* increases. Loss of disc height results in 'offsetting' of the superior and inferior articular processes, accompanied by inadequate capsular and ligamentous support in the posterior columns (Kirkaldy-Willis *et al.* 1978). Frequent bouts of lumbar pain, with apparently normal lumbar function in the intervening periods, are experienced.

If 'offsetting' and degenerative hypertrophy of the facet joints worsen, the intervertebral foramina are narrowed, and sciatica due to *lateral canal stenosis* may ensue. Although the age group

(a)

(b)

FIG. 5.7 (a) A stress fracture in the lumbar spine (spondylolysis) affects the isthmus (pars interarticularis) of the neural arch at L5, L4, or occasionally L3. A scottie dog with a collar is seen on the oblique X-ray. (b) A tomogram reveals a spondylolysis at L4

(b)

Fig. 5.8 Spondylolysis is more common in those sports in which hyper-extension of the lumbar spine is repetitive, for example (a) back walkovers in gymnastics and (b) Fosbury flop in high jumping.

(a)

(55 years and over) is at the upper range for indulgence in vigorous sporting activity, nevertheless it is not uncommon to see patients whose symptoms arise during recreational exercise such as badminton or sailing.

Chronic ligamentous insufficiency may occur in the young athlete, when it is usually associated with hypermobility. Assessment may be made by the use of a scoring system that refers to mobility of the trunk, elbows, little fingers, thumbs, and knees (Beighton *et al.* 1973). In respect of forward flexion of the trunk, hypermobility may be primary or secondary; in the latter case ligamentous stretching results from specific exercises required to promote flexibility in activities such as ballet and gymnastics. In either event, low backache may become increasingly troublesome, though usually it is not felt during exercise. Prolonged immobility—for example, sitting or standing for some time—is painful. Therefore ligamentous insufficiency is often referred to as the 'cocktail party' or 'theatre-goer's' syndrome.

Ligamentous insufficency may also be associated with progressive degenerative changes in the posterior columns. Sports such as squash, which necessitate considerable twisting and turning, may cause premature degenerative changes in the facet joints at a relatively early age—for example, in the fourth decade. Peri-articular ossification around the L4/5 or L5/S1 facet joints may

develop as a reaction to stress (Fig. 5.9), and has been noted by the author in relatively young sportsmen such as professional footballers. Symptoms from nerve root entrapment as well as exercise-related low back pain may result. At a later age frank *arthrosis* of the facet joints may give rise to stiffness and discomfort, which are particularly noticeable after immobility such as prolonged sitting—the more so when provoked by injudicious exertions on the squash court or in the garden. The 45–60 year-old is principally affected; such degenerative change is a direct consequence of the commitment to vigorous exercise over the previous decades.

Morning stiffness in the younger age group raises the possibility of *sacroiliitis* associated with one of the spondyloarthritides, such as ankylosing spondylitis. Low backache and alternating sciatic ache, bearing little relationship to posture or exercise, are the main features. It is not unusual for the presentation to be as a sports injury, as the patient often assumes that symptoms are due to physical strain.

Although backache in the older age group may be due to more serious pathology, patients do not usually present with exercise related pain: indeed the feature of chronic infective and malignant conditions is one of nagging persistent pain that is unrelated to posture or exercise.

FIG. 5.9 Periarticular ossification (around the L5 posterior apophyseal joints) in this professional soccer player is a reaction to repetitive rotational stress: (a) PA X-rays, (b) oblique X-rays.

Examination

Gait and posture. A patient walks, sits, and stands awkwardly when in severe pain from an acute lumbago or sciatica.

Standing. Pelvic tilt or sciatic scoliosis may be observed (Fig. 5.10). Neck flexion assesses dural irritation. Active forward flexion, extension, and lateral flexions are attempted. Range, pain, and abnormal rhythms are observed. Since the examiner may not have a record of the normal range of motion, particularly flexion, the degree of movement may be recorded with a note of whether the patient feels this is normal for him/her. Alternatively, the Schober test may be used: the distance

FIG. 5.10 A marked pelvic tilt is associated with a sciatic scoliosis due to a lumbar HNP.

(identified by tape measure) between skin markers over the L1 and S1 spinous processes is recorded in the upright position and in the fully flexed position. Deviation on forward flexion is typical of an L4/5 protrusion. An arc of pain or 'hitch' on recoil from flexion indicates segmental instability. The lower lumbar spine may be palpated for the existence of a ledge indicating spondylolisthesis. The sacroiliac mobility test is performed by asking the patient to stand on one leg and flex the opposite hip. Inferior movement of the posterior superior iliac spine (PSIS) on the side of the flexed hip is the normal response. If the sacroiliac joint is dysfunctional the PSIS does not descend (Fig. 5.11).

The one-legged hyperextension test may be performed if there is a suspicion of recent spondylolysis (Fig. 5.12). While standing on one leg the spine is extended: the test is positive if pain is felt on the weightbearing side. Extension may be reinforced by rotation (as in the Fitch catch test in which the raised heel is touched by the opposite hand).

Isometric paraspinal muscle contraction may be tested (by resisting lateral flexion) and is found, even with intense muscle spasm, to be painless—primary muscle tears are most unusual. An exception is a fracture of a lumbar transverse process which as a consequence of its muscle attachments, behaves as a muscle.

Assessment of calf power (S1/2) is made by asking the patient to stand on tip-toe on each leg in turn.

Sitting. Neural tension may be estimated by the 'slump' test: with the patient seated and the trunk flexed, the neck is gently flexed by the examiner (thereby increasing dural tension). In the

FIG. 5.11 Unilateral sacroiliac mobility may be assessed by noting the inferior movement of the PSIS (posterior superior iliac spine when the patient flexes his ipsilateral hip in the standing position: normal (left); abnormal (right).

FIG. 5.12 The unilateral hyperextension test is positive (indicating a possible spondylolysis) if pain is reproduced when the patient flexes his ipsilateral hip and extends his lumbar spine.

FIG. 5.14 The lumbosacral stress test is positive (indicating the presence of a lesion in either the sacroiliac or lumbosacral joints) if pain is reproduced on passive bilateral SLR.

FIG. 5.13 The position of the examiner and patient on performing the slump test.

(a)   FIG. 5.15 The lumbar apophyseal joints may be stressed by passive flexion and rotation of the spine as demonstrated: (b)
(a) to the right; (b) to the left.

presence of dural irritability—for example, secondary to disc pro-lapse—lumbar pain is reproduced. If sciatica is predominant the test may be modified (after Troup 1986) by extending the knee of the affected leg (Fig. 5.13). Sciatic pain is then reproduced.

Supine. The passive range of hip movements is determined. Straight leg raising (SLR) is performed for each leg individually and then together, as the lumbosacral (LS) stress test.

Experience of the normal end-feel of unilateral SLR should be gained. The usefulness of the SLR has occasionally been questioned, because there are determinants other than root compression responsible for the discomfort felt towards the end of range—for example, sacroiliac ligament strain and hamstring

tightness. However, unilateral SLR does remain a most useful test, particularly when comparison with the normal side is made, and may be performed without the need for refinements such as the bowstring or Lasègue test. A significant degree of restriction is usually due to stretching of the dura mater secondary to disc herniation.

The lumbosacral (LS) stress test is performed by passively raising both legs simultaneously, thereby stressing the sacroiliac and lumbosacral facet joints (Fig. 5.14). Pain and restricted range are indicators of dysfunction. Further stress may be applied to the facet joints by performing passive flexion and rotation/lateral flexion from a baseline position of bilateral hip and

FIG. 5.16 Daily lumbar traction of 80–140 lb for 20 minutes is an effective treatment for lumbar disc prolapse without neurological signs.

knee flexion (Fig. 5.15). Sacroiliac stress may be applied unilaterally by passive axial compression of the adducted and flexed hip. Additional sacroiliac stress and mobility tests are described by Grieve (1976) and Lewit (1985).

While in the supine position, neurological examination is made by reference to motor function, as determined by isometric contraction:

Hip flexors	L2/3
Extensor hallucis longus (EHL)	L4/5
Tibialis anterior	L4
Peronei	L5

Additionally, the knee jerk (L3/4) is assessed, and the Babinski response determined.

Prone. Once more, hip movements may be examined and passive rotations recorded with the hip extended. The femoral stretch test (FST) is painful with L3/4 root compression (or in a lesion of the quadriceps muscle). Segmental compression (performed by a downward thrust on each spinous process when grasped between thumb and forefinger) is painful when there is facetal dysfunction, acute or chronic. Tenderness may be palpated over the posterior sacroiliac ligaments in chronic sacroiliac ligamentous insufficiency. The proximal gluteal attachments may also be tender. Further neurological assessment is made by isometric contraction:

Glutei	S1
Hamstrings	S1
Quadriceps	L3/4
Ankle jerk	S1/2

Interpretation and Management

Mechanical dysfunction gives rise to the partial (non-capsular) articular pattern, in which some movements are painful and may be restricted, whereas others are not. HNP is characterized by painful restriction of forward flexion of the lumbar spine and positive dural stretch tests (restricted SLR at the L4/5 and L5/S1 levels, restricted FST at L3/4). In the presence of a substantial protrusion at either of the two lowest intervertebral levels, particularly L4/5, both ipsilateral and contralateral SLR may be restricted, and deviation is noted on attempted trunk flexion. A pelvic tilt or sciatic scoliosis may be observed. Side flexion towards the painful side is usually restricted and neurological signs, in a strict dermatomal distribution, are commonly found when there is sciatic root compression. Prolapse at the L3/4 level often gives rise to a reversed pattern—that is, to limitation of extension (possibly a fixed flexion posture) and less limitation of flexion. Management of a prolapsed disc is by sustained lumbar traction which is given daily as an outpatient procedure for two weeks (Fig. 5.16). In the presence of neurological signs, caudal epidural injections of 25–50 ml of 0.5 per cent procaine HCl are indicated: the addition of steroid—for example, triamcinolone hexacetonide 20 mg—is logical for reduction of the inflammatory reaction at the disc–dura interface. A positive response, manifested by improvement of both symptoms and signs, is to be expected in over 80 per cent of cases.

Investigation by X-ray is conventionally performed, although nothing is gained other than exclusion of bony pathology. If conservative management fails to control the symptoms, or improve the signs of sciatic root compression, further investigation by CT scan or particularly by MRI (which has largely overtaken the myelogram) is necessary. Referral to an orthopaedic surgeon or neurosurgeon for consideration of discectomy is indicated in the presence of a substantial HNP and unremitting sciatica. Chemonucleolysis is an alternative approach: if suitable diagnostic criteria are satisfied (more leg pain than back pain, restricted SLR, neurological deficit, and positive imaging), a success rate of over 70 per cent is achieved, and the long-term results are as good as or better than surgery.

Lumbar facet dysfunction is characterized by discomfort on flexion (possibly with a 'hitch' on recoil), extension, and lateral flexion away from the painful side. SLR is of full range. The LS and facet stress tests are painful. Segmental pressure is painful. The treatment of choice is segmental manipulation (see Fig. 12.7, p. 211), which may be combined with ultrasound to the affected facet joint. If symptoms persist, infiltration of steroid and local anaesthetic along the posterior aspect of the relevant facet joints (usually L4/5 or L5/S1) is useful. Intra-articular facet injection under fluoroscopic screening may be performed though it is unnecessary, in the author's experience, for therapeutic response.

In *sacroiliac dysfunction* the articular signs on the conventional trunk mobility tests in the standing position are often unremarkable. However, the sacroiliac mobility test reveals an abnormal rhythm, and internal rotation of the hip is often uncomfortable and slightly limited (see p.112 for further tests). Normal sacroiliac joint mobility is restored by manipulation (see Fig. 12.8, p. 211). Reassessment at the end of a week is advisable, and further manipulative procedures should be undertaken, if necessary, at weekly intervals until resolution of dysfunction is established. Recurrent dysfunction may be treated by sclerosant injections (see *Chronic ligamentous insufficiency*).

Minor articular signs are detected in a recent *spondylolysis*; extension is uncomfortable, and rotations variably so. Increased discomfort is felt on the one-legged hyperextension test and on the Fitch catch test. X-rays, including obliques, are necessary if there is suspicion of spondylolysis. The mere presence of lytic defects on X-ray, however, does not indicate the vintage of the lesion: a bone scan is required to confirm a recent stress fracture. (Read (1994) has advised the use of single photon emission computed tomography (SPECT) scanning to detect very early cases). In the presence of a positive scan, rest from sport is compulsory in any attempt to achieve satisfactory healing. Although the lysis may not necessarily be expected to heal by bony union, a sound fibrous union is required.

Three to six months' rest may be necessary, and twice that length of time is not unusual. If progress, as determined by lessening discomfort on movement, is not in evidence after six months, it is advisable to seek an orthopaedic surgical opinion from a spinal specialist. Surgical stabilization may be required. Occasionally spondylolisthesis develops, and requires specialist advice. Listhesis is an *early* complication after lysis, and is unlikely to develop at a later stage (Fig. 5.17). A slip of 25 per cent is considered acceptable; a 50 per cent slip increases the likelihood of incapacitating symptoms and a cosmetically undesirable posture. A fusion is normally required for this degree of slip in a child.

Biomechanical assessment of sport technique may be helpful in rehabilitation (and indeed in prophylaxis). Hardcastle *et al.* (1992) analysed the delivery techniques of a group of Western Australian fast bowlers and concluded that a 'mixed' action (combining features of both side-on and front-on actions) gave rise to considerable spinal rotation and a relatively high incidence of spondylolysis.

Lumbar instability (or 'segmental instability') is characterized by recurrent bouts of acute low back pain, and is a difficult problem to influence. More often than not, the bouts appear to

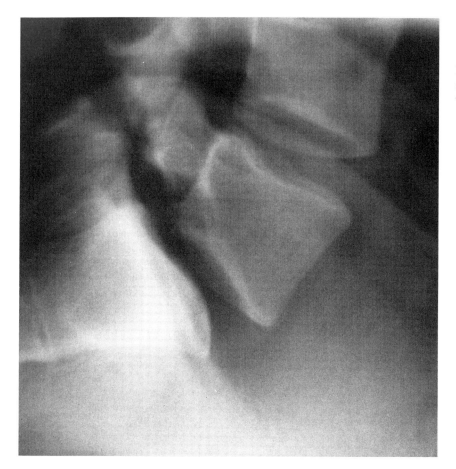

FIG. 5.17 A spondylolysis at L5 is associated with a grade I spondylolisthesis in this professional cricketer.

bc provoked by relatively trivial incidents, unconnected with sport, such as reaching forward. Paradoxically the patient comments that he is often able to indulge his back in vigorous pursuits without necessarily incurring any derangement. Acute bouts tend to last for several days, and are often helped by manipulation. The signs are usually of facet dysfunction (discomfort on flexion and/or extension, normal SLR, and pain on LS and facet stress tests), though more dominant discogenic signs may predominate (pelvic tilt, restricted flexion, and restricted SLR). X-ray is usually unhelpful, and examination between attacks is normal.

The major management problem relates to the recurrent nature of the condition. Prior to the establishment of an appropriate rehabilitative policy for an individual patient, the following biomechanical fact-file should be taken into account.

1. There is good evidence that the likelihood of recurrence is lessened by improved physical fitness (Nachemson 1984). This applies to those patients who indulge in recreational sport only, such as golf, rather than those who keep fit by more energetic means.

2. Muscle imbalance, particularly inadequacy of the abdominals, may be present. An appropriate strengthening regime should be prescribed (see p. 189).

3. Although the patient may improve his dynamic stabilizers, and therefore the dorsilumbar fascial tone, by such a regime of exercises, he can do little about the capsular, lumbosacral, and sacroiliac ligaments. A course of sclerosant injections (25 per cent dextrose and 2 per cent phenol) to these ligaments should

be considered. Referral to an orthopaedic physician or sports injury specialist is indicated for treatment by sclerotherapy.

In the mature athlete who is unwilling to 'hang up his boots' at an appropriate time, degenerative changes (*arthrosis*) in the facet joints are a source of low back and posterior thigh pain. The signs that accompany the typical post-exercise discomfort and stiffness are restriction of all lumbar movements (the capsular pattern), discomfort on LS and facet stress, and positive segmental pressure. Although localized steroid injections to the posterior capsular ligaments of the facet joints (or even intra-articularly under X-ray screening) give temporary relief, and sclerosant injections more prolonged relief, there is likely to be recurrence unless appropriate reduction in biomechanical stress is achieved. Despite this perfectly valid and rational approach, a lack of compliance with such guidance and the search for a 'cure' by exercise fanatics is not unusual. Participation in squash and (to a less extent) other racket sports is ill-advised. Swimming and cycling may usually be tried, and therefore prescribed, without adverse effect. Degenerative disease in the hip is a common concomitant to low back stress, and should always be considered during examination.

Chronic ligamentous insufficiency is characterized by discomfort on prolonged immobility and an absence of articular signs. Discomfort may be elicited on the sacroiliac stress test if the sacroiliac ligaments are significantly involved. Tenderness overlying the sacroiliac joints may be detected; otherwise there is little to find clinically, and any further investigations are negative. Despite the absence of positive signs discomfort may be substantial. Sclerosant injections to the lumbosacral and sacroiliac ligaments are the treatment of choice, and may be repeated every few years if necessary. Ongley *et al.* (1987) have recorded improvement in chronic low back pain using the technique of sclerosant ('proliferant') injections preceded by steroid injection to the gluteus medius origin.

There remains one further condition—*unexplained sciatica* (with or without backache)—that appears to be related to exercise in the young adult. This is often associated with middle-distance or long-distance running. However, there are few, if any, signs on examination. In the older age groups, central or lateral spinal stenosis should be considered, and the spinal diameter assessed by X-ray or CT scan. This does not appear to be the cause of sciatica in the younger age group: although conjectural, the presence of dural irritation secondary to facet joint stress or previous disc herniation may be postulated. An empirical approach by the use of epidural injections may be employed, and is often found to be successful.

Sacroiliitis gives rise to the characteristic examination findings of negative lumbar function tests (although the spine subsequently becomes progressively more stiff as spondylitis develops) and pain on sacroiliac stress tests. X-rays reveal the typical features of sclerosis of the joint margins (see Fig. 6.9, p. 108). A positive HLA B27 antigen test adds further weight to the diagnosis. Sacroiliitis is considered further in Chapter 6.

Summary of Examination Procedures

Cervical Spine

Standing:

1. Observation
   - torticollis
   - muscle wasting (in pectoral girdle)
2. Active movements
   - flexion
   - extension
   - rotation
   - side flexions
3. Passive movements
   - flexion
   - extension
   - rotations
   - side flexions
4. Resisted muscle contractions (neck)
5. Neurological—motor function in upper limbs.
6. Neural tension test
7. Trigger points—particularly superior scapular fixators

Supine

1. Joint play
   - A–P glide
   - lateral glide
   - side bending
2. Palpation
   - facet joints, overlying muscle tension
   - interspinous ligaments

Thoracic Spine

Standing

1. Observation
   - kyphosis/kyphus
   - scoliosis
2. Neck flexion (dural stretch)
3. Active movements
   - flexion
   - extension
   - rotations
   - side flexions
4. Deep inspiration/rib cage compression

Sitting:

1. Passive movements
   - rotations
   - side flexions
2. Resisted muscle contraction—rotations
3. Palpation—rib cage/sternum

Prone

1. Palpation—interspinous ligaments
2. Segmental compression
3. Skin rolling

Lumbar spine and sacroiliac joints

Standing:

1. Observation
   - posture/lordosis
   - flexion deformity
   - pelvic tilt
   - gait
2. Neck flexion (dural stretch)
3. Active movements
   - flexion (hitch, deviation)
   - extension
   - side flexions
   - sacroiliac mobility
   - unilateral hyperextension/Fitch catch
4. Resisted muscle contraction (lumbar)
5. Calf strength
6. Palpation—ledge

Sitting

1. Slump test
2. Sacroiliac stress/mobility

Supine:

1. Hip examination
2. Sacroiliac stress
3. SLR
4. Bilateral SLR (LS stress)
5. Facet stress
6. Neurology
   - muscle function
   - knee jerk
   - Babinski

Prone

1. FST
2. Neurology
   - muscle function
   - ankle jerk
3. Palpation
   - segmental compression
   - tenderness (interspinous ligaments, facet joints)
   - trigger points (glutei)

Injuries to the spinal cord

F. R. I. MIDDLETON

Introduction

This subchapter deals primarily with injury to the spinal cord. This leash of central nervous system tissue, which runs from the brain stem in the region of the foramen magnum of the skull to just above the upper border of the second lumbar vertebra, comprises mainly pathways for nervous impulses, but also a considerable number of neurones with an uncertain amount of intrinsic processing activity. Occasionally damage to the well-protected cord occurs without evident damage to the supporting structures, but in most instances the forces involved are so great that major injuries ensue, often combining instability of the spine with other injuries to internal organs or to the limbs. Brain injury may also occur, and in any unconscious patient following injury it must be assumed that cord injury exists in addition to brain injury, and appropriate precautions must be taken. It can be appreciated that the cord is a direct continuation from the brain, and that, even in the absence of overt brain injury, an insult to the cord sufficient to disrupt its function is likely to have some effect on the brain. These effects have been measured and documented using formalized psychometric testing (Wilmot *et al.* 1985) and have some importance in terms of further management, particularly during the rehabilitation stage for spinal cord injury.

Spinal cord injury is one of the greatest disasters that can befall the human organism; interruption of control mechanisms to muscle groups and other essential organs results in devastating loss of function and disability. Even worse, the loss of functions of sensation and feedback from these muscles and other organs creates even greater problems in terms of maintaining the organism as a whole.

Incidence

In the United Kingdom some fifteen to twenty new cases of spinal injury per million of population occur each year (Crockard 1981), that is about one thousand new cases annually. Despite the introduction of seat-belts, the alteration of rules, the introduction of protective head-gear in sport, and improvements in the health and safety code at work, this incidence has not altered significantly over the past twenty years. However, there now appears to be a greater percentage of cervical injuries (lesions involving nerve roots T1 and above which cause tetraplegia) compared with paraplegia, and more incomplete lesions (where some residual motor or sensory function remains below the level of injury) compared with complete lesions. Most injuries occur at the sites of maximal potential movement in the spine—lower cervical and thoracolumbar regions. Road traffic accidents and sporting injuries (rugby, gymnastics, trampoline, diving) tend to produce cervical injuries, whereas falls and jumping from heights more commonly cause thoracolumbar lesions.

There is an increasing awareness of more disabled people in wheelchairs in our communities owing to the increasing prevalence of the condition (now some forty thousand persons across the UK). This increase in awareness is in some part due to the increasing acceptability of people with disability in the community and to greater access to public buildings for those who are mobility-impaired, but is primarily due to a dramatic increase in life expectancy over the past forty years. When Sir Ludwig Guttmann began his work at the Stoke Mandeville Hospital in the early 1940s, cervical cord injury resulted in virtually one hundred per cent mortality within a couple of months. Patients with lower cord injuries resulting in paraplegia had a life-expectancy of approximately two years (death resulting within that time from complications affecting the kidneys, bowel, or skin). A major increase in life expectancy resulted from Sir Ludwig's work of devising management programmes to maintain activity (Guttmann 1954) and to minimize the development of secondary complications. Nowadays paraplegics have a very nearly normal life expectancy, while tetraplegics can expect a diminution of approximately ten years (Geisler *et al.* 1983). When one considers that between a third and a half of all spinal cord injuries occur to young people in the age group sixteen to twenty-five, it is not surprising that the prevalence is increasing. There is also about a four to one male to female ratio, presumably owing to the nature of the usual underlying causes of spinal cord injury.

Aetiology of Spinal Injury Relating to Sport

Statistical analysis over the last fifteen years in the United Kingdom has revealed that some fifty-five per cent of all spinal cord injuries result from road traffic accidents, either to the occupants of vehicles or to pedestrians. The introduction of seat belts has made little impact on the overall numbers occurring, though this may be due to more survivors with spinal cord injury amongst those who would previously have been killed by their head injury. Great controversy still rages about the potential benefits of increasing the range of speed-limits, and also about alterations in the design and manufacture of motor vehicles.

Falls from heights or downstairs are the second most common category of injuries. Deliberate jumps from height remain a small but consistent group, at around five per cent. Falling injuries are approximately equally distributed between home and place of work, and again health and safety regulations do not appear to have made any significant impact on reduction in the numbers.

Sport regularly comprises about twenty per cent of spinal cord injuries. Diving into shallow water, both into swimming pools and the sea, is the most common cause. Equestrian sports

Table 5.1. Aetiology of spinal cord injury: cause of injury in 250 consecutive admissions to the Spinal Injuries Unit, Royal National Orthopaedic Hospital, Stanmore, 1983–88

Road traffic accident		
Driver	22%	
Passenger	12%	
Motorcycle	10%	= 50%
Bicycle	2%	
Pedestrian	4%	
Falls		
Fall from height	12%	
Fall down stairs	4%	= 27%
Fall/trip	5%	
Jump from height	6%	
Assault		2%
Heavy weight/crush		3%
Sport		
Diving	5%	
Gliding		
Skiing		
Horse riding	6%	= 11%
Jet ski		
Rugby		
Trampoline		
		7%
Other		100%

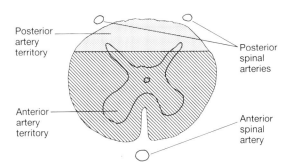

FIG. 5.18 Blood supply to the spinal cord. The anterior spinal artery is particularly vulnerable in the lower cervical and lower thoracic regions.

produce a large number of injuries considering the overall numbers taking part.

The increasing interest and participation in gymnastics and trampolining (Torg and Das 1985) has been paralleled by an increase in the numbers of serious injuries sustained in those sports. Rugby football continues to produce a few dramatic injuries each year (Silver and Gill 1988). It would appear that changes in the laws of the game have led to a decrease in cord injuries over the past five years. However, injuries continue to be caused by scrums collapsing, scrum 'collisions', or the practice of 'popping' (trying to drive the opposing front row upwards). Injuries also occur by axial loading, when players' heads are driven into the ground during mauls or rucks, in 'spearing' in American football, and in multiple or unskilled tackling. The small number of tragedies each year remains an unacceptable hazard, and more needs to be done by rugby authorities (Burry and Calcinai 1988). There has been increasing awareness among the organizing bodies of many sports and among schools and young people's organizations that proper rules and regulations, attention to equipment and environment and appropriate supervision are essential if this small but enormously important cause of injury is to be reduced. Recent trends are encouraging: analysis of two hundred and fifty consecutive admissions to the Spinal Injuries Unit at the Royal National Orthopaedic Hospital, Stanmore, between 1983 and 1988 reveals a smaller percentage (11 per cent) resulting from sport (Table 5.1). The inculcation of a responsible attitude to taking part in sporting activities will increase the pleasure resulting from the sport and will certainly help to diminish injuries.

Pathology

Accurate pathophysiology of the spinal cord injury remains a poorly investigated and understood subject. Detailed definition of the anatomy of injury and alteration of function are extremely difficult to carry out, and further mention will be made of this in the section on accident and emergency centre management. Much of what we know results from the work of Griffiths and Kakulas (Kakulas 1988) in Perth, Australia, during the sixties and seventies. It is known that in injuries in which the individual survives it is rare for the cord to be transected or cut across. The majority of injuries to the cord result from crushing of nervous tissue by surrounding bones and ligaments. This pressure, which may be momentary or prolonged, may also cause interference with the blood supply, and it is this feature which is thought to lead to the further secondary pathology (Fig. 5.18). It is convenient to divide the pathology into *primary*, or that resulting directly from the force of the injury, and *secondary*, or that due to those processes which are the result of biochemical and vascular changes.

The effects of altering or shutting off blood-supply to major areas of tissue result in necrosis of variable amounts of the cord, proximal and distal to the site of injury. This loss of tissue may occur over a number of segments, and result in quite major cavitation of the cord. If there is subsequent blockage to cerebrospinal fluid flow then further syrinx formation (classical syringomyelia) may occur, and may result in further damage to the cord and loss of function if the syrinx ascends proximally. This may occur within a few months of injury, or more frequently some years after injury.

In the immediate period following injury the clinical development of neurological deficit is of some importance. It may be that there is a complete loss of function instantaneously below the site of the lesion. Not infrequently, however, patients and witnesses describe purposeful movement occurring shortly after the injury in limbs which subsequently have become paralysed. This may give some clue as to the primary or secondary nature of the injury, and particularly in the second situation one must be guarded about eventual prognosis. The prognosis in someone who has just undergone spinal cord injury is further complicated by the presence of *spinal cord shock*. This is a condition in which there is cessation of conduction of electrical activity through the cord tissue as a result of the injury to the cord. It may last from a few seconds to several weeks or perhaps even months, and in its presence it is impossible to be certain as to the eventual outcome. Return of reflex activity in paralysed limbs and the return of tone in muscle below the level of the injury indicate the passing off of shock, and when this occurs a clear indication of outcome can be given.

However, not all injuries result in total loss of function temporarily or indeed permanently after injury, and clinically lesions are said to be *complete* or *incomplete*, depending on whether there is any motor or sensory function below the level of the lesion. This distinction between complete and incomplete is made difficult because of the presence of spinal shock as outlined above. Nowadays it is further complicated by the development of electrophysiology in the form of *somatosensory and motor evoked potentials*. This is an investigation in which one intentionally passes electrical current from the periphery through the spinal cord and records it through the skull over the appropriate cortical area. The reverse can also be carried out, stimulating the motor cortex through the skull and recording at the periphery. When these recordings are carried out it is sometimes seen that, in those who have apparently clinically complete lesions, some electrical activity is capable of being transmitted along certain pathways in the cord. The importance of this situation is that the prognosis is markedly different when any degree of incompleteness remains.

The ability to measure what is occurring in the cord following injury is also of major importance when deciding whether or not surgical intervention should be carried out. Surgery may be carried out for several reasons; first, to stabilize the spine, thus allowing the individual to be mobilized some ten days after injury, rather than having to remain flat in bed for some three months; secondly, to attempt to relieve pressure around the spinal cord at the site of injury, removing fragments of bone or disc etc. from the spinal canal. Controversy has existed for many years as to whether real benefit is obtained from such interventions, and until better means of measurement are available it is likely that such arguments will continue. However, the development of MRI (Fig. 5.19) and more sophisticated computer-based somatosensory evoked potentials is leading to a capability of better measurement. The application of such investigations to those with spinal cord injury sufficiently early after the injury remains a problem area, and certainly places even greater importance on the immediate care at the injury site, the transport to accident and emergency facilities, and the speed at which these processes are carried out and investigations are instigated.

FIG. 5.19 MRI is particularly valuable in demonstrating early syrinx formation in the cord. In this patient a crush fracture of the body of C5 (suggested by the X-ray and confirmed by the scan) is associated with cord damage (revealed by a depressed signal in the adjacent cord).

Immediate Care at Site—First Aid

The first problem in first-aid management is *recognition* that a spinal cord injury has occurred. This recognition is more likely if there is a high level of suspicion and awareness of the circumstances in which such injuries may occur. Usually the injury itself has been very significant, and the immediate response must be one of saving life by maintaining vital systems—breathing and circulation. Clearly, if cardiac massage has to be carried out, the patient will have to be positioned supine. When there is an obvious misalignment of the cervical spine, that is, when there is a marked lateral flexion or rotation, the head should be brought back gently into the neutral position, and a gentle traction should be maintained. This can be achieved either in the supine position, when it will be particularly necessary to pay attention to the position of the tongue if the patient is unconscious, or in full side-lying with the upper knee flexed and the head supported on the underneath arm.

The next principle which should be applied is that once the patient is in a satisfactory position and vital signs have been restored, *no further unnecessary movement should be allowed.* The patient should be kept in that position until further expert help and equipment arrives. Sandbags may be used to maintain the head position if the patient is inclined to be restless, but one person should remain at the head maintaining a neutral position at all times, if necessary by exerting gentle traction. Most ambulances and many sports centres and places of work now maintain basic equipment for removing people with spinal injury. The most commonly used are a Hines Frame for cervical injuries, or a scoop stretcher, which may be inserted beneath the patient on the ground without the need for further adjustment of position. If such a stretcher is not available, the patient will need to be lifted from the ground on to a suitable firm well-supported well-padded stretcher. This lifting procedure will require at least four people, with one maintaining the head in the neutral position and the others ensuring that the rest of the body remains in line throughout the procedure. One person should act as the team leader and give instructions on the moment to lift, lower, etc.

Once the patient is in the ambulance or helicopter, his position needs to be maintained throughout the journey. Attention must continue to be paid to breathing and circulation, and, because of an early specific complication of spinal cord injury, to the protection of anaesthetic skin. Accordingly, hard objects etc. should be removed from the pockets of the individual, as skin damage sufficient to cause complete ulceration subsequently may occur within ten to fifteen minutes (well within the time that it takes for an ambulance to arrive at the scene of an accident, and a far shorter time than that taken by most subsequent journeys to hospital). It is tragic when a cervical cord injury is complicated by a massive pressure sore, which may take several months to heal, and which may well delay and dictate the course of any rehabilitation process for some considerable time.

At the site of injury the existence of spinal cord injury is likely either to be immediately apparent or else extremely difficult to detect. The conscious patient may report the loss of movement and sensation in the legs, and simple examination will confirm this. Any further attempts at diagnosis at the site of injury are unwarranted and probably dangerous, and it is better that such actions should be reserved for the hospital accident and emergency department.

Assessment and early management

Following any significant insult to the spinal cord a situation of conduction block of the nerve tissue is likely to be present. There will be an absence of intrinsic electrical activity in the cord, resulting in loss of afferent and efferent impulses, and loss of reflexes. Once the patient is in hospital one cannot overemphasize the importance of proper documentation of the clinical signs on a regular basis. From a clinical point of view at this stage, when absence of movement, absence of sensation, and loss of reflexes are demonstrated, it is possible only to say that the patient is in *spinal shock*. Therefore, it is crucial that a proper and full examination of the nervous system is carried out, with particular attention to defining the neurological level of the injury and the presence or absence of reflexes, including the bulbocavernosus, the cremasteric, and the anal responses (Table 5.2). The division of the lesion clinically into complete or incomplete will also occur at this stage; and this must be expressed both from a motor and a sensory point of view.

Table 5.2. Evaluation of reflexes: reflexes which should be tested routinely during the assessment of the spinal cord injured patient

Biceps	C5/6
Supinator	C6
Triceps	C7
Abdominal	T8–12
Cremasteric	L1
Knee	L3/4
Ankle	S1/2
Bulbocavernosus	S3/4
Anal	S5
Plantar	

Early management strategies require the patient to be placed on a well-padded firm supported surface and a size of 12 or 14 indwelling urinary catheter inserted. The presence or absence of ileus is noted, and a subsequent decision made on the need to pass a nasogastric tube. Assessment of respiration, chest injuries, and other complications should be carried out at this stage, and measurements made of pulse and blood-pressure. Once these systems are under control, investigation can then proceed.

Further investigations

X-rays of the spine and chest should be carried out to define the bony injury. In cases of thoracic and lumbar injury a cervical spine X-ray should also be carried out to exclude cervical injury. (In ten per cent of cases of damage to the spinal cord no bony injury is demonstrated, and in a further ten per cent bony injuries occur at multiple levels.) In any unconscious patient, a lateral X-ray of the cervical spine should be carried out. The primary decision at this stage is whether the spine is *stable* or *unstable*; instability should be assumed until further information is available. The most common injuries are due to flexion–rotation or hyperextension forces (Fig. 5.20). In the rugby scrum hyperflexion of the neck may occur, with or without rotation. A flexion injury will produce a wedge fracture of the vertebral body concerned, and may be associated with dislocation or fracture of the facetal joints. This combination is always unstable, as

FIG. 5.20 Fracture—dislocation at C6/7 is demonstrated on the lateral X-ray of this patient who sustained a hyperextension injury.

severe ligamentous damage will inevitably be present. A 'burst' fracture of the vertebra implies an element of vertical compression in the force causing injury. This commonly arises in American football and rugby when axial loading results from the head-on tackle. Hyperextension injuries occur mostly in the cervical region, and much of the damage to the underlying cord is frequently caused by vascular compression, particularly in the elderly. Once the bony and neurological lesions have been defined and deficits demonstrated, the appropriate specialist spinal injuries unit should be contacted. The next stage of management will depend on the facilities available in the hospital concerned. CT scanning of the spine and cord may define the bony lesion, and may also demonstrate the presence of retropulsed disc material or bony fragments lying in the spinal canal. The significance of such material, in regard to the cord injury or its potential for continuing cord injury, is difficult to evaluate, and operative decisions taken on the basis of such pictures may not produce the beneficial results expected.

From a surgical point of view MRI scanning of the cord, with its better definition of nervous tissue, may be a better examination on which to base any future intervention (Fig. 5.19). However, decisions taken purely on demonstration of the anatomical situation are bound to be controversial, and have been the source of much argument over the years. Residual function in the cord, or potential for improvement of function, may bear little relationship to the resulting anatomical structure. Inability to define underlying cord function clearly at this stage following injury means that such arguments and controversy are likely to continue for some time into the future. The

development of somatosensory and motor evoked potentials (SSEPs and MEPs) has given some encouragement towards a better functional definition, but this examination is extremely difficult to carry out in the environment immediately following a spinal cord injury; the recording of such minute amounts of electrical current is likely to be lost within the vast array of electrical equipment which now surrounds the acutely injured patient in the accident and emergency department. Also, the positioning of the patient, and the necessity of not moving him, make it difficult to apply good contact electrodes in the required positions. The application of skull tongs (which may well have been carried out at this stage in order to provide traction on the cervical spine in T1 lesions and above) will also inhibit electrode access to the skull over the required sensory areas. To date no significant series of early spinal cord injury SSEP recordings have been published, almost certainly because of the lack of availability of such equipment and the personnel to operate it in accident and emergency departments, and also because of the great difficulty of achieving adequate recordings. Therefore few clinical surgical decisions have been taken in the early stage of spinal cord injury management on the basis of evoked potential examinations. The need for a good functional measurement of cord activity to parallel the demonstration of anatomic structure remains. As a result the great difficulty in surgical decision, as to whether to decompress around the spinal cord to prevent secondary injury from compression or hypoxia, also remains.

The decision on whether to carry out surgical internal stabilization of the spine, or to proceed with a conservative approach, is based on more clearly defined criteria. However, the decision to carry out such decompression and/or stabilization procedures is either best left to the specialist spinal cord injury unit, or carried out in conjunction with that unit as such surgical interventions will play an important role in the future management of the patient.

The next stage involves the transfer of the patient to the specialist spinal unit or to the specialist unit within the district general hospital pending transfer.

Rehabilitation

This stage in the management of the majority of spinal cord injuries takes place in a spinal injury centre. The process of rehabilitation is frequently subdivided into psychological, social, and physical aspects (Mair 1972); attention to the psychological aspects in the early stages of rehabilitation is crucial. The centre should have a comprehensive team with a broad range of skills and experience appropriate to the complex task of minimizing disability, and thereby minimizing handicap for the patient. In this setting it is likely that the team will be led by a physician or surgeon, and the members will comprise nurses, physiotherapists, occupational therapists, nurse educators, a social worker, a resettlement officer, a psychologist, special education and appropriate administration officers, and back-up support. Such a complexity of structure and expertise requires an appropriate system of ensuring that the available skills and experience are used in the most purposeful and effective way. A system of goal-planning with short-term targets within those goals can provide such a framework (Kennedy 1989), and can be a useful means of enabling the patient, his relatives, and the team to make necessary achievements. It can also provide motivation for both patient and staff in what may be an extremely difficult time in the life of the patient, when such non-productive emotions as anger, denial, or depression may dominate the situation.

Rehabilitation is essentially a learning process. During the first few months after spinal cord injury (a catastrophic event) anxiety will be high, the environment will be unfamiliar, and there may be associated high-level brain dysfunction consequent upon insult to the central nervous system. In this situation it is inevitable that learning ability will be low. There should be an availability of psychological expertise to the patient and relatives for a significant and substantial period following the injury, certainly for at least two to three years.

Social handicap resulting from spinal cord injury may be catastrophic at the worst, and is always major. As previously stated, the commonest group sustaining spinal cord injury is the age group 18–28, comprising a population who are attempting to establish themselves as adults in the community, independent of their parents. They are at an extremely vulnerable time in their lives, and the immense problems which spinal cord injury may present, in addition, may result in a total inability to achieve this independence without major help and support. Experience shows that relationships which are long-standing and structured are likely to continue, but that those which are rather more short-lived and dependent on the ability of both parties to change together are very much less likely to survive the trauma of severe physical disability. The formation of new relationships of importance is unlikely to occur within the two years or so following injury, until the injured person has come to terms with his new identity.

With modern physical management of spinal cord injury, the period of hospitalization is becoming shorter and, although this reduces the serious danger of institutionalization, this means that the finding of suitably accessible accommodation assumes great importance. For the majority this will involve moving from their present home or having major adaptations carried out within it. Achieving outdoor mobility is also crucial. Re-establishing driving skills in a suitably adapted vehicle should have a high priority. The lack of employment of disabled people is one of the more depressing aspects of our society today. It is likely that only some ten per cent will return to gainful employment following severe injury, and that, of those ten per cent, the majority will return to their previous occupation.

Therefore the use made by spinal-cord-injured people of their leisure time and their participation in sporting activities assume great importance, as it is these activities which may well dictate the future quality of life of disabled persons (Creek *et al.* 1988). In the USA leisure education is one of the major components of any rehabilitation programme. In this country, as yet, we have not organized it into a structured and researched programme (Smith 1989). However, some research is progressing at the present time in this field, and it may well be that a more formal approach and structure develop during the next few years.

Sport for the disabled, on the other hand, has become quite highly developed in this country, led by the International Sports Centre for the Disabled at Stoke Mandeville Hospital (Fig. 5.21). The international paraplegic games have achieved considerable recognition in the primary sports of swimming, basketball, archery, and track and field, revealing extraordinary levels of quality at the higher national and international levels. Participation in sport can be an extraordinary confidence-builder, and help along the road to adaptation for the disabled person.

Nowadays there are developments of sporting facilities which cater for both able-bodied and disabled. Such centres can provide environments where the disabled can achieve real social integration with able-bodied people, and provide for many their most useful activity in re-achieving a meaningful place in society.

The re-expression of sexuality may be achieved in such an environment, and it is therefore of paramount importance that the re-establishment of sexual function and identity have been sought and hopefully achieved during the period of rehabilitation. The majority of those with spinal cord injury are physically able, given certain compromises, to achieve satisfactory sexual physical relationships. It is likely that the majority do not, and this must reflect a great failure on the part of rehabilitation services.

Physical Rehabilitation

The primary aims of physical rehabilitation are to maximize the individual's residual abilities and to prevent the development of complications. The essence of this aspect is in the combination of skills from physiotherapy, occupational therapy, nursing, and psychology, which must be blended together in order to achieve the best possible outcome. The setting of realistic goals, and appropriate targets prior to full achievement, is of vital importance in maintaining purposefulness in the team and motivation for the patient. For the patient with a complete neurological lesion, the outcome objectives can be set at a relatively early stage, and some indication of the sort of time-scale that it is likely to take can be given in terms of weeks. For the patient with an incomplete lesion, this is more difficult, as outcomes have to be frequently updated in terms of the changes taking place in neurological status. In this situation it is also more difficult for individuals to maintain motivation towards seeking abilities of a lower level when the expectation is one of significant improvement.

In the early stages, while the bony spine is still unstable, the main roles of the therapists involve maintenance of range of movement in joints, the acquisition and maintenance of a satisfactory respiratory situation in the tetraplegic, and, as the patient comes out of spinal shock, the control of increasing spasticity.

Once the spine is stable and the phase of mobilization commences, a broader range of activities can be commenced with the goals of strengthening existing muscles, seeking and achieving mobility, achieving independence in a wheelchair, and seeking independence in the necessary activities of everyday living. When mobilization commences, the assuming of an upright posture will reveal lack of function within the autonomic nervous system, causing significant and distressing hypotension. Sitting up after a spinal cord injury even for quite short periods may take several days to achieve. In most patients this problem diminishes over a period of weeks or months, and for most ceases to be a major problem. At this stage the physiotherapist will concentrate on the acquisition of new skills, achieving sitting balance, and learning to carry out transfers from bed to wheelchair and vice versa, and will then move on to wheelchair skills. The achievement of a standing posture on a daily basis will also be sought because of its metabolic benefits, primarily in keeping calcium in the bones and also in terms of kidney and bladder drainage. The continuance of maintaining range of movement in joints, stretching muscle groups, assuming more normal postures, and achieving weight-bearing while standing will all contribute to controlling spasticity, which in

(a)

(b)

(c)

FIG. 5.21 (a) Wheelchair table-tennis, (b) archery, and (c) marathoning. Involvement in sport can be a positive beginning of re-integration into the community

some patients may become an extremely important problem, preventing even the simplest activities. At present, available oral drug regimes based on Baclofen or Dantrolene are not particularly effective, and the mechanical aspects of physiotherapy or electrical stimulation provide the most hopeful means of control. The earlier that these regimes are instituted the more likely satisfactory control will be maintained. The development of intrathecal delivery systems for Baclofen now offers a further and potentially highly successful treatment for spasticity. As yet this management is only available in certain specialist centres

where its development is being carefully monitored as the system is not without hazards.

During this phase of rehabilitation there will be a gradual development of new skills and the re-acquisition of old abilities. It is essential that these abilities are translated from demonstration of muscle strength and range of movement in the physiotherapy department to carrying out necessary tasks in everyday living in the real world. The role of the occupational therapist becomes paramount, as also does that of nurses, with whom patients spend the majority of their day. The achievement of independence in everyday living skills can be approached in a logical manner, with attempts being made initially to re-achieve basic activities by utilizing the patient's remaining motor and sensory abilities. If this is not possible, the therapist will attempt to teach the patient new ways of achieving the required skill. It may be necessary to introduce splints and aids with which the individual may then achieve an independent result. The alteration of a patient's environment in order to achieve independence, with the use of simple measures, such as provision of ramps and the regulation of the heights of working surfaces, alongside the use of modern technology in the shape of the development of computer-based environmental controls, has become one of the major roles of occupational therapy.

If altering the environment still fails to achieve satisfactory independence, then it becomes necessary to introduce attendants trained in the support situation.

In very-high-level tetraplegics, who require continuing ventilatory support, and in those who have cognitive deficits associated with brain damage, long-term hospitalization may remain the only option. Fortunately this is a relatively rare situation.

Although the re-achievement of independence probably remains the apparent goal of those who have sustained spinal cord injury, it is extremely important to balance the compromises necessary for such independence with some cognizance of quality of life. Frequent human contact and reassurance are important elements in providing a meaningful and satisfactory quality of life.

Education and Prevention of Complications

Until the 1950s, and the successful development of the Stoke Mandeville National Spinal Injuries Centre by Sir Ludwig Guttmann, the development of serious complications following spinal cord injury was inevitable, as was progression to a fatal outcome, usually within a couple of years. The most frequent and devastating of these complications were massive decubitus ulceration and the combination of infection and increase in pressure within the bladder, leading to hydronephrosis and destruction of the kidneys. The presence of an indwelling urethral catheter implies a permanent route for bacteria to the bladder from the atmosphere, and a constant pressure upon the urethral mucosa, causing changes in that complex structure which may result in perineal ulceration. The presence of such a foreign body in the bladder, associated with infection and an increased calcium availability consequent upon absence of bony stress, frequently led to stone formation, which aggravated bladder inflammation and renal destruction. The loss of calcium from bones also frequently led to pathological fractures which further exacerbated the problems of skin ulceration. These complications of injury to the spinal cord should now be looked on as preventable in the vast majority of patients, and modern spinal injury units exist to prevent such complications. They have been helped in this regard by the development of investigations such as video cystourethrography, which enable the clinician to have a clear picture of the anatomy and functioning of the neurogenic bladder. The use of intermittent catheterization programmes helps to maintain a more normal bladder function—an important aspect as the availability of electronic implantable bladder-controllers increases (Brindley et al. 1986).

Although a number of complications are preventable, a number of others remain which are not dependent upon the patient's education or discipline in managing his various systems. One of the causes of mortality in the first year of tetraplegia is autonomic dysreflexia, a condition where massive, and potentially fatal, hypertension can rapidly occur consequent upon stimulation of the unopposed sympathetic nervous system (McGuire and Kumar 1986). Such stimulation arises most frequently from a distended bladder, but may result from severe constipation or indeed a severely inflamed ingrowing toenail, all of which are common situations in the tetraplegic patient. The simple manoeuvres of sitting the patient up and passing a urinary catheter in this situation may be life-saving.

Complications of late bony instability leading to kyphosis or scoliosis may require surgical intervention to prevent unacceptable skeletal compromise. Such bony instability in adults is relatively rare (Bedbrook and Edibam 1973); however, it is the rule in children, leading to serious deformity.

There are three major complications which occur from within the damaged cord itself: central pain, spasticity, and ascending disabilities associated with syrinx formation (dilatation of the central canal). The development of severe persistent *central pain* may be one of the most destructive aspects of spinal cord injury; fortunately it remains relatively rare, but less severe degrees of pain are common and distressing. Such severe central pain responds poorly to the more commonly used analgesics, yet the use of a more powerful opiate analgesia is to be avoided except in an extreme case. Therefore the first treatment of choice, for most patients, is transcutaneous nerve stimulation, which can be remarkably successful in more than sixty per cent of cases. This may be supplemented with the use of various forms of acupuncture, or nerve- or ganglion-blocking techniques. It should be remembered that central pain of this type tends to diminish over months, and its impact on the individual is greatly dependent upon mood state and on general activity.

The demonstration of *syrinx formation*, now more commonly diagnosed as a result of CT and MRI scanning, requires surgical intervention to relieve a pressure drainage problem. It has already been stated that the drugs available for the control of *spasticity* are disappointing in their effects and in the frequency with which they produce unacceptable side-effects. Physiotherapy techniques remain the main management choice, supplemented with electrical stimulation techniques and, more recently but still rarely, the use of dorsal column stimulation or insertion of an intrathecal Baclofen pump, which delivers, at a controlled rate, antispasmodic drugs directly to the central nervous tissues involved. Despite these measures there remain a number of spinally injured patients whose spasticity remains uncontrolled and uncontrollable, and in whom contractures and trophic problems eventually supervene. The next research developments in spinal cord injury management are likely to take place within these fields, and to result in better management of these types of complications.

Discussion

The rehabilitation process today emphasizes the importance of the multidisciplinary involvement of an adequate range of skills, and the effective and efficient education of the patient, his relatives, and his carers. Measurement of success in rehabilitation is difficult, as parameters of outcome are so extraordinarily variable. However, it is likely that the success of an education programme and a rehabilitation process can be judged by the absence of development of avoidable complications. Clearly it is of enormous importance to the individual to avoid complications, but it is also of importance to the specialist spinal cord injury centres, where, if much of their work and bed capacity is taken up with the management of preventable complications, they inevitably have less time and ability to deal with those with acute injuries, and also have less ability to develop and apply to patients new developments such as bladder controllers. The development of more sophisticated calipers, of computer-controlled muscle stimulation, and of implantable motor-function controllers requires resources in terms of personnel, equipment, and facilities. With the increasing life expectancy for those with spinal cord injuries, the likelihood of such developments becoming applicable to them is also increased.

References

Bedbrook, G. M. and Edibam, R. C. (1973). The study of deformity in traumatic spinal paralysis. *Parapelgia*, **10**, 321–35.

Beighton, P., Solomon, L., and Soskolne, C. L. (1973). Articular mobility in an African population. *Ann. Rheum. Dis.*, **32**, 413–18.

Bogduk, N. and Twomey, L. T. (1987). *Clinical anatomy of the lumbar spine*. Churchill Livingstone, Melbourne.

Brindley, G. S., Polkey, C. E., Rushton, D. N., and Cardoza, L. (1986). Sacral anterior root stimulators for bladder control in paraplegics. *J. Neurol. Neurosurg. Psych.*, **49**, 1104–14.

Burry, H. C. and Calcinai, C. J. (1988). The need to make rugby safer. *Br. Med. J.*, **296**, 149–50.

Cailliet, R. (1981). *Low back pain syndrome* (3rd edn). F. A. Davis, Philadelphia.

Colachis, S. C., Warden, R. E., Bechtol, C. O., and Strohm, B. R. (1963). Movement of the sacroiliac joint in the adult male. *Arch. Phys. Med. Rehabil.*, **44**, 490.

Creek, G., Moore, M., Oliver, M., Salisbury, V., Silver, J., and Zarb, G. (1988). *Personal and social implications of spinal cord injury—a retrospective study*. Thames Polytechnic, London.

Crockard, H. A. (1981) Spinal injuries. In *Trauma care* (ed. N. Odling-Smee and H.A. Crockard), p. 224, Academic Press, London.

Cyriax, J. (1982). *Textbook of orthopaedic medicine*, Vol. 1 (8th edn). Baillière Tindall, London.

Cyriax, J. and Russell, G. (1984). *Textbook of orthopaedic medicine*, Vol. 2 (11th edn). Baillière Tindall, London.

Elliott, S., Hutson, M. A., and Wastie, M. L. (1988). Bone scintigraphy in the assessment of spondylolysis in patients attending a sports injury clinic. *Clin. Radiol.*, **39**, 269–72.

Elvery, R. L. (1986). Treatment of arm pain associated with abnormal brachial plexus tension. *Aust. J. Physiother.*, **32**(4), 225–30.

Farfan, H. F. (1973). *Mechanical disorders of the low back*. Lea and Febiger, Philadelphia.

Fitch, K. (1981). Controversial issues in sports medicine. Proceedings of the Australian Sports Sports Medicine Federation National Scientific Conference, Adelaide, Vol. 1, pp. 282–5.

Fredrikson, B., Baker, D., McHolick, W. J., Yuan, H. A., and Lubickly, J. P. (1984). The natural history of spondylolysis and spondylolisthesis. *J. Bone Jt. Surg.*, **66A**, 699–707.

Geisler, W. O., Jousse, A. T., Wynne-Jones, M., and Breithaupt, D. (1983). Survival in traumatic spinal cord injury. *Paraplegia*, **21**, 364–73.

Grieve, G. P. (1976). The sacroiliac joint. *Physiotherapy*, **62**(12), 384–400.

Guttmann, L., (1954). Statistical survey of one thousand paraplegics and initial management of traumatic paraplegia. *Proc. R. Soc. Med.*, **47**, 1099–1103.

Hardcastle, P., Annear, P., Foster, D. H., Chakera, T. M., McCormick, C., Khangure, M., and Burnett, A. (1992). Spinal abnormalities in young fast bowlers. *J. Bone Jt. Surg.*, **74B**, 421–5.

Holden, D. L. and Jackson, D. W. (1985). Stress fracture of the ribs in female rowers. *Am. J. Sports Med.*, **13**, 342–8.

Jackson, D. W., Wiltse, L. L., and Cirincione, R. J. (1976). Spondylolysis in the female gymnast. *Clin. Orthop. Relat. Res.*, **117**, 68–73.

Jackson, D. W., Wiltse, L. L., and Dungeman, R. D. (1981). Stress reactions involving the pars interarticularis in young athletes. *Am. J. Sports Med.*, **9**, 304–12.

Kakulas, A. (1988). The applied neurobiology of human spinal cord injury: a review. *Paraplegia*, **26**, 371–9.

Kennedy, P. (1989). Psychological approaches to the management of spinal cord injury. *J. Hol. Med.* **4**(4), 169–76.

Kirkaldy-Willis, W. H., Wedge, J. H., Yong-Hing, K., and Reilly, J. (1978). Pathology and pathogenesis of lumbar spondylosis and stenosis. *Spine*, **3**, 319–28.

Lewit, K. (1985). *Manipulative therapy in rehabilitation of the motor system*. Butterworth, London.

McGuire, T. J. and Kumar, V. N. (1986). Autonomic dysreflexia in the spinal cord injured. *Postgrad. Med.*, **80**, (2), 81–4.

Mair, A. (1972). *Report of the subcommittee of the Standing Medical Advisory Committee, Scottish Health Services Council, on medical rehabilitation*. HMSO, Edinburgh.

Maitland, G. D. (1986). *Vertebral manipulation* (5th edn). Butterworth, London.

Mennell, J. McM. (1960). *Back pain: diagnosis and treatment using manipulative techniques*. Little, Brown, Boston.

Nachemson, A. L. (1984). Prevention of chronic back pain. The orthopaedic challenge for the 80s. *Bull. Hosp. Jt. Dis. Orthop. Inst.*, **44**, 1–15.

Nachemson, A. and Elfstrom, G. (1970). Intradiscal dynamic pressure measurements in lumbar discs. *Scand J. Rehabil. Med.*, **Suppl**. 1, 1–40.

Ongley, M. J., Klein, R. G., Dorman, T. A., Eek, B. C., and Hubert, L. J. (1987). A new approach to the treatment of chronic low back pain. *Lancet*, **8551**, 143–6.

Poster, R. W., Hibbert, C. S., and Wicks, M. (1978). The spinal canal in symptomatic lumbar disc lesions. *J. Bone Jt. Surg.*, **50B**, 485–7.

Read, M. T. F. (1994). Single photon emission computed tomography (SPECT) scanning for adolescent back pain. A *sine qua non*? *Br. J. Sports Med.*, **28**(1), 56–7.

Silver, J. R. (1993). Spinal injuries in sports in the UK. *Br. J. Sports Med.*, **27**(2), 115–20.

Silver, J. R. and Gill, S. (1988). Injuries of the spine sustained during rugby. *Sports Med.*, **5**, 328–34.

Smith, G. (1989). Use of leisure time by spinal cord injured. *Leisure Education Bulletin*, June.

Stallard, M. C. (1980). Backache in oarsmen. *Br. J. Sports Med.*, **14**, 105–8.

Stoddard, A. (1980). *Manual of osteopathic technique (3rd edn)*, Hutchinson, London.

Sward, L., Hellstrom, M., Jacobsson, B., Nyman, R., and Peterson, L. (1991). Disc degeneration and associated abnormalities of the spine in elite gymnasts: a magnetic resonance imaging study. *Spine*, **16**, 437–43.

Torg, J. S. and Das, M. (1985). Trampoline injuries. *Clin. Sports Med.*, **4**(1), 45–60.

Troup, J.D.G. (1986). Biomechanics of the lumbar spinal canal. *Clin. Biomech.*, **1**(1), 31–43.

Wilmot, C. B., Cope, D. N., Hall, K. M., and Acker, M. (1985). Occult head injury: its incidence in spinal cord injury. *Arch. Phys. Med. Rehabil.*, **66**, (4), 227–31.

6 Pelvic injuries

M. A. HUTSON

Introduction

Apart from compression injuries sustained in sports such as motor racing or equestrian events, most injuries to the pelvis are to the soft tissues, principally the joints, muscle attachments, and bursae. They are caused principally by overuse. Symptoms may sometimes be accurately localized by the patient (for instance, to the groin in adductor strains), though quite often they are more diffuse in nature. The association of groin pain with pain felt in the lower abdomen, in the testes, around the 'hips', and into the anteromedial thighs is common. The combination of groin pain with backache suggests a spinal cause: occasionally difficulties in diagnosis arise when groin pain from a spinal lesion exists without coexisting backache. Lesions at the thoracolumbar junction, as well as the lumbar spine and sacroiliac joints, may refer pain to both the groin and the thigh.

Clicking or 'clonking' may be complained of, particularly by the adolescent athlete. The young dancer, for instance, may complain either of clicking due to movement of the iliotibial tract over the greater trochanter, or (more anteriorly) clonking due to snapping of the iliopsoas over the lesser trochanter, the iliopectineal eminence, or the anterior inferior iliac spine (Schaberg 1984). Patients may need to be reassured of the benign nature of these irritating conditions. When stress injury occurs in the region of the pelvis, much patience is required by the patient (and his physician!), as conditions tend to be refractory to specific therapeutic modalities; spontaneous resolution often occurs over many months.

Applied anatomy and biomechanics

The pelvis is a ring structure, a fact that is just as relevant to a study of overuse injury as it is to the management of pelvic fractures. Stress or weakness at one site in the ring (of which the lumbosacral joint as well as the sacroiliac joints should be considered to be an integral part) will inevitably impart stress to the remaining structures. The hip joints are central to the study of the biomechanics of the pelvis, as an essential function of the pelvis is to provide a mechanism for transmission of forces and mobility from the lower limbs to the trunk.

There are no muscles which are attached to both the sacrum and the ilium. The erector spinae, iliopsoas, and piriformis muscles overlie, and therefore exert an influence on, the sacroiliac joints (SIJs). The SIJs are also influenced indirectly by other powerful muscles (for instance, the glutei and abdominals) acting on the lumbar spine and pelvis to reduce the lumbosacral angle. The sacroiliac joints are synovial joints, well supported by tough ligaments: anterior sacroiliac, posterior sacroiliac, and interosseous (Fig. 6.1). Additional strength is provided by the sacrospinous and sacrotuberous ligaments. The iliolumbar ligament also may be considered to be functionally supportive. The surfaces of the joint are made up of irregular humps and hollows, which contribute to its stability. Joint mobility has been studied extensively: both Weisl (1955), who used cineradiographic studies, and Colachis et al. (1963), who embedded Kirschner wires into the posterior iliac spines, found approximately 5 mm of movement.

Posterior rotation (nutation) of the ilium on the sacrum results in elevation of the anterior superior iliac spine (ASIS) and depression of the posterior superior iliac spine (PSIS) (Grieve 1976). Anterior rotation (contranutation) results in a reversal of these movements. The plane of movement is usually described as posteromedial to anterolateral. Such rotational movement is important in gait when reciprocal rotation in a figure-of-eight pattern occurs with each leg movement. Equal movements of the sacroiliac joints occur in trunk flexion and rotation: in flexion, for instance, there is a relative posterior movement of the ilia on the sacrum.

When there is persistent unilateral posterior rotation, pelvic torsion (or 'distortion') occurs. Lewit (1985) states that, in this (one-sided nutational) situation, rotation of one ilium occurs around a horizontal axis, and rotation of the other ilium occurs around a vertical axis. He considers it to be a common condition. During posterior rotation the acetabulum rises, and functional leg shortening occurs. This apparent leg-length inequality (as determined by the relative positions of the medial malleoli) is observed in the supine position; leg lengthening occurs in the sitting position

The natural history of the mobility of the SI joints is for them to become stiffer, with gradual obliteration of the synovial joint with increasing age. However, *hypermobility* may be a problem in younger athletes. As a result of ligamentous incompetence, increased rotation occurs and may give rise to acute *dysfunction*, in which apparent *hypomobility* may be demonstrated. Dysfunction in which an SIJ is 'stuck', most often in posterior rotation, responds to manipulation, though the basic hypermobility problem remains, with the additional risk of symptoms from chronic ligamentous strain. The innervation of the posterior ligaments is from L5, S1, and S2; thus pain may be referred to the posterior leg as far as the heel. The anterior ligaments have a more extensive innervation, from L3 to S1. Symptoms may then be felt in the groin.

The pubic symphysis is a cartilaginous joint, with the joint surfaces separated by a fibrocartilaginous disc. There are no muscles overlying the symphysis, though several muscles attach

FIG. 6.1 The sacroiliac joints are well supported by ligaments: (a) anterior view; (b) posterior view; (c) transverse section at S2

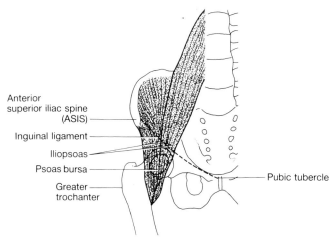

FIG. 6.2 The surface anatomical markings of the hip joint (overlaid by the psoas bursa).

is also found at the midpoint of an imaginary horizontal line from the pubic tubercle to the greater trochanter. An anterior approach to the hip joint for intra-articular injection or aspiration may be made lateral to the femoral neurovascular bundle (see Fig. 12.20, p. 219). Alternatively a lateral approach immediately above the greater trochanter may be used. The term femoral anteversion refers to the angle made by the femoral neck to the femoral condyles—that is, the degree of forward projection of the neck from the coronal plane (Fig. 6.3). Excessive ('fetal') anteversion in the adult leads to excessive medial femoral rotation and squinting patellae (see Fig. 11.6, p. 188). It is one of a number of aetiological factors involved in overuse injury in the lower limb.

The capsular pattern of the hip, indicating articular pathology, is early restriction of medial rotation, flexion, and abduction. The loss of some degree of medial rotation, in particular, is a sensitive guide to early degenerative disease. The powerful muscles acting upon the hip arise from the pelvis and lumbar spine. Hip flexion is largely controlled by iliopsoas, with additional support from rectus femoris. The iliopsoas tendon is immediately adjacent to the anterior aspect of the hip joint, separated from it by a bursa (Fig. 6.2). The buttock muscles control hip extension (in which they are aided by the hamstrings) and abduction. There is an extensive attachment of gluteus medius to the femur distal to the greater tuberosity. These are strong postural muscles; medius and minimus help to stabilize the hip

to each pubic bone. The triad of joints making up the pelvic ring (that is, SIJ—pubic symphysis—SIJ) have a strong shock-absorbing function. The hip joint, formed from three separate centres of ossification (ilium, ischium, and pubis) is a ball-and-socket joint, allowing movement in all directions. The strengthening of the capsule by ligaments positioned anteriorly (iliofemoral ligament) and medially (pubofemoral ligament) helps restrict overextension and abduction. However, the main stability arises from the depth of the acetabulum and the strength of the muscles acting upon the joint.

Familiarity with the position of the hip joint from surface anatomical markings should be gained (Fig. 6.2). The head of the femur is positioned immediately inferior (and posterior) to the middle one-third of the inguinal ligament. The femoral head

FIG. 6.3 Axial view of right femur. Femoral anteversion refers to the angle made by the femoral neck to the femoral condyles — that is, the degree of forward projection of the neck from the coronal plane.

FIG. 6.4 The hip adductors are a powerful group of muscles involved in kicking and running.

Pectineus
Adductor brevis
Adductor longus
Adductor magnus
Gracilis

in running, and maximus is active in the backward thrust of the leg in uphill running. Injuries to the gluteal muscle bellies occur infrequently; insertional tendinitis (particularly of gluteus medius) and bursitis (between the muscle layers) are rather more common. Tensor fascia lata, which inserts into the iliotibial tract, is also an abductor: bursitis, caused by repetitive movement of the tract over the underlying bone at a proximal level (overlying the greater trochanter) or distal level (overlying the lateral femoral condyle), may reflect its tightness.

The adductors are a powerful group of muscles arising from the pubis and puboischial rami; they are inserted into the linea aspera, adductor tubercle of the femur (adductor magnus), and the medial tibial condyle (gracilis) (Fig. 6.4). Adduction of the thigh is one of a sequence of movements that takes place in running and kicking; the adductors flex and internally rotate the thigh as well as adduct, movements which are carried out vigorously in kicking a football. The combination of kicking, the sudden movements which take place in change of direction, and the stress applied in tackling are responsible for the relatively high incidence of chronic adductor strain and anterior pelvic strain in footballers. Internal rotation is produced as an accessory function by the iliopsoas, the adductors, and the glutei; external rotation is produced by the smaller muscles (gemelli, piriformis, and obturators).

There are a few acute injuries giving rise to localized symptoms, and a large variety of overuse injuries which give rise to more diffuse ache in the lower abdomen, anteromedial thigh, buttock, or trochanteric region.

Acute injury

'Groin strain'. In the skeletally mature, the most common acute injury to the soft tissue attachments to the pelvis is a strain of the origin of adductor longus. The patient feels a sudden pain in the groin on stretching the thigh into abduction and external rotation—for example, on turning quickly in soccer (Fig. 6.5). Discomfort is felt on attempted pivoting, sprinting, or kicking. The examination findings are discomfort on passive abduction of the thigh, and pain on resisted adduction. Tenderness is localized to the origin of the cord-like adductor longus tendon from the inferior pubic ramus. The essentials of management are to allow this potentially chronic injury to heal fully, and to postpone resumption of training until a full painless range of abduction is achieved and normal adduction power is regained. A minimum period of three weeks is usually required. Steroid injections should not be used for fear of weakening the tendon.

Rupture of the adductor longus may occur at its origin, midbelly, or insertion on the linea aspera. Weakness and pain, if rupture is incomplete, are elicited on resisted adduction; usually soft tissue swelling and bruising become extensive in the medial

FIG. 6.5 Injuries to the adductors of the thigh are common in soccer players.

FIG. 6.6 Myositis ossificans in the femoral attachment of the adductor longus

FIG. 6.7 Gluteal muscle tears may result from forced hip flexion in accidents at high speed, such as may occur in water-skiing.

and posterior thigh. Healing without complications may be anticipated unless premature resumption of activity is allowed, in which case myositis ossificans may occur, either proximally or distally (Fig. 6.6). At a later stage, the defect and proximal muscle swellings are palpable, though adductor function is unaffected. Symeonides (1972) advocates a surgical approach for midbelly and distal ruptures. In the author's experience, however, an uneventful recovery may be expected following a conservative approach.

Acute strain of iliopsoas also occurs—the pain is felt in the groin on hip flexion—for example, during walking or attempted running. Passive hip extension is uncomfortable. The pain is reproduced on resisted flexion and medial rotation of the thigh. Deep tenderness is felt over the musculotendinous junction which is in close proximity to the anterior aspect of the hip joint. For accurate localization the hip should be supported in slight flexion. Uneventful recovery is to be expected inside two weeks or so.

Muscle tears in the gluteal group are uncommon. They normally result from forced hip flexion in accidents at high speed—for example, while water-skiing (Fig. 6.7). However, the hamstrings are more likely to be injured under these circumstances (see Chapter 9).

Overuse injury

A plethora of conditions exist, for the assessment and management of which a knowledge of aetiological factors is necessary.

Chronic adductor strain. An enthesitis at the origin of the adductor longus may develop from an acute strain that has been inappropriately managed, either by the patient or his physician. Alternatively, a more insidious onset is recorded in the absence of an acute phase. Hockey and soccer players are primarily affected. Pain is felt in the groin and medial thigh on sprinting, turning quickly, or kicking. The signs are similar to an acute sprain: there is no capsular pattern, merely signs of a lesion in a contractile structure. It is tempting to inject steroid around the tendon origin though, if this is done, it is imperative that adequate stretching and strengthening exercises continue to be undertaken for several weeks thereafter. If an acute-on-chronic strain occurs, the underlying condition may take many months, even a year, to respond. X-ray and bone scan are advisable in the refractory case, to distinguish from stress fracture of the puboischial rami. Adductor tendinitis due to chronic overload may occur also at the origin of gracilis and adductor brevis. In patients who do not respond to a conservative regime partial tenotomy appears to be a viable alternative management (Martens *et al.* 1987). Ectopic ossification in the adductor longus tendon ('rider's thigh') is a response to overactivity, and is seen particularly in horse-riders.

Osteitis pubis ('pubic symphysitis'). The earlier descriptions of this condition associated it with chronic urinary or prostatic infection, hence the '-itis'. As a sports injury, the condition is manifested by exercise-dependent pain felt in the lower abdomen and medial thighs, gradually increasing in severity and eventually preventing exercise. It is due to excessive stress from those activities which involve running and twisting, and is precipitated particularly by overuse of the abdominal muscles, principally the rectus abdominis. Adams and Chandler (1953) postulate that recurrent microtrauma causes thrombosis and aseptic necrosis of the bone and cartilage. There is evidence that the condition is more likely to arise in the presence of restricted movement and/or reduced resistance to stress in other parts of the pelvis. Muckle (1982) has drawn attention to the association between osteitis pubis and spinal abnormalities. Williams (1978) has noted an association with tilt deformity of the femoral head. The author's experience is of a high correlation between degenerative change in the hip joint and osteitis pubis.

When taking a history it is necessary to determine the extent of abdominal muscle activity that preceded the onset of symptoms. A typical patient is a sportsman who augments his daily long-distance running by several games of squash and sessions of circuit training each week, with additional daily sit-ups and press-ups performed at home—by no means an unusual situation. Females may substitute aerobics for circuit training, and develop the same overload problem. The examination signs are those of chronic strain at the pubic attachments of both the abdominal and adductor muscles: pain on resisted contraction and discomfort on stretch. Although there is some tenderness at the adductor attachments to the inferior pubic rami, *maximal* tenderness is found on palpating the pubic symphysis. Instability of the symphysis may develop in a severe case owing to shear forces secondary to powerful muscle contraction, particularly of the adductors.

AP X-rays of the pelvis taken while weightbearing, first on one leg and then the other (flamingo views), will reveal any supero-inferior instability. Gross irregularity, moth-eaten erosions, and sclerosis of the margins of the symphysis pubis are stress-related changes; however, they correlate poorly with the presence or severity of symptomatology. Severe changes may be found on routine X-ray—for example, during pre-employment examinations in professional soccer players in the absence of symptoms (Fig. 6.8). In one review Harris and Murray (1974) found that radiographic changes at the symphysis were present in 76 per cent of professional soccer players on routine X-rays. In a group that included footballers and other athletes, sacroiliac stress changes were also present in 55 per cent. Bone scan is a supplementary test: increased uptake at the symphysis is shown in symptomatic cases.

Management is by stress reduction, which may, in the fully developed syndrome, necessitate complete rest from sport for several months. Localized treatment is initially to little avail, although steroid injections to the superior aspect of the pubic symphysis may be helpful at a later stage. Flexibility exercises, particularly for the hip joints and the muscles acting upon them, are instituted once symptomatic improvement has been gained. Very occasionally, surgical stabilization of the symphysis may be considered if symptoms persist for over six months in the presence of demonstrable instability. More often, even in the presence of instability, symptoms gradually resolve during six to twelve months.

Stress fractures. Stress fractures of the puboischial rami or the femoral neck may present as gradually worsening exercise-dependent pain in the groin. The importance of diagnosis in the case of femoral neck fracture is the possibility of the development of a frank fracture, with its inevitably more serious consequences. There is often no particular pattern of discomfort on hip movement. Localized tenderness may be detected in an anterior pelvic stress fracture. X-rays may not be positive for a couple of months: bone scanning is essential for diagnosis. Treatment is again by complete rest from exercise for three to six months.

Sacroiliitis. Sacroiliitis may occur as an inflammatory condition—for instance, as a component of one of the spondyloarthritides such as ankylosing spondylitis. It is not a mechanical problem, though is mentioned here to differentiate from sacroiliac stress. Although most common in young men, it may also occur in females. The history, of low backache, alternating sciatica, and morning stiffness which are uninfluenced by exercise, should raise suspicions. Sacroiliac stress tests are positive, and the diagnosis confirmed by the typical features on X-ray and a positive HLA B27 antigen test (Fig. 6.9). Referral to a rheumatologist is advised: spinal flexibility exercises are the main-stay of management.

Sacroiliac stress has a biomechanical aetiology. The shock-absorbing function of the sacroiliac joint may become inade-

Fig. 6.8 'Osteitis pubis'. These severe erosive changes at the pubic symphysis were found at routine pre-employment screening in a professional soccer player.

F<small>IG</small>. 6.9 Sacroiliitis: the typical erosive changes associated with sclerosis at the sacroiliac joints.

quate as a result of repetitive stress involved in sports such as the steeplechase in athletics. Although there is presently little supporting evidence, it is possible that muscle imbalance may play a part—for instance, greater strength of the rectus femoris and relative weakness of the gluteals, giving rise to chronic anterior rotational strain. Discomfort is felt typically over the SIJ, radiating through the buttock to the thigh and lower leg, and commonly also to the groin. Unlike the inflammatory condition of sacroiliitis, the symptoms are aggravated by exercise and arise progressively earlier during exercise as the condition worsens. Stress tests are painful, and X-rays reveal increased sclerosis (though no other changes) around the SIJs. Serological testing is negative. Intra-articular steroid injections may be helpful. However, reduced stress is necessary for some months, and muscle imbalance requires correction if present.

Conjoined tendon strain. The conjoined tendon is formed principally from the inferior fibres of the internal oblique and the aponeurosis of the transversalis; it is inserted medially into the pubis, and reinforces the posterior aspect of the superficial inguinal ring. A strain of the medial attachment should be considered with a history of discomfort in the inguinal region, extending to the perineum, felt during and after activity. There are no definite signs on hip movement or resisted muscle contraction. However, there is localized tenderness at the pubic tubercle and in adjacent soft tissues. The integrity of the fibromuscular components of the walls of the inguinal canal should be specifically determined; impulse bulge, tenderness, and dilatation of the superficial inguinal ring following finger invagination of the scrotum indicate the development of Gilmore's groin, in which there is a torn external oblique aponeurosis and a dehiscence between the inguinal ligament and the torn conjoined tendon. X-rays and bone scan are negative. Rest and a steroid injection may help the relatively minor injury, but the more established case requires surgical repair. Occasionally, a frank hernia is detectable by impulse swelling. Inguinal and femoral

hernias in athletes should always be referred for surgery, whether symptomatic or otherwise.

Psoas bursitis. Excessive bouts of exercise requiring hip flexion are the causative factors. This may be seen in hurdling and in ultramarathon running. Discomfort is localized to the anterior aspect of the groin and thigh for instance, and, when severe, may be accompanied by soft tissue swelling. Because of its anatomical proximity to the anterior aspect of the hip, it needs to be differentiated from pathological conditions arising from the hip joint. In psoas bursitis, passive hip flexion is painful because the bursa is squeezed in this position. In addition, other passive movements, such as external rotation, may be uncomfortable, though a non-capsular pattern prevails. Resisted muscle contraction is painless. Tenderness is present over the anterior aspect of the hip. In the less pronounced case, induction of local anaesthesia may be necessary to establish a diagnosis. The addition of steroid is therapeutic: ultrasound also helps.

Hip conditions. 'Sprains' of the hip joint manifesting as synovitis are uncommon, unless accompanied by other pathology—for example, osteoarthritis. When confronted by symptoms and capsular signs suggesting intra-articular pathology, investigation by X-ray and blood tests should be undertaken to exclude conditions which, if unrecognized, are potentially disastrous. Thus Perthes' disease between the ages of five and twelve, slipped femoral epiphysis between twelve and sixteen, and relatively uncommon conditions such as avascular necrosis in the adult should all be considered. Occasionally inflammatory joint disease, such as that associated with ankylosing spondylitis, is present. In the adult a 'frozen hip' analogous to 'frozen shoulder' has been described (Chard and Jenner 1988). Nevertheless, synovitis is usually an accompaniment of early degenerative change, and may be caused by excessive exercise.

Hip pain is felt principally in the groin and anterior thigh. Patients commonly fear that discomfort felt over the greater trochanters ('the hips') indicates hip disease; they need reassurance, should hip pathology be excluded, that this is not the case. The capsular pattern (in which loss of medial rotation is an early feature—see p. 104) is found on examining the passive range of movements in a patient with synovitis of the hip. Resisted muscle contraction is painless. There may be slight tenderness overlying the hip joint. Aspiration for microscopy and culture, erythrocyte sedimentation rate, and white-cell count may be necessary to exclude infection. In the absence of any other significant pathology an intra-articular steroid injection (on a 'one off' basis) may be useful. Resolution, aided by stress reduction, usually takes place over several months; non-steroidal anti-inflammatory drugs may be tried, though the results are disappointing. Shortwave diathermy may be helpful.

Osteoarthritis (OA) of the hip is a condition that is primarily seen in the over-45s, though it is by no means uncommon in athletic males in their thirties. In the relatively young, this may be due to old Perthes' disease or previous trauma. Although the aetiology is incompletely understood, it is logical to assume that repeated physical stress, probably stemming from childhood, is a major factor. Males who have played team sports such as soccer for many years, particularly at professional level, appear to be at much greater risk than long-distance runners, in whom the increased risk appears minimal. Athletes with symptomatic degenerative disease should be counselled, as the symptoms, and possibly the progression of the condition, may be controlled. However, it is notoriously difficult to prognosticate on either the level of symptomatology or its progression from radiological analysis. Some patients with radiological changes of advanced OA complain of nothing more than a little stiffness; others have pain associated with early degenerative changes only (Fig. 6.10). If there is a history of sharp twinges, a loose body should be considered in the diagnosis.

Established OA increases the likelihood of low back problems. Sports such as squash, which demand repetitive flexion and rota-

tory movements of the trunk and lower limbs, are particularly demanding on the lumbar spine if hip mobility is reduced. Patients should be encouraged to take up non-weightbearing exercise such as swimming and cycling. In the early case, stretching exercises may be helpful, and a few weeks of treatment by shortwave diathermy may give relief for a longer period of time.

Nerve entrapment: lateral cutaneous nerve of thigh. Entrapment may occur at the level at which the nerve passes under the lateral aspect of the inguinal ligament; repetitive pressure or direct trauma is the usual cause in athletes. Paraesthesiae and numbness are felt over the anterolateral aspect of the thigh; this condition is known as *meralgia paraesthetica*. There is no motor involvement, and spontaneous resolution is anticipated.

Gluteal bursitis. Haemorrhagic bursitis has been recorded, possibly secondary to muscle trauma. More commonly, gluteal bursitis is due to overuse, and occurs particularly in long-distance runners. It is more common in the mature athlete. Discomfort is felt in the buttock, with occasional reference to the posterior thigh, and is most troublesome after exercise. Prolonged sitting is often very uncomfortable. Examination reveals what Cyriax has labelled 'the sign of the buttock': pain on both passive hip flexion and on the straight leg raise test (Cyriax 1982). There may be discomfort on performing other passive hip movements, though in no particular pattern. Resisted muscle contraction is usually painless. Deep tenderness is usually present, though may be difficult to find: it may be necessary to locate by injection of a large volume of dilute anaesthetic—for example, 50 ml of 0.5 per cent lignocaine or procaine.

Gluteal bursitis is a difficult condition to treat. Deep frictions, ultrasound, laser therapy, and localized injections may all be tried. Reduction of exercise intensity is required, and a flexibility programme for the hip joint and the hip extensor muscles in particular is instituted.

Fig. 6.10 Osteoarthritis of the hip: the typical early features of narrowing of the joint space, subchondral sclerosis, and osteophytes.

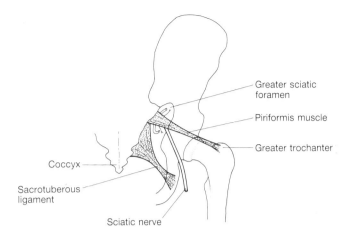

Fig. 6.11 Posterior view of the pelvis: in the piriformis syndrome tenderness may be detected on palpation of the muscle medial to the greater trochanter.

Piriformis syndrome. This condition is probably due to stretching and tearing of fibres of the piriformis muscle (Kirkaldy-Willis 1983). Pain is felt in the buttock and posterior thigh. On isometric contraction of the external rotators, pain and weakness are found. Tenderness is present on palpation of the muscle medial to the greater trochanter (Fig. 6.11). Marked tenderness of the muscle may also be detected by rectal or vaginal palpation just medial to the ischial spine. Treatment is by localized injection of local anaesthetic and deep transverse friction massage, subsequently progressing to graded stretching exercises. In the past the author has not recognized the existence of the condition as frequently as it is purported to occur in a number of other texts.

Trochanteric bursitis. This is a common condition, usually an overuse injury, and is found in both young and old. It is prevalent particularly in long-distance runners and in ballet dancers. Discomfort is felt in the lateral buttock and trochanteric region, and is often referred to the posterolateral thigh. Examination

reveals a full painless range of passive movements of the hip except for pain on adduction in flexion. The iliotibial tract may be shown to be taut on Ober's test, in which passive adduction in 0° hip flexion is assessed in the side-lying position (Fig. 6.12). There is no pain on resisted muscle contraction. Tenderness is extremely well localized to the superolateral aspect of the greater tuberosity. Although conventional physiotherapeutic modalities may be employed, there tends to be a better response to localized steroid injections—for example, 10 mg triamcinolone hexacetonide mixed with 4 ml of 1 per cent lignocaine, combined with regular stretching exercises for the iliotibial tract (see Fig. 11.14, p. 199). The cause of trochanteric bursitis in ballet dancers may be training regimes which favour flexibility in abduction, external rotation, and flexion (Reid *et al.* 1987). A more balanced stretching programme, which includes adduction and medial rotation flexibility exercises, may be necessary.

Ischial bursitis. This is a friction bursitis, and does not occur too often in athletes. In the same region a *chronic strain of the origin of the hamstrings* from the ischial tuberosity is more common. In this condition discomfort is felt in the inferior buttock and posterior thigh, and must be differentiated from sciatic root pain. Both are painful on straight leg raise. In hamstring-origin strain, however, some degree of weakness and discomfort on resisted knee flexion will be found. In addition, localized tenderness is present. Occasionally an acute tear at the origin fails to settle adequately, and develops into a more chronic injury. Alternately overload, and/or excessive stretching of the hamstrings, may give rise to a traction injury. X-rays are usually negative, though they occasionally reveal a localized erosion in the tuberosity (Fig. 6.13). Diagnostic ultrasound and bone scanning may be helpful to differentiate from sciatic root irritation. Surgical excision of granulomatous and fibrotic tissue at the muscle origin may be required to promote healing.

Puranen and Orava (1988) have coined the term 'hamstring syndrome' to describe a condition of persistent pain felt over the inferior buttock and radiating down the back of the thigh, which resulted from tight tendinous structures within the hamstring attachment to the ischial tuberosity. Surgical division of these

Fig. 6.12 The position of the examiner and patient on performing Ober's test (assessment of tautness of the iliotibial tract) are demonstrated.

Fig. 6.13 Pelvic X-ray revealing an ischial erosion due to stress at the hamstring origin.

structures resulted in complete relief in fifty-two out of fifty-nine patients. They suggested that the condition may be secondary to excessive stretching.

The differentiation from sciatic pain is worthy of further comment. Occasionally a situation arises when an athlete is disabled by exercise-related posterior thigh pain, though examination reveals no definite signs. Diagnostic caudal epidural injections of procaine may be required to assist in the diagnosis. Students of musculoskeletal medicine used to be taught that chronic hamstring pathology does not exist, and that posterior thigh pain should be considered to be sciatica unless proved otherwise. Clearly, in athletic injury, this is not the case. Taking a thorough history is desirable, as an acute incident may be recalled by the athlete when the hamstring is at fault.

Adolescent injuries. The apophyses of the pelvis are sites of traction injury in the adolescent (Fig. 6.14). The patho-anatomical lesion is basically an avulsion fracture (traction

separation) of the apophysis (Metzmaker and Pappas 1985). Injuries occur at the following sites:

iliac crest—origin of gluteus medius and oblique abdominal muscles
ASIS—origin of sartorius
AIIS—origin of straight head of rectus femoris
ischial tuberosity—origin of hamstrings (see Fig. 1.13, p. 13)
lesser trochanter—insertion of iliopsoas.

Avulsion results from the same intrinsic stress (vigorous muscle contraction during lengthening) that causes intramuscular injury in the adult. The signs on examination are those of acute injury to a contractile structure: restricted passive stretch, and pain on resisted contraction of the affected muscle. Localized tenderness and firm swelling are found: X-rays confirm. These injuries heal quickly, and almost invariably without complications. The length of time required for healing prior to resumption of early training is approximately four to six weeks.

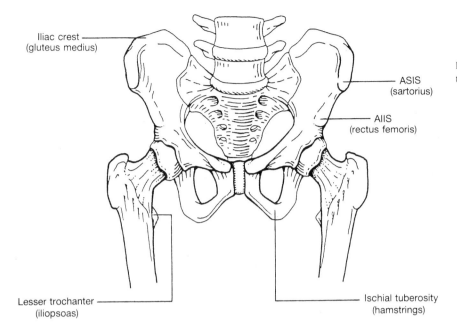

Iliac crest
(gluteus medius)

ASIS
(sartorius)

AIIS
(rectus femoris)

Lesser trochanter
(iliopsoas)

Ischial tuberosity
(hamstrings)

FIG. 6.14 The pelvic apophyses are sites of traction injury in the adolescent.

Summary of examination procedures

Initially a suitable examination of the thoracolumbar junction and lumbar spine should be undertaken to determine any loss of segmental mobility or exacerbation of pain on movement (see Chapter 5).

Examination of the pelvis

Gait
Antalgic
Trendelenburg

Standing
- Observation of the relative heights of ASIS and PSIS
- Sacroiliac mobility (gliding of ilium):
  - loss of ipsilateral downward movement of the PSIS on hip flexion occurs when the SIJ is 'hypomobile' (see Fig. 5.11, p. 88)
  - ipsilateral PSIS is higher on flexion of the trunk when 'hypomobile'
- active weightbearing hip movements
  - squat (hip flexion)
  - groin stretch (abduction)
- cough impulse (inguinal hernia)

Supine
Passive hip movements
- flexion
- abduction in flexion
- adduction
- medial rotation in 45° flexion
- lateral rotation in 45° flexion

Sacroiliac stress
- backward pressure on ASISs
- passive adduction of the flexed hip

Sacroiliac mobility (sitting up with legs outstretched and leaning forward)

- Piedallu sign: PSIS is elevated ipsilaterally on leaning forward when the SIJ is hypomobile (Piedallu 1952)
- apparent leg-length inequality in the supine position, reversed in the sitting position, is noted when the SIJ is hypomobile

Resisted muscle contraction (hip):
- flexors
- abductors
- adductors
- medial rotators (in flexion)
- lateral rotators (in flexion)
- abdominals (bilateral SLR/sit up)

Tenderness:
- pubic symphysis/pubic tubercle/conjoined tendon (± defect)
- puboischial rami
- anterior aspect of hip joint
- adductor origin and muscle belly

Prone
Passive hip movements:
- extension
- medial rotation
- lateral rotation

Resisted muscle contraction (hip):
- extensors
- medial rotators
- lateral rotators

Resisted muscle contraction (knee):
- extensors (quadriceps)
- flexors (hamstrings)

Tenderness
- overlying SIJ
- lateral sacral margin
- gluteal
- ischial tuberosity

Side-lying

- iliotibial tract tautness: the degree of adduction of the hip under gravity (Ober's test)
- tenderness of the tensor fascia lata, trochanteric bursa, and proximal lateral femur (insertion of gluteus medius)

References

Adams, R. J. and Chandler, F. A., (1953). Osteitis pubis of traumatic aetiology. *J. Bone Jt. Surg.*, **35A**, 658.

Chard, M. D. and Jenner, J. R. (1988). The frozen hip: an underdiagnosed condition. *Br. Med. J.*, **297** (6648), 596.

Colachis, S. C., Warden, R. E., Bechtol, C. O., and Strohm, B. R. (1963). Movement of the sacroiliac joint in the adult male. *Arch. Phys. Med. Rehabil.*, **44**, 490.

Cyriax, J. (1982). *Textbook of orthopaedic medicine*,Vol. 1 (8th edn). Baillière Tindall, London.

Grieve, G. P. (1976). The sacroiliac joint. *Physiotherapy*, **62** (12), 384–400.

Harris, N. H. and Murray, R. G. (1974). Lesions of the symphysis in athletes. *Br. Med. J.*, **4**, 211–14.

Kirkaldy-Willis, W. H. (1983). *Managing low back pain*, pp. 96–7. Churchill Livingstone, Edinburgh.

Lewit, K. (1985). *Manipulative therapy in rehabilitation of the motor system*. Butterworth, London.

Martens, M. A., Hansen, L., and Mulier, J. C. (1987). Adductor tendinitis and musculus rectus abdominis tendopathy. *Am. J. Sports Med.*, **15**(4), 353–6.

Metzmaker, J. N. and Pappas, A. M. (1985). Avulsion fractures of the pelvis *Am. J. Sports Med.*, **13**, 349–58.

Muckle, D. S. (1982). Associated factors in recurrent groin and hamstring injuries. *Br. J. Sports Med.*, **16**(1), 37–9.

Piedallu, P. (1952). Problèmes sacro-iliaques. Homme Sain, no. 2. Bière Édition, Bordeaux.

Puranen, J. and Orava, S. (1988). The hamstring syndrome. *Am. J. Sports Med.*, **16**(5), 517–21.

Reid, D. C., Burnham, R. S., Saboe, L. A., and Kushner, S. F. (1987). Lower extremity flexibility patterns in classical ballet dancers. *Am. J. Sports Med.*, **15**, 347–52.

Schaberg, J. E., Harper, M. C., and Allen, W. C. (1984). The snapping hip syndrome. *Am. J. Sports Med.*, **12**, 361–5.

Symeonides, P. P. (1972). Isolated traumatic rupture of the adductor longus muscle of the thigh. *Clin. Orthop. Relat. Res.*, **88**, 64–6.

Weisl, H. (1955). The movements of the sacroiliac joint. *Acta Anat.*, **23**, 80–91.

Williams, J. G. P. (1978). Limitation of hip joint movement as a factor in traumatic osteitis pubis. *Br. J. Sports Med.*, **12**(3), 129–33.

7 Injuries to the knee joint

M. A. HUTSON

In this chapter acute injuries to the knee joint are considered; overuse problems are dealt with in Chapter 9. The majority of acute knee injuries presenting to the sports physician result from a valgus and/or twisting strain. Most commonly they involve the medial joint structures and the anterior cruciate ligament, which has a crucial role in the functional integrity of the tibiofemoral joint. Other types of strain exist, however, so that no ligament is exempt from injury. The menisci and patellofemoral joint mechanism are also frequent sites of injury. The use of the arthroscope for diagnostic and therapeutic purposes has improved knowledge and aided management considerably in acute knee injuries. However, it should not be assumed that all painful knee conditions which give rise to an effusion warrant arthroscopy. Although recognition of the different types of ligamentous instability demands some experience, it should be within the capabilities of the sports physician to make a provisional diagnosis in the 'acute knee' and to determine when referral to a specialist knee surgeon is necessary. A thorough examination regime should be adopted for all patients, and this is summarized at the end of the chapter.

Applied anatomy and biomechanics

The *tibiofemoral joint* is a modified hinge joint that allows a restricted amount of gliding and rotation in addition to flexion/extension. Lateral rotation of the tibia takes place in the 'screw-home' mechanism at the extreme of extension. The synovium communicates with many of the bursae around the joint, and is so arranged internally that the cruciate ligaments are extrasynovial. Folds of synovium known as 'plicae' are present in most knees, and are classified as suprapatellar, mediopatellar, or infrapatella (Hardaker *et al.* 1980). When traumatized a plica may become symptomatic and give rise to a condition known as the plica syndrome (see Chapter 9).

The menisci are attached to the tibia, held in place peripherally by the coronary (meniscotibial) ligaments. They act as shock-absorbers, dispersing stress over the articular cartilage, and make the joint surfaces more congruent (Fig. 7.1). Together with the collateral and cruciate ligaments, they play an important part in the provision of stability to the knee: the combination of meniscectomy and anterior cruciate ligament loss is often disastrous in respect of functional instability, and leads to early degenerative change.

The medial (tibial) collateral ligament (MCL) is composed of a superficial layer and a deep layer (the medial capsular ligament) (Fig. 7.2). It is further strengthened by the posterior oblique ligament that merges with the posterior capsule. The superficial

FIG. 7.1 Right tibial plateau from above: the lateral meniscus is circular and is not attached to the capsule and the medial meniscus is C-shaped and is attached to the capsule and medial ligament: ACL, attachment of anterior cruciate ligament; PCL, attachment of posterior cruciate ligament.

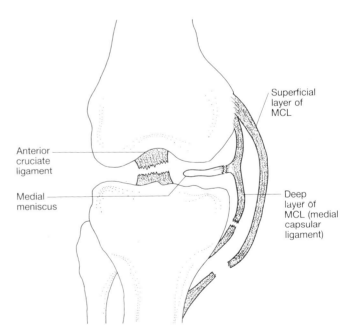

FIG. 7.2 The medial collateral ligament (MCL) is composed of superficial and deep layers. O'Donoghue's triad is shown: rupture of MCL and ACL, and tear of medial meniscus.

layer of the MCL extends from the adductor tubercle of the medial femoral condyle to the tibial metaphysis, approximately 6 cm below the joint line. The deep layer is composed of meniscotibial and meniscofemoral elements. The lateral collateral liga

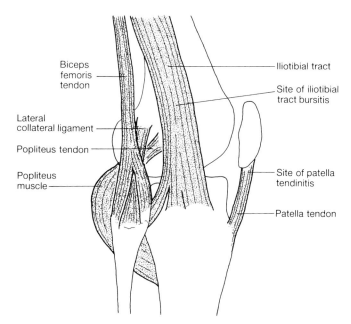

Biceps femoris tendon
Lateral collateral ligament
Popliteus tendon
Popliteus muscle

Iliotibial tract
Site of iliotibial tract bursitis
Site of patella tendinitis
Patella tendon

FIG. 7.3 The lateral ligamentous complex of the knee. The sites of overuse injury also are shown.

ment (LCL) is attached superiorly to the lateral femoral epicondyle and inferiorly to the head of the fibula. It is rounded, and may be felt in one's own knee when sitting with the lateral aspect of the ipsilateral ankle resting on the contralateral knee, allowing the thigh to rotate laterally, in which position it is prominent. The lateral ligamentous complex (Fig. 7.3) comprises the LCL reinforced by the iliotibial tract, the biceps femoris tendon, the popliteus tendon, and the arcuate ligament (a thickening of the capsule). The anterior and posterior cruciate ligaments are named by the relationship of their attachments to the tibia (Fig. 7.1). The anterior cruciate ligament (ACL) is composed of an anteromedial and posterolateral bundle positioned in a spiral fashion. The specific functions of the ligaments, as determined by their actions as primary restraints, have been outlined by Marshall and Rubin (1977). A working knowledge helps with interpretation of physical signs, and provides an understanding of the type of instability found upon rupture.

Medial stability is provided initially by the superficial MCL then by the ACL and, in extension, by the posterior capsule. The deep MCL appears to play a minor role.

Lateral stability is provided by the LCL and its associated structures within the lateral ligamentous complex, reinforced by both cruciates.

Anterior stability (that is, restraint against anterior displacement of the tibia on the femur) is provided principally by the ACL.

Posterior stability is provided by the PCL.

Hyperextension stability is provided principally by the ACL, supported by the posterior capsule and PCL.

External rotation stability is provided principally by the superficial MCL and the ACL.

Internal rotation stability is provided by both the ACL and PCL and, to a lesser extent, the lateral supporting structures. In extension, the ACL is the main restraint.

From the foregoing it can be seen that the anterior cruciate ligament must be taut in most, if not all, positions of the joint. This is explained by the fact that it is a multifascicular structure, with two identifiable portions which are distinguishable both anatomically and functionally. The anteromedial bundle is taut in flexion and is the primary restraint to anterior stress, whereas the posterolateral bundle is taut in extension.

The patellofemoral joint. The main biomechanical function of the patella is to increase the effective lever arm of the quadriceps in effecting knee extension, or resisting knee flexion, by distancing the patella tendon from the axis of movement (Hungerford and Barry 1979). It allows the components of the quadriceps muscle to act under as stable a situation as possible in the intercondylar groove of the femur, thereby functioning effectively as a frictionless pulley. The articular cartilage on the back of the patella withstands high compression loads—stresses that tendon is poorly designed to withstand (Ficat and Hungerford 1977). It has been estimated that a pressure of seven times bodyweight is exerted upon the patellofemoral joint during a deep knee bend (Cailliet 1983). A similar pressure may be applied on *descending* stairs, compared with a twofold increase on ascending stairs. The patella also protects the anterior aspect of the tibiofemoral joint from direct trauma.

Studies on patellofemoral loading reveal different contact areas on the patella facets in different degrees of flexion (Goodfellow *et al.* 1976; see also Fig. 9.6, p. 145). The overall contact area is increased with greater degrees of flexion. It is of some significance that extension resistance exercises performed in the sitting position (that is, from knee flexion to extension) have been shown to load the articular cartilage in a non-physiological fashion. However, loading in extension—that is, straight leg raising against resistance—creates no patellofemoral compression and provides the basis for strengthening exercises in patellofemoral problems (see Chapter 11, Quadriceps femoris exercises, p. 190).

Stability of the patella is provided by the vastus medialis (or vastus medialis obliquus (VMO)) and the congruency between the lateral patella facet and the articular surface of the lateral femoral condyle (Wiberg 1941). The Q-angle (see Fig. 9.5, p. 145) is the angle between the quadriceps muscle (measured by a line from the anterior superior iliac spine to the midpoint of the patella) and the patella tendon (measured from the midpoint of the patella to the tibial tubercle). The normal range is stated to be 13°–18°. An increase in the Q-angle is often associated with patellofemoral disorders.

Haemarthrosis

It is essential to distinguish between a haemarthrosis and a serous joint effusion. The initial clue lies in the history: swelling that occurs within an hour or two of injury, giving rise to a feeling of joint tightness, is most likely due to bleeding—that is, a haemarthrosis. However, a joint effusion develops overnight, and is noticed by the patient the morning after injury. The size of the joint swelling is another factor—a haemarthrosis is a tense joint containing up to 100 ml of blood. Unless the patient has a chronic or recurring rheumatological problem, a serous effusion associated with osteochondritis dissecans or a torn meniscus for instance is much smaller.

When haemarthrosis of the knee results from acute injury in sport the likely diagnoses are rupture of the ACL, peripheral meniscus tear, or patella dislocation. Of these the most common is ACL rupture. Noyes *et al.* (1980) found that ACL rupture occurred in 72 per cent of cases of traumatic haemarthrosis without significant collateral ligament injury on clinical examination. Clues to the nature of the intra-articular pathology may be obtained from the history—for example, recognition by the patient of patella dislocation and relocation. A 'pop' from within the joint may be experienced if the ACL tears. Clinical examination is followed by X-rays looking particularly for evidence of osteochondral injury to the patella, when small avulsed fragments may be observed (see Fig. 10.16, p. 177), and for evidence of avulsion fracture of the distal attachment of the ACL to the tibia. Management strategies are dependent upon establishment of the underlying cause of the haemarthrosis. Aspiration may be performed for confirmation of the haemarthrosis and/or for patient comfort. The presence of fat globules within the aspirate indicates an intra-articular fracture.

In the differential diagnosis of a swollen knee due to trauma, the presence of substantial soft tissue swelling may indicate that the joint derangement includes collateral ligament (and therefore capsular) rupture, allowing extravasation of blood into the subcutaneous tissues. ACL rupture remains the most likely diagnosis when the examiner is faced with traumatic haemarthrosis (and therefore with an intact capsule) and negative X-rays.

Patella dislocation

Lateral dislocation of the patella is usually caused by valgus stress to the knee. Although it is often an isolated injury, it may be associated with more extensive derangements of the knee joint such as MCL tear. Normally patients are taken to the nearest accident and emergency department, particularly when relocation has not occurred spontaneously. However, relocation often occurs before medical attention is sought, and the patient presents with a history of valgus or rotational stress, pain over the anterior aspect of the knee, and swelling. The presence of a haemarthrosis is noted, and signs of recent patellofemoral (PF) trauma (due to osteochondral injury) are present.

1. Manipulation of the patella provokes discomfort.
2. There is marked tenderness along the length of the medial retinaculum that has torn during lateral dislocation.
3. Attempts at gentle laterally directed pressure upon the patella evoke discomfort and apprehension.
4. There is tenderness of the medial margin of the medial articular facet of the patella.

If the injury was ignored or unrecognized initially, and the patient presents some weeks or months afterwards, the signs of *patellofemoral dysfunction* may still be present.

(a) Positive patella compression. Manual compression of the patella against the femur is painful.
(b) Tenderness on palpating the margins of the patella facets, particularly the medial facet. This should be differentiated from adjacent tenderness, which is more likely to indicate a painful plica or resolving retinaculitis.
(c) Positive Clarke's sign. Contraction of the quadriceps while the examiner presses the patella into the trochlea causes pain. It is an insensitive test.
(d) Pain on attempting the squat position may be helpful in identifying PF pain when other tests are largely negative. It

is unnecessarily painful for confirmation in recent injury or in PF arthritis.
(e) Positive patella apprehension. The patient is apprehensive that further dislocation or subluxation will occur when the examiner exerts a laterally directed force on the patella with the knee slightly flexed. It is pathognomonic of patella instability, or at least recent dislocation.

A thorough examination of the tibiofemoral joint is made to exclude additional injury. Further assessment is by X-rays—AP, lateral, and patella (skyline) views should be requested. The presence of an intra-articular fragment indicates the need for referral for a surgical opinion. The combination of a relocated patella and a haemarthrosis may otherwise be managed by joint aspiration followed by application of a POP cylinder, from groin to ankle, for three weeks, to allow the torn medial retinaculum to heal. For aspiration a 50 ml syringe and a 20 G 2 inch needle are required. Although there are a number of suitable puncture sites, including the suprapatellar pouch and over the lateral joint line, a recommended and reliable route is the medial approach. The needle is inserted approximately 1 cm posterior to the midpoint of the medial border of the patella and directed laterally (see Fig. 12.21, p. 220).

Physiotherapy is instituted after cast removal. The emphasis initially is on isometric muscle contraction and range of motion exercises. Considerable care is taken not to introduce isotonic exercises too quickly, to reduce the risk of chronic patellofemoral pain.

Tears of quadriceps expansion and patella tendon

Complete loss of extensor function results from a tear of the quadriceps expansion or complete tear of the patella tendon (syn. quadriceps tendon, infrapatellar tendon, patella ligament). The mechanism is the same as that causing quadriceps muscle-belly tear: vigorous contraction, usually against resistance, from the flexed position. The supportive function of the quadriceps in the stance phase is lost and the leg collapses. Diagnosis is normally straightforward, as straight leg raise is impossible. Loss of muscle strength is due to intrinsic muscle dysfunction, and not pain inhibition. There may be a palpable gap at the level of the tear, though surrounding soft tissue swelling may obscure this. When the patella tendon is ruptured X-rays often reveal a 'high-riding' patella (see Fig. 10.5, p. 171). Surgical referral is indicated.

Medial collateral ligament injury

The commonest injury to the knee is to the MCL, resulting from the combination of valgus and external rotation force. In certain sports such as alpine skiing and rugby football MCL sprain represents a significant proportion of recorded lower limb injuries. It represents 25 per cent of all recorded alpine ski injuries in some statistical surveys. External rotational forces are magnified by the presence of the attached ski, invoking risk of injury despite improvements in binding-release in recent years (see Fig. 1.7, p. 5). A common cause is 'catching an inside edge'. External rotation is then augmented by reduction in speed and altered direction of the ski, whilst forward body momentum remains unchecked. In rugby football a blow to the lateral aspect of the knee in a tackle creates a valgus stress to the medial aspect of the joint.

There are three grades of MCL injury.

Grade I: Sprain of the superficial MCL in which there is no demonstrable laxity.

Grade II: Partial tear of the superficial MCL in which laxity may be demonstrated though the deep layer is intact (a firm end-point on valgus stress in 30° flexion).

Grade III: Complete tear of the MCL, involving both superficial and deep layers. A mushy end-point is felt on valgus stress in 30° flexion; frequently over 15° of laxity is present.

The secondary restraints against medial instability—the ACL and the posterior capsule with the knee extended—may also be injured. Therefore examination of the knee includes relevant tests for the PF joint, the cruciate and collateral ligaments, and both menisci, as indicated in the examination summary at the end of the chapter. The significant findings in MCL injury are described further.

Grade I injury

There is no effusion or it is minimal. A full range of movement is found, with discomfort only at the extreme of flexion. On stressing the MCL in 30° flexion there is discomfort, though no instability. Tenderness and minimal soft tissue swelling are present at the site of the sprain (usually the femoral attachment). Treatment by anti-inflammatory modalities, resisted quadriceps contraction, and early range of motion exercise may be instituted without the need for structural support. Immobilization, for instance in a splint which restricts knee flexion, is contraindicated.

Grade II injury

The signs on examination depend upon the length of time which has elapsed since the injury. The traumatic synovitis causes a small effusion and restriction (to 90°) of passive flexion of the knee, maximal on day 2, resolving over ten days. Extension is initially uncomfortable. The knee is stable to valgus stress in extension. In 30° flexion there is medial laxity of 10°–15° (increased medial joint opening up to 10 mm) with a firm painful end-point. There is a small swelling, approximately the size of a half walnut, overlying the tear, usually at the femoral attachment. Tenderness is localized to the tear; diffuse tenderness along the whole length of the MCL is more likely to indicate grade III injury. Quadriceps wasting is not as profound as when the knee is locked, though it is sufficient to warrant isometric exercises as soon as passive extension is comfortable. X-ray examination is advisable, and in the child may be combined with stress films to detect epiphyseal injury.

Management principles are common to collateral ligament injuries at both knee and ankle. The combination of functional support for acute ligamentous instability and early mobilization are the cornerstones of therapy. An ambulatory cast-brace may be used: a suitable arrangement is a thigh cast connected through medial and lateral knee hinges to a lower leg cast that in turn is connected to a plastic heel cup (see Fig. 12.1, p. 204). Thereby valgus/varus and rotational movement at the knee are controlled. This should be maintained for three weeks, and then the cast-brace should be removed and the patient referred for flexibility, strengthening, and proprioceptive exercises.

In a less severe grade II injury crutches may be used for several days, during which time range of motion exercises are instituted

and isometric quadriceps contraction commences as soon as possible (within 48 hours). Local therapeutic measures include the use of ice and ultrasound. Normally isometric contraction against resistance is commenced within a few days. A cycling programme may be started as soon as a full range of motion has been regained (usually inside a week), and isokinetic exercise soon afterwards. A progressive rehabilitation programme is continued until full power and endurance have been regained.

If mobilization following grade II injury is allowed to take place without functional support, there is a risk of the development of ectopic calcification at the site of the injury—namely, the femoral attachment of the MCL (see Fig. 9.10, p. 149). This condition, the Pelligrini-Steida syndrome, is associated with mild laxity of the MCL and may be intermittently painful. However, it usually responds to localized steroid injections. When untreated or unrecognized the presence of MCL laxity increases the likelihood of further injury, and when combined with ACL rupture it often results in functional instability.

Grade III injury

This may be an isolated injury, although frequently it is associated with medial meniscus tear, ACL tear, or patella dislocation (Fig. 7.2). The patient is aware of significant functional disturbance, and finds that the knee tends to give way unless locked into extension. Diffuse swelling due to bleeding and oedema forms periarticularly. The additional features which suggest a complete tear are an empty feeling—that is, a mushy end-point—on performing the valgus stress test in 30° flexion. However, the knee is stable in full extension, unless the posterior cruciate or posterior capsule has been disrupted. Tenderness is often felt along the entire length of the MCL.

If stress X-rays in valgus are taken, medial laxity is found to be 15° or more. Referral should be made to an orthopaedic surgeon for further management. A surgical approach is usually chosen, although cast immobilization alone for four to six weeks is an alternative management. A peripheral meniscus tear is often associated with complete MCL rupture. Therefore a minimal therapeutic requirement is a period of immobilization sufficient to allow healing of a secondary structure. Intensive physiotherapy follows (see under ACL tear).

Anterior cruciate ligament tears

Recognition of the incidence of ACL tears has been facilitated by the widespread use of arthroscopy and/or MRI (see Fig. 10.18(a), p. 178). It is a common injury, though frequently missed by inexperienced clinicians (Noyes et al. 1985). Unfortunately it gives rise to considerable morbidity following initial injury, followed by a significantly increased risk of symptomatic instability and early joint degeneration. A study of the restraining function of the ACL allows an understanding of the biomechanical stresses which are involved in the acute tear. The two commonest situations are first rotational stress applied to the flexed knee and secondly excessive hyperextension. There are a number of sports in which flexion–rotation stress is common, particularly when the participant descends from a jump and is then jostled, either 'legally' or 'illegally', as, for example, in soccer, rugby, netball, and basketball. ACL tears are also common in skiing. Sometimes a 'popping' sensation is experienced at the moment of injury. Rapid onset of swelling (haemarthrosis) is a further feature.

Assessment of the injury, following the history, is made by a full examination of the knee. Positive physical signs in the acute case are as follows.

1. The presence of a haemarthrosis.

2. The signs of an intense traumatic synovitis: passive flexion restricted to approximately 90° and loss of full extension. This pseudolocking in, for example, 10° of flexion mimics the true locking found in bucket-handle tears of the medial meniscus, and may not be fully differentiated until arthroscopy.

3. Positive Lachman's test. Anterior displacement of the tibia is detected in approximately 10° of flexion (Fig. 7.4). This test relies on the ability of the physician to grasp the patient's thigh above the knee with one hand and the lower leg just below the tibial tuberosity with the other, and thus is not easy for doctors with small hands or in patients of heavy build. Alternatively, it can be performed with both hands cupping the upper calf and an assistant stabilizing the thigh.

4. Positive pivot shift or jerk test (Hughston *et al.* 1976; Ireland and Trickey 1980). Demonstration of anterolateral instability depends on anterior subluxation of the lateral tibial plateau (Fig. 7.5). This is a rotatory movement. The patient's leg is internally rotated, and a valgus force applied to the knee. Passive flexion and extension are then performed. A positive pivot shift is recorded by a thud when the lateral tibial plateau is relocated when passing from the fully extended position through approximately 20° flexion. A positive jerk test relies on manoeuvring the knee from flexion into extension: at approximately 20° a jerk is recorded when subluxation and then relocation are felt and observed. The test is facilitated by forward pressure on the fibula head by the examiner's thumb (Fig. 7.6). The critical degree of flexion is the one at which the function of the iliotibial band changes from a restraint to flexion to a restraint to extension (or vice versa). Positive Lachman's and jerk tests are usually obtainable in the acute knee with careful handling of the patient. They are pathognomonic of ACL deficiency.

FIG. 7.4 (a) The positions of the examiner and patient when performing Lachman's test are demonstrated. (b) The position of the examiner's hands is shown.

(a)

(b)

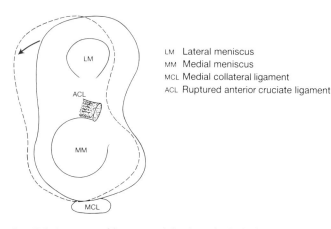

LM   Lateral meniscus
MM   Medial meniscus
MCL Medial collateral ligament
ACL Ruptured anterior cruciate ligament

FIG. 7.5 Anterior subluxation of the lateral tibial plateau occurs in anterolateral (rotatory) instability.

FIG. 7.6 The jerk test is facilitated by forward pressure on the fibula head by the examiner's thumb.

FIG. 7.7 The position of the examiner and patient when performing the anterior and posterior drawer tests in 90° knee flexion are demonstrated.

5. Positive anterior drawer sign at 90° flexion (Fig. 7.7). The anterior drawer test, performed with the knee in 90° flexion (maintained by sitting on the patient's feet) and the tibia in neutral rotation, assesses the integrity of the ACL. An abnormal degree of anterior laxity, due to anterior subluxation of the *lateral* tibial plateau, indicates ACL insufficiency. This laxity is also present in external rotation of the tibia, though it is reduced in internal rotation. Interpretation may not always be clear-cut, however. It is sometimes difficult to decide whether anteroposterior instability is due to a positive posterior drawer sign (indicating injury to the posterior cruciate ligament) or to a positive anterior drawer sign. Anterior subluxation of the *medial* tibial plateau with the tibia in neutral (anteromedial instability) indicates MCL injury; this is accentuated when the anterior drawer test is performed with the tibia in external rotation. It is further accentuated by combined ACL and MCL insufficiency.

It should be recognized that an ACL tear is often associated with injury to the menisci or collateral ligaments (Hughston 1983). Therefore a combination of a grade II or III MCL and an ACL tear is not uncommon. Debate in the past has centred upon whether it is feasible biomechanically for an isolated ACL tear to exist. Although the author believes this to be the case, nevertheless the knee should be examined fully for the existence of other injuries. The coexistence of additional injury increases the likelihood of functional disability at a later stage.

Full assessment necessitates the use of conventional X-rays of the knee prior to consideration of referral for arthroscopy and joint wash-out. X-rays may detect a bony fragment representing avulsion of the distal attachment of the ACL from the tibial intercondylar eminence; a surgical opinion should be sought, as internal fixation is often the treatment of choice. Arthroscopy, if available, is useful to determine the extent of the intra-articular injury; otherwise MRI may be required to confirm the presence of an additional injury such as a meniscus tear. When used principally for confirmation of diagnosis, it should be borne in mind that preliminary clinical examination may reveal just as much (or more!) information, particularly when the arthroscopist is inexperienced and the cruciate ligaments are poorly visualized.

Management strategy is based on the following facts.

(a) A haemarthrosis requires draining or washing out to facilitate rehabilitation.

(b) Over 50 per cent of patients with ACL deficiency recover sufficiently to participate in sport without surgical intervention (McDaniel and Dameron 1980). However, there is evidence that although the initial functional disability of ACL insufficiency may be minimal, the natural history of the condition is for progressive degenerative change some years later, and for a significantly increased risk of further injury such as meniscus tear (Noyes *et al.* 1983). Thus primary repair has its advocates; however, the consensus of opinion in the UK is to eschew primary repair and to achieve functional stability through intensive rehabilitation.

(c) Surgical repair or reconstruction should be considered on failure of conservative management after six months—that is, on the presence of the symptoms of functional instability (the knee 'giving away').

After aspiration the knee should be given functional support until full extension and adequate quadriceps/hamstring tone have been regained. In this acute phase there is danger of further damage to the knee. The use of a cast-brace should be considered (Bassett *et al.* 1980); failing this the use of crutches is advisable for two to three weeks, during which time range of motion and muscle-strengthening exercises are instituted. Initially isometric exercises are emphasized (straight leg raises and sets of static quadriceps contractions). Isotonic exercises for the quadriceps may be started in the seated position when an adequate range of motion has been restored (Fig. 7.8). Repetitions using light weights—for example, 2–5 lbs—are used at the outset; concentric contraction is achieved on slow extension, and eccentric contraction on slow flexion. For rehabilitation of the knee flexors the patient lies prone or stands, and performs both concentric and eccentric work using a similar range of weights (Fig. 7.9).

The subsequent muscle rehabilitation programme concentrates on the redevelopment in the knee flexors and extensors of strength, power, and endurance. Rapid isotonic repetitions with light weights are necessary to build up power and endurance. Isokinetic exercise may be performed after a few weeks (see Fig. 11.11, p. 193). The capacity of the dynamometer to improve the characteristics of strength (slow speeds—for example, 60° to 90°), power (fast speeds—for example, 240° to 300°), and endurance (repetitions at fast speeds) in both the flexors and extensors makes it a most valuable piece of equipment. In the ACL-deficient knee it is imperative that the knee flexors (hamstrings) in particular are fully rehabilitated. Inadequate muscle balance in favour of the quadriceps increases the likelihood of functional instability by contributing to anterior subluxation of the tibial plateau.

Subsequently bicycling, swimming, and then jogging are added to the programme. Care must be taken by the athlete at this stage—around two months after injury—to avoid any cutting movements. Participation in activities including such movements and start–stops should not be allowed until quadriceps and hamstrings are nearly equal in strength to the normal limb, and flexion has been restored to full range ± 5°. During rehabilitation constant evaluation is made, and adaptations to the muscle-strengthening programme are executed if necessary—for example, to accommodate the onset of patellofemoral pain. After sport is resumed a maintenance programme of exercises should be prescribed to prevent the insidious development of muscle deficit or imbalance. Modification of the intensity of participation in specific types of activity and/or a reduction in competitive standard may be necessary if there are subjective feelings of insecurity or instability.

Established functional instability, manifested by recurrent giving way, pain, and effusion, requires surgical assessment. First, the presence of an associated meniscus tear or mechanical interference by a stump of the ACL should be excluded at arthroscopy. The type of surgical reconstruction for ligamentous insufficiency depends on the exact nature of the anterior instability. Anterolateral rotatory instability (ALRI) due to isolated ACL rupture, or anteromedial rotatory instability due to a

FIG. 7.8 Isotonic exercise for the quadriceps is demonstrated

FIG. 7.9 Isotonic exercise for the hamstrings is demonstrated: (right) prone, (below) standing.

advantage of the use of autografts is the retention of proprioceptive function. A recent vogue is the use of the synthetic material, Gore-tex; an advantage appears to be a reduction of rehabilitation time (although concern is expressed about the presence of intra-articular foreign material). During rehabilitation the early use of hamstring-strengthening exercises and the cautious use of quadriceps exercises have been advocated by Renstrom *et al.* (1986). The importance of a prolonged well-balanced rehabilitation programme that allows adequate healing and strengthening of the ligament is stressed by Rovere and Adair (1983).

As an alternative to surgery, or in patients who have not benefited from surgery, a knee brace should be considered. Various knee braces are commercially available, including some with derotational constructions such as the Lenox Hill brace (see Fig. 12.2, p. 205). Hunter (1985) states that 'these braces attempt to limit rotation and prevent hyperextension, thereby minimising forward subluxation of the tibia on the femur ... but it is virtually impossible for any brace to mechanically substitute for the function of the cruciate ligaments and prevent excessive rotation of the tibia on the femur ... other braces provide patients with comfort and a feeling of support and serve merely as a reminder to the wearer to exert caution in sport activity.' Normally surgical reconstruction should be a logical first step in the reversal of functional instability.

Current surgical practice in the management of the torn anterior cruciate ligament—a personal view
John Ireland

The management of acute injuries of the ACL, and also of the chronic instability that often follows, remains controversial. A number of developments have occurred in recent years.

Acute ACL rupture is increasingly being recognized as the common cause of knee haemarthrosis resulting from contact and non-contact injury during sporting activities. The diagnosis can usually be made satisfactorily by detecting a positive Lachman sign at the time of primary presentation. Aspiration of the haemarthrosis often facilitates clinical examination and

combination of MCL tear and ACL rupture, require different techniques. Autogenous materials such as split grafts from the patella tendon have been used widely for ACL reconstruction; the basic procedure involves passing the graft through a drilled tibial tunnel to the lateral femoral condyle. Paterson and Trickey (1986) have reported good results, and advocate the addition of a MacIntosh extra-articular tenodesis in young sportsmen. An helps to confirm the diagnosis. The usually normal X-ray appearance unfortunately misleads the inexperienced casualty officer, who tends to adopt a reassuring stance, when a caution for the patient and a specialist referral are required.

An informed but conservative approach is the accepted practice in the UK when this injury concerns patients whose sporting interests are purely recreational. Arthroscopy is not generally needed in the early stages unless there is undue persistence of a block to full extension of the knee, or the relatively early development of symptoms which suggest an associated meniscal lesion.

Probably the most important therapeutic event at the outset is the advice for these patients that they should NOT attempt an early return to their sport. This must be delayed until as full a recovery as possible has occurred, and in the ideal situation it would only be with the approval of an experienced specialist. Premature attempts to return to the football field or squash court often precipitate early instability when a giving-away episode completes what may have been a partial anterior cruciate rupture.

When high-class or professional athletes present with an acute anterior cruciate tear a rather different approach is called for. If their livelihood or lifestyle is threatened by possible instability, early arthroscopy to establish the full diagnosis is advisable. If a worrying degree of instability is confirmed on examination under anaesthesia, primary ligamentous surgery may well have to be considered. Simple anterior cruciate repair has not been shown to have significant advantage. Nowadays, primary reconstructions are usually performed by the same techniques as those used in chronic anterior cruciate instability, but more often without an additional lateral tenodesis. Because of the increased likelihood of serious stiffness and the problems of 'arthrofibrosis', immobilization has largely been abandoned as an adjunct to anterior cruciate reconstruction when this is undertaken within six weeks of the causative injury.

Primary reconstructions may also be indicated where the anterior cruciate is torn in association with complete rupture of medial structures in a severe valgus-type injury. In this situation, central reconstruction would be undertaken without surgical repair of the medial ligament, and early mobilization would still be the rule.

In patients presenting with symptoms and signs of chronic knee instability, the high incidence of associated and significant meniscal lesions (75–78 per cent) must be remembered. Some 10 per cent of these will have an asymptomatic posterior peripheral separation of the medial meniscus. These particular meniscal lesions can be demonstrated satisfactorily by a high-quality double-contrast arthrogram. It must be stressed that the arthrography must be of the very highest quality. Poor-quality radiography is widespread in this field, and has often been counterproductive and confusing. Its usefulness is probably being superseded by MRI, although this technique does not always clarify the crucial site at the posterior periphery of the medial meniscus.

Arthroscopy is invariably the primary surgical investigation for the majority of these patients. There is very little place nowadays for open meniscal surgery in the management of the unstable knee. When ligamentous laxity has been detected, even the straight-forward removal of a displacing bucket-handle tear should be dealt with by a competent arthroscopic surgeon. It is not reasonable to remove such a lesion by open surgery when there is a considerable chance that it may only partly relieve the patient's symptoms and it may aggravate his instability complaint.

In a recently reviewed series of over a hundred unstable knees, substantial symptomatic improvement occurred in 40 per cent following complete arthroscopic treatment of associated meniscal lesions.

Only approximately 25 per cent of patients presenting with chronic anterior cruciate instability are likely to require a stabilizing operation. The vast majority of such patients are aged below 30. The precise anatomical diagnosis of the instability is crucial before any operative procedure is advised. This type of surgery should only be carried out by experienced surgeons with a strong interest in knee surgery. It is not for surgeons who deal with knees on an occasional basis.

The majority of knees requiring stabilization will need both central replacement of the deficient ACL and additional reinforcement of the stretched peripheral structures. The ideal choice of material for the central reconstruction remains unresolved. At the time of writing, there is no place in a primary stabilizing procedure for the use of a purely prosthetic ligament. The use of prosthetic ligaments may be justified in occasional cases of persisting instability when conventional autogenous techniques have failed. The use of a prosthesis may also be permitted in certain centres and under close scientific scrutiny for operations in which it is used as an 'augmentation' for an autogenous tissue reconstruction. The prosthesis may be seen as providing initial protection for the autogenous graft and may allow earlier mobilization than would otherwise have been possible. A major national review of the use of prosthetic ligaments has indicated an unacceptably high level of complications and of secondary operative procedures. While it is accepted that in some patients a satisfactory result may be obtained in the short term, the long-term effects of foreign material within the knee joint remain unknown. The unpredictable occurrence of disabling synovitis is another problem that has yet to be resolved. When infection of a prosthetic implant occurs, it is a devastating complication and cases have been reported where arthrodesis of the knee has been required following complications of prosthetic ligament surgery.

Most surgeons favour the use of the central third of the patellar tendon with bone blocks securely fixed in bony tunnels. Perhaps the importance of striving to achieve precise isometry has been overemphasized. There has been gradual refinement of the instrumentation for these techniques from most manufacturers. Controversy remains as to whether there is significant advantage in undertaking bone–tendon–bone reconstruction with arthroscopic assistance and whether the single-scar technique, introducing the femoral fixation screw into a blind-ending tunnel from within the joint, has advantages other than the obvious cosmetic one. Surgeons who favour this method will be less inclined to reinforce their reconstruction with an additional lateral tenodesis, and it is of concern that there appears to be a wave of enthusiasm for this type of surgery before the availability of satisfactory long-term results.

It is the author's opinion that an additional lateral tenodesis should be available in cases of severe chronic instability, particularly when the jerk sign is very obvious and increased in tibial internal rotation. This would imply stretching out of the secondary restraints on the lateral side of the joint, and it is surely unreasonable to expect an isolated central reconstruction to replace the function of these deficient structures as well as that of the originally torn ligament.

A less popular recent development is the use of pes anserinus tendons centrally in the joint as an alternative to the patellar tendon. Of course, by their very nature, tendons cannot be fixed as satisfactorily as bone blocks can with interference screws. However, techniques have been developed which are sufficiently robust to allow relatively early mobilization and thus largely to avoid the patellofemoral complications associated with immobilization and particularly with the former use of patellar tendon grafts.

In summary, therefore, a cautious and conservative approach is advocated in the management of most acute ACL ruptures. In chronic instability precise anatomical diagnosis is of paramount importance. A two-stage approach to the problem is advocated, first dealing with associated meniscal lesions by closed arthroscopic means. Those patients who subsequently require a stabilizing operation should be concerned about the unpredictability of outcome if any prosthetic materials are to be used in their reconstruction. Conventional autologous ligament reconstruction using patellar or pes anserinus tendons can produce satisfactory results in the vast majority of cases. These operations will require additional gestures to reinforce deficient peripheral ligamentous structures. This type of surgery should be carried out under close scientific scrutiny and in special centres where the surgeon is concerned predominantly with knee problems of this nature.

Posterior cruciate ligament tears

The PCL has a most important stabilizing function. Unlike the ACL, it is taut principally in the midrange of motion (maximally at 30° flexion). Its primary restraining function is to check posterior displacement of the tibia. When the ligament is ruptured symptoms are often sufficiently disabling to prevent involvement in body contact sports. Injury is relatively uncommon in sport, however—collision impact to the region of the tibial tuberosity with the knee in flexion is the usual cause. PCL rupture may also be part of a combination injury involving other structures secondary to severe valgus, varus, or rotational stress. The PCL is thus at considerable risk in roadtraffic accidents (by collision impact against the dashboard) and in those sports in which frontal impact occurs, such as American football.

Immediate pain is felt, and difficulty experienced in weight-bearing. Early swelling is a feature, with the type being dependent upon the extent of the injury. It is not uncommon for concomitant damage to occur to the posterior capsule or collateral ligaments, giving rise to posterolateral or posteromedial instability. The initial findings are extensive periarticular swelling and bruising. In the early stages there is considerable traumatic synovitis, and corresponding restriction of movements, particularly flexion. The signs that indicate posterior cruciate tear are as follows.

1. Posterior sag sign. With the patient supine, the hip flexed to 45° and the knee flexed to 90° the tibia drops back on the femur (Fig. 7.10). If both the hip and the knee are flexed to 90° and the heel is supported by the examiner or upon a plinth, the sag may be observed again.

2. Positive posterior drawer test. Posterior laxity is demonstrated when AP stress is applied to the knee maintained in 90° flexion. There is no excessive movement in 0°–10° flexion (negative Lachman's test).

3. Posteromedial or posterolateral instability tests.

   (a) Posterorotatory subluxation of the respective tibial plateaux when posterior stress is applied during rotation with the hip flexed to 45° and the knee flexed to 90°.

   (b) External rotation/recurvatum test. When the legs are held by the toes and lifted off the couch the affected knee slips back into hyperextension and the tibia rotates laterally (giving the appearance of genu varum). A positive test indicates posterolateral instability.

   (c) Reverse pivot shift test (for posterolateral instability). The affected limb is held in a similar way to that in

FIG. 7.10 The sag sign is demonstrated in a PCL tear.

which anterolateral instability is demonstrated, though in external rather than internal rotation. The posterior subluxation of the lateral tibial plateau that exists in 90° knee flexion is suddenly reduced as the knee is brought into approximately 30° flexion.

It may not be easy to distinguish clinically between a PCL and ACL tear if the signs of rotatory instability are difficult either to elicit or to interpret. In the presence of abnormal AP laxity at 90° and stability at 10° one suspects PCL deficiency. X-rays should be taken, as a posterior intercondylar fracture of the tibia may result from PCL avulsion, in which case an urgent surgical opinion should be sought. Management accords to the guidelines for ACL tears. At a later stage a surgical opinion is required if functional instability develops. It is unusual for the PCL-deficient knee to be compatible with contact sports, particularly those requiring sudden twisting and turning such as soccer, hockey, rugby football, and American football.

Lateral collateral ligament injury

This injury is also relatively uncommon, as varus stress occurs less frequently than valgus/external rotation stress. The supporting structures to the lateral collateral ligament may also be torn—for example, the biceps femoris tendon and the popliteus tendon. If the injury occurs in extension, the ACL is often torn in addition and demands surgical appraisal.

Varus stress tests are employed in both extension and in 30° flexion (see Fig. 1.11, p. 10). If laxity is found in extension there is associated cruciate ligament damage. If present at 30° flexion only the lateral structures are torn. Cast-brace management of lateral tears with intact cruciates may be considered along similar lines to those discussed for MCL tear.

Injury to the superior tibiofibular joint

A fall onto the flexed knee with the leg adducted under the body and the ankle inverted may derange the superior tibiofibular joint. Partial disruption of the proximal tibiofibular ligaments allows anterolateral dislocation of the fibular head to occur. The head of the fibula is found to be excessively prominent and may, in an acute presentation, be relocated by posterior pressure when the knee is flexed. In the subacute case the patient may accept the presence of minimal symptoms. Turco and Spinella (1985) suggest exclsion of the fibula head in patients who suffer from recurrent pain from the lax joint. Irritation of the lateral peroneal nerve that winds round the fibula head may be an additional complication.

Meniscus tears

Meniscal tears take many forms, from peripheral tears to midsubstance tears, and from full to split thickness in depth (Fig. 7.11). A vertical tear is common in young athletes; a horizontal tear is more likely with advancing age. Not all tears cause symptoms, particularly in degenerate menisci. The stabilizing function of the menisci has become increasingly recognized, so that if it is possible to leave the damaged meniscus *in situ* and repair the tear, or at least perform partial arthroscopic meniscectomy rather total meniscectomy, the likelihood of increasing instability (and of long-

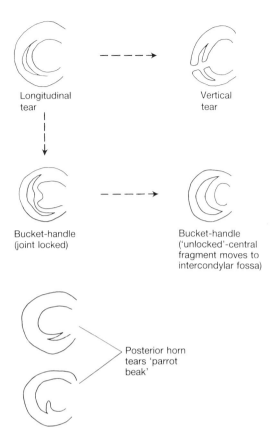

FIG. 7.11 Different types of meniscus tear may be found.

term OA) is reduced. This is particularly important when a meniscus tear arises in the already ACL-deficient knee. The combination of simultaneous ACL rupture and peripheral or posterior horn tear of the medial meniscus is common in an acute injury. The incidence of degenerative change when meniscectomy is performed in an ACL-deficient knee has been referred to already. Jackson (1968) has identified the incidence of degenerative changes twenty years after meniscectomy. In a prospective study Jørgenson *et al.* (1987) have highlighted the frequency of complaints and incidence of definite OA after meniscectomy for an isolated meniscus injury in an otherwise normal knee.

Injuries to the menisci, of which the medial is considerably more common than the lateral, usually occur when substantial rotational strains are applied to the flexed knee. A common situation is one in which a foot is fixed to turf by a studded boot (in soccer for instance), and thereupon rotational stress is imposed on the leg by the rest of the body. Sudden pain accompanied by a click is felt. A common sequence of events is for there to be initial recovery, followed by further episodes of painful giving way of the joint on twisting. Usually an effusion develops, which gradually resolves but recurs with each acute painful episode. There is often a subjective sensation of inability to extend the knee fully, with a subsequent return of movement on self-manipulation. With a history of this type of instability the examiner may make a tentative diagnosis of meniscus tear giving rise to bouts of intra-articular derangement.

However, it is necessary to ask for clarification when a patient describes the affected knee as 'giving way' or 'letting him down', as the following circumstances may apply:

(a) meniscus tear (pain on turning);
(b) ACL insufficiency (gives way on turning);
(c) patellofemoral syndrome (anterior pain on weightbearing flexion, such as descending stairs);
(d) loose body (sharp twinges of pain and/or fleeting locking).

As previously recorded, a detached fragment of meniscus may give rise to intra-articular locking and unlocking. In a bucket-handle tear the joint remains locked—that is, with loss of 5°–10° extension. This situation is not necessarily incompatible with walking or running: regrettably patients may experience considerable delay before appropriate management is instituted. The diagnosis may have been missed on initial attendance at a busy accident and emergency department, and the patient encouraged to exercise; alternatively the patient may have deferred attendance for advice until some time after the initial incident.

Less dramatic histories may be given by the middle-aged patient who complains principally of recurrent pain; commonly horizontal tears are found. The meniscus rim is then palpable at the joint line, and occasionally is capable of being reduced by digital pressure. Alternatively a flap is formed that is free to become trapped inside the joint. When this occurs in the lateral meniscus a type of flap known as a 'parrot beak' may be seen at arthroscopy. Degenerate tears of the menisci, usually the lateral meniscus, may be associated with the formation of a cyst that becomes palpable at the joint line.

Assessment

A history of acute rotational strain and recurrent bouts of pain and swelling is particularly important when a patient has a 'quiescent' knee at the time of examination. When present, the positive signs are due to the mechanical derangement within the knee on meniscus detachment, the associated coronary ligament sprain that inevitably occurs when a meniscus is torn, and the accompanying synovitis. These signs are as follows.

1. A small effusion if injury is recent.
2. A loss of 5°–10° extension with a springy block indicating locking. (Flexion is usually full, though possibly uncomfortable owing to accompanying synovitis). It may not be possible to differentiate from pseudo-locking in acute ACL tear without arthroscopy.
3. Restricted rotation, particularly external rotation.
4. Localized tenderness and thickening of the coronary ligament on the affected side. (In posterior tears these localizing signs are less definite.)

Other signs are particularly unreliable: the McMurray test relies on a click or 'clonk' on passive internal and external rotation of the knee in different positions of flexion, and is more likely to be positive with a posterior tear. The Apley test is performed with the patient lying prone and the knee flexed to 90°. The patient's thigh is firmly anchored to the couch by the examiner's knee. Using the patient's foot as a lever, his lower leg is subjected to internal and external rotation, first with distraction and then with compression (Fig. 7.12). Pain during distraction suggests ligamentous injury: pain on compression or 'grinding' suggests meniscus tear. X-rays are advisable to exclude other pathology, such as osteochondral injury. If there is doubt about the diagnosis, particularly in a patient with a quiescent knee and a history of recurrent pain and swelling, an *arthrogram* or (particularly) an MRI may give positive information (see Fig.

Fig. 7.12 The positions of the examiner and patient when performing Apley's test are demonstrated.

10.19, p. 179). Unfortunately a negative arthrogram does not definitely exclude meniscus injury, and *arthroscopy* may be required in any event.

Management

In the presence of a locked knee, probably due to a bucket-handle tear, immediate referral to an orthopaedic surgeon is needed. The patient should be supplied with crutches to avoid weightbearing, for comfort, and to reduce further damage prior to surgery. The practice of manipulation, particularly manipulation under anaesthesia, should be eschewed. Even if successful in moving the intra-articular detachment to a position in which extension is freed, the tear is still present and requires excision, not adjustment.

A *peripheral tear* is capable of healing (not so a tear in the avascular body of the meniscus). It is often associated with collateral and ACL tear. When the injury is isolated, there is often a history of a recent twisting strain and the principal complaint is of pain on certain activities. The signs are a trace or small effusion, localized joint-line tenderness and induration, and discomfort in the last 5° of extension. Nevertheless extension is of full range. A localized steroid injection to the coronary ligament soon restores painless extension, and quadriceps-strengthening exercises are commenced. Healing may be expected in approximately eight weeks. The practice of prescribing provocative exercises to establish a diagnosis should be abandoned, or otherwise a peripheral tear that is capable of healing may be converted into a more substantial tear that requires surgery.

Surgical management for a suspected tear through the body of the meniscus may be initiated by arthroscopy. Coexisting damage to the ACL may be noted, and a suitable strategy determined. Suture of a peripheral tear, if found, or trimming of the meniscus, rather than extensive meniscectomy, should be employed whenever possible. Modern management is based on the policy of attempting to save the meniscus, and thus maintain its shock-absorbing and stabilizing function if at all possible.

Coronary ligament sprain

The coronary (meniscotibial) ligaments are inevitably sprained during peripheral meniscal tear. However, rotational stress may give rise to coronary ligament sprain without meniscal involvement. Management is as described for peripheral meniscus injury. Coronary ligament sprain, particularly medially, is common in the middle-aged, when there is often no history of acute trauma. Pain is felt during activities requiring frequent knee rotation, such as golf or squash. It is not uncommon for the condition to continue to exist for many months, even if the provocative stress is withdrawn.

On examination the signs of medial coronary ligament sprain are discomfort on full extension (and sometimes on flexion and external tibial rotation) and very localized tenderness associated with slight thickening along the joint line. There is no effusion (and no history of swelling) and the quadriceps tone is well maintained. Treatment is by localized injection of steroid (for example, 10 mg triamcinolone hexacetonide (see Fig. 12.22, p. 220)) or by friction massage. If an injection is given the effect is dramatic: the pain usually disappears entirely within three days. Sport may be resumed within ten days.

Another cause of anteromedial or anterolateral joint line pain is *Hoffa's disease*, in which the alar fat pads adjacent to the patella tendon are traumatized. Tenderness and fullness may be detected on either side of the patella, extending to the anterior joint line, in knee extension. Surgical excision or trimming is occasionally required if symptoms are unremitting.

Osteochondritis dissecans

This condition in juveniles and young adults, in which an area of subchondral bone and overlying articular cartilage becomes non-viable and liable to separation, has been known for centuries. However, the aetiology (and to some degree the management) remains subject to differing views. The consensus of opinion appears to be that the primary fault in osteochondritis dissecans is a fatigue fracture in the subchondral bone. The favoured site in the knee is the lateral surface of the medial femoral condyle, although it may occur elsewhere, including the articular surface of the patella. It affects predominantly the adolescent, whose symptoms are of recurrent swelling owing to effusion, and aching in the knee. A direct relationship to exercise may not be apparent. If separation takes place, with the formation of a loose fragment, symptoms of intra-articular locking may occur. Such a history of locking (owing to a loose body) tends to be different from that caused by a meniscus tear, in that

the experience is fleeting, painful, and quickly reversed by a shake of the knee.

Diagnosis relies on an awareness of the possible existence of the condition in an adolescent or young adult with a knee effusion, as localizing signs are absent on examination. Radiological confirmation is necessary to establish the diagnosis (see Fig. 10.17, p. 177), although plain films alone do not reveal the capacity for healing. Scintigraphy (radioisotope scanning) is helpful: the healing potential can be gauged by the level of activity.

Management is by appropriate reduction of stress: weightbearing sports should be excluded. The patient should be monitored by serial X-ray or bone scan over a period of some months. Failure of conservative treatment and/or the establishment of separation are indications for surgery. Revascularization of the fragment by internal fixation is attempted, followed by early joint motion.

Indications for arthroscopy

Arthroscopy may be performed for diagnostic and therapeutic reasons. Referral to an orthopaedic surgeon experienced in the arthroscopic technique may be made for one of the following indications.

Diagnostic

To confirm the presence of a torn meniscus.

To confirm the presence of an ACL tear (partial or complete).

To confirm the extent of an osteochondral lesion.

To confirm the presence of a loose body.

To elucidate the cause of a haemarthrosis.

To elucidate the cause of an unexplained effusion.

To elucidate the cause of unremitting and unexplained knee pain (caused, for example, by a chondral defect).

Therapeutic

To excise or trim a torn meniscus.

To excise a stub of ACL (causing mechanical interference in joint action).

To remove loose bodies or a small osteochondral fragment.

To carry out synovial biopsy (in persistent or unexplained synovitis).

To repair damage to articular cartilage.

Summary of examination procedures for evaluation of acute knee injuries

The following information should be treated as a guide to the procedures to be adopted. As usual, a suitable examination routine should be based on the principles of motion, stress tests, resisted muscle contraction, and then palpation. The division of the knee into tibiofemoral and patellofemoral joints necessitates some overlap during each sequence.

History

Mechanism of injury
Pain location
Locking/unlocking

Giving way
Initial 'pop'
Swelling (immediate/late)

Examination

Standing/walking
Observation
- fixed flexion
- swelling
- limp

Supine
1. Observation
- fixed flexion
- swelling? intra-articular or extra-articular
- bruising
- femorotibial alignment
- patellofemoral alignment

2. Assessment of effusion
- nil (0), trace (1), small (2), moderate (3), tense (4)

3. Range of motion
- flexion, extension, and hyperextension
- nature of 'end-feel'

4. Extensor mechanism
- manipulation of patella
- tenderness of patella articular surfaces
- tenderness of medial retinaculum
- compression test
- Clarke's sign
- apprehension test
- isometric quads: VMO tone
- straight leg raise

5. Ligament stress tests
- valgus/varus at 0°
- valgus/varus at 30° flexion
- Lachman's test
- anteroposterior stress at 90° flexion in neutral, external rotation, and internal rotation
- pivot shift/jerk test
- posterior sag sign
- reverse pivot shift
- external rotation/recurvatum test

6. Meniscal stress tests
- McMurray's test
- limitation of/pain on rotations

7. Palpation
  a) tenderness
  - joint line
  - collateral ligament
  - elsewhere

  b) extra-articular swelling
  - joint line or collateral ligament
  - periarticular haematoma
  - swelling elsewhere, e.g. Baker's cyst
  - periosteal swelling

8. Mobility assessment of superior tibiofibular joint

Prone
1. Meniscus stress test
- Apley's test

2. Muscle function (isometric contraction)
- resisted knee extension (quads)
- resisted knee flexion (hams)

3. Range of motion
- confirmation of range of passive flexion

Radiology

AP, lateral, and patella films are requested (augmented if indicated by tunnel views), with particular reference to the following:
- intercondylar area of tibia (avulsion fracture at cruciate attachment)
- tibial plateaux (compression fracture)
- osseous fragments (osteochondral fracture of the patella or osteochondritis dissecans)
- femoral condyles (fracture sprain of MCL or osteochondritis dissecans)

Aspiration

(of haemarthrosis)
- observe blood/fat globules

Arthroscopy

if necessary (referral to orthopaedic surgeon)
- wash out joint
- diagnostic
- arthroscopic surgery

References

Bassett, F. H., Beck, J. L., and Weiker, G. (1980). A modified cast brace: its use in nonoperative and postoperative management of serious knee ligament injuries. *Am J. Sports Med.*, **8**(2), 63–7.

Cailliet, R. (1983). *Knee pain and disability* (2nd edn). F. A. Davis, Philadelphia, PA.

Ficat, R. P. and Hungerford, D. S. (1977). *Disorders of the patello-femoral joint.* Williams and Wilkins, Baltimore, MD.

Goodfellow, J. W., Hungerford, D. S., and Zindel, M. (1976). Patellofemoral mechanics and pathology. *J. Bone Jt. Surg.*, **58B**, 287–91.

Hardaker, W. T., Whipple, T. L., and Bassett, F. H. (1980). Diagnosis and treatment of the plica syndrome of the knee. *J. Bone Jt. Surg.*, **62A**, 221–5.

Hughston, J. C. (1983). Editorial: Anterior cruciate deficient knee. *Am. J. Sports Med.*, **11**(1), 1–2.

Hughston, J. C., Andrews, J. R., Cross, M. J., and Moschi, A. (1976). Classification of knee ligament instabilities. *J. Bone Jt. Surg.*, **58A**, 159–79.

Hungerford, D. S. and Barry, M. (1979). Biomechanics of the patellofemoral joint. *Clin. Orthop. Rel. Res.*, **144**, 9–15.

Hunter, L. Y. (1985). Braces and taping. *Clin. Sports Med.*, **4**(3), 439–54.

Ireland, J. and Trickey, E. L. (1980). MacIntosh tenodesis for antero-lateral instability of the knee. *J. Bone Jt. Surg.*, **62B**, 340–5.

Jackson, J. P. (1968). Degenerative changes in the knee after meniscectomy. *Br. Med J.*, **5604**(2), 525–7.

Jørgensen, U., Sonne-Holm, S., Lauridsen, F., and Rosenklint, A. (1987). Long-term follow-up of meniscectomy in athletes. *J. Bone Jt. Surg.*, **69B**, 80–83.

McDaniel, W. J. and Dameron, T. B. (1980). Untreated ruptures of the anterior cruciate ligament. *J. Bone Jt. Surg.*, **62A**, 696–705.

Marshall, J. L. and Rubin, R. M. (1977). Knee ligament injuries—a diagnostic and therapeutic approach. *Orthop. Clin. North Am.*, **8**(3) 641–68.

Noyes, F. R., Matthews, D. S., Mooar, P. A., *et al.* (1983). The symptomatic anterior cruciate deficient knee. Part I: The long-term functional disability in athletically active individuals. *J. Bone Jt. Surg.*, **65A**, 154–62.

Noyes, F. R., Bassett, R. W., Grood, E. S., and Butler, D. L. (1980). Arthroscopy in acute traumatic haemarthrosis of the knee. *J. Bone Jt. Surg.*, **62A**, 687–95.

Noyes, F. R. *et al.* (1985). The anterior cruciate deficient knee. *Orthop. Clin. North Am.*, **16**(1), 47–67.

Paterson, F. W. N. and Trickey, E. L. (1986). Anterior cruciate ligament reconstruction using part of the patellar tendon as a free graft. *J. Bone Jt. Surg.*, **68B**, 453–7.

Renstrom, P., Arms, S. W., Stanwyck, T. S., Johnson, R. J., and Pope, M.H. (1986). Strain within the anterior cruciate ligament during hamstring and quadriceps activity. *Am. J. Sports Med.*, **14**(1), 83–7.

Rovere, G. D. and Adair, D. M. (1983). Anterior cruciate-deficient knees: a review of the literature. *Am. J. Sports Med.*, **11**(6), 412–19.

Turco, V. J. and Spinella, A. J. (1985). Anterolateral dislocation of the head of the fibula in sports. *Am. J. Sports Med.*, **13**(4), 209–15.

Wiberg, G. (1941). Roentgenographic and anatomic studies of the patellofemoral joint. *Acta Orthop. Scand.*, **12**, 319–410.

8 Injuries to the ankle and foot

M. A. HUTSON

The common acute soft tissue injuries to the ankle and foot are described here. Overuse injury is described in Chapter 9. Ligamentous injuries are particularly common; it has been estimated that over five thousand inversion injuries of the ankle are seen each year in the Accident and Emergency Department at the University Hospital, Nottingham, alone (Muwanga *et al.* 1986). Although the majority are capable of healing naturally and uneventfully, it is often (incorrectly) assumed that the 'sprained ankle' may be safely managed by strapping or Tubigrip support. The frequency of injury is such that complications contribute significantly to the workload of the sports physician. The 'weak ankle syndrome' is common. This, and other conditions which result in a prolonged period of rehabilitation, are potentially avoidable, however.

Applied anatomy and biomechanics

The foot and ankle combine flexibility with stability, thus providing two main functions—propulsion and support. The propulsion that is required in walking, running, and jumping takes place in the various joints of the foot as a result of a complicated series of movements involving rotation and gliding. Stability is offered by the ankle and the foot in its pronated position. The *inferior tibiofibular* joint is a fibrous joint supported by the anterior tibiofibular, posterior tibiofibular, and inferior transverse ligaments and the interosseous ligaments. Although the move-ments are minimal, there is a little expansion when the ankle joint is fully dorsiflexed.

The ankle (talocrural) joint is a hinge synovial joint, consisting of the articular surfaces of the medial malleolus, distal tibia and lateral malleolus of the fibula (forming a mortise), and the articular surface of the talus. The talus is wedge-shaped, being approximately 2.4 mm wider anteriorly than posteriorly, thus allowing little or no inversion or eversion at the ankle joint in dorsiflexion. The lateral malleolus is situated posterior to the medial malleolus, thus creating an axis of rotation that is approximately 18° to the coronal plane. A greater range of dorsiflexion than plantarflexion is found. The capsular pattern of the ankle joint is more limitation of plantarflexion than dorsiflexion. Medially the joint is supported by the deltoid (medial collateral) ligament, and laterally by the three components of the lateral ligament.

The *subtalar (talocalcanean) joint* is a synovial joint, allowing movements around an average axis of motion that is 42° to the transverse plane and 16° to the sagittal plane (Fig. 8.1). It is supported by medial and lateral ligaments, in addition to the interosseous talocalcanean ligaments. Inferior to the medial malleolus may be palpated the sustentaculum tali (a projection of the os calcis), immediately above which is the medial opening of the sinus tarsi; this canal divides the joint into anterior and posterior parts. The lateral opening is found below the lateral malleolus. The triplanar movements that take place are as follows:

FIG. 8.1 The subtalar joint: axes of motion are 42° to the transverse plane and 16° to the sagittal plane.

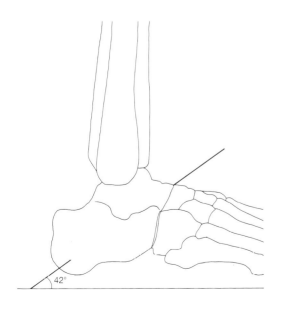

(i)   inversion/eversion in the coronal plane;
(ii) abduction/adduction in the transverse plane;
(iii) dorsiflexion/plantarflexion in the sagittal plane.

Pronation of the foot is a combination of eversion, abduction, and dorsiflexion. Supination is a combination of inversion, adduction, and plantarflexion. Clinically the degree of eversion/inversion at the subtalar joint may be gauged by moving the calcaneum when the ankle joint has been locked into dorsiflexion.

The *midtarsal joint* consists of the talonavicular joint medially and the calcaneocuboid joint laterally. The two axes (longitudinal and oblique) allow pronation and supination of the forefoot on the rearfoot to take place (Fig. 8.2). The oblique axis makes an angle of 52° from the transverse plane, and 57° from the sagittal plane. The longitudinal axis angulates 15° from the transverse and 9° from the sagittal planes. The midtarsal joint is functionally 'unlocked'—that is, a greater range of movement is allowed, thereby enabling the forefoot to accommodate to uneven surfaces, when the subtalar joint is pronated. At the interconnecting joints with the cuneiform bones further gliding and rotational movements occur. In the forefoot are the tarsometatarsal joints, at which gliding occurs, the intermetatarsal joints (gliding only), the metatarsophalangeal joints, which allow flexion, extension, abduction, and adduction, and the interphalangeal joints, at which flexion and extension take place.

Inversion Injury

The provocative stress is usually a combination of plantarflexion and inversion, although true adduction stress may occasionally occur. The primary restraints at the ankle are the ligaments of the lateral ligament complex (Fig. 8.3): the anterior talofibular ligament, the calcaneofibular ligament (intimately bound to the peroneal tendon sheath), and the posterior talofibular ligament. Threatened instability occurs in plantarflexion, when the relatively narrow posterior part of the dome of the talus becomes positioned in the ankle mortise. Up to 10° of talar tilt into inversion may be seen in the plantarflexed position in the normal

ankle—thus it is important when considering abnormality to compare with the contralateral normal side.

The initial injury at the ankle as a result of inversion is a sprain of the anterior talofibular ligament; with increasing stress rupture occurs, followed by rupture of the calcaneofibular ligament (Fig. 8.4). Further rupture of the posterior talofibular ligament results in dislocation. The importance of the establishment of an accurate diagnosis lies in the fact that untreated or mistreated ligament rupture may give rise to mechanical instability, proprioceptive insufficiency, or persistent capsulitis. Prolonged rehabilitation and/or the weak ankle syndrome are the consequences.

Assessment

A patient with a moderately severe ankle sprain may hobble or be carried into the consulting room on a stretcher. The stoic may attend with a flat-footed limp. However, a patient who retains a heel-toe gait has not sustained a recently ruptured ankle ligament. A history of the ankle 'going over' into inversion is usually obtained, although the ankle that is injured in an 'over the ball' tackle on the soccer field may suffer from direct trauma from an opponent's boot as well as indirect strain, and the history may be somewhat inexact. Early swelling and bruising, difficulty in weightbearing, and pain felt throughout the ankle region, though tending to be maximal laterally, are features.

Observation of the ankle and foot when the patient is comfortable in the supine position reveals swelling over the lateral aspect of the ankle extending into the forefoot, and bruising in the same region often extending to the toes. Soft tissue swelling may be seen circumferentially around the ankle due to infiltration of oedema. The active ankle movements are uncomfortable and limited in range. Examination of the passive movements of the ankle in the sagittal plane reveals restriction of both dorsiflexion and plantarflexion, particularly the latter, due to traumatic synovitis. All findings are compared with the non-injured side, which should be examined first.

The *anterior stress test* is then employed to assess the integrity of the anterior talofibular ligament. One of the examiner's hands firmly grasps the leg above the ankle whilst the other grips the

FIG. 8.2 The midtarsal joint. There are two axes of motion, oblique and longitudinal: O, oblique axis; L, axis longitudinal axis.

Anterior talofibular ligament

Posterior talofibular ligament

Peroneal tendons

Calcaneofibular ligament

FIG. 8.3 The lateral ligamentous complex of the ankle joint. The peronei are superficial yet intimately bound to the calcaneofibular ligament.

FIG. 8.4 Diagrammatic representation of inversion and eversion injuries at the ankle. (a) Inversion injury: rupture of calcaneofibular ligament. (b) Eversion injury: the possibilities are

- rupture of deltoid ligament
- rupture of tibiofibular ligament
- oblique fracture of fibula
- fracture of medial malleolus
- wide joint space on X-ray.

heel, so that with the foot in the neutral position force is applied to draw the heel (and therefore the talus and the rest of the foot) anteriorly (Fig. 8.5). If the anterior talofibular ligament has been sprained, the anterior stress test provokes discomfort, though it does not reveal excessive laxity. If the ligament has been ruptured, however, the *anterior drawer sign*, in which anterior displacement of the talus in the ankle mortise leads to laxity which is both seen and felt, is positive. In common with the findings on clinical stress tests of complete ligament tears in other joints, there is often minimal discomfort on stress-testing a ruptured anterior talofibular ligament; on careful examination the experienced examiner is often confident in his judgement in the non-anaesthetized patient. The *inversion stress test* determines the integrity of the calcaneofibular ligament (Fig. 8.6). In moderate plantarflexion the foot is passively inverted. This is painful for the patient with a sprain, and is often uncomfortable when the ligament is ruptured, possibly as a result of further traction on adjacent structures. Nevertheless, with experience, laxity may be detected by the examiner. Alternatively, anaesthesia (for

FIG. 8.5 Examination of the ankle: the anterior stress test assesses the integrity of the anterior talofibular ligament.

FIG. 8.6 Examination of the ankle: the inversion stress test (for the integrity of the calcaneofibular ligament) may require a peroneal nerve block or local anaesthesia.

example, peroneal nerve block or extensive local anaesthesia) may be necessary: should this prove to be the case it should be combined with stress radiography.

Resisted muscle contraction is used to detect abnormality of the peroneal tendons. Even if the peroneal tendon sheath is ruptured, as happens in association with rupture of the calcaneofibular ligament, there should be full painless muscle power (resisted eversion of the foot). However, when examining a patient with a 'subacute ankle', that is, one recovering from previous injury, it may be found that the evertors are weak. One of the differential diagnoses in the recurrently painful ankle is subluxation of the peroneal tendons anteriorly over the lateral malleolus, owing to rupture of the restraining retinaculi, and this should be excluded.

Palpation reveals maximal tenderness over the lateral ligamentous complex, although the associated capsulitis often results in additional tenderness felt medially. Tenderness in the surrounding tissues—for example, those overlying the distal fibula—is usually due to extravasation of blood and oedema, though at least AP and lateral X-rays may be required to exclude a fracture. Since there is capsular rupture in severe ligamentous injury and much soft tissue swelling in any event, the

determination of haemarthrosis is irrelevant and intra-articular aspiration is pointless. However, if there is little soft tissue swelling or bruising in the presence of diffuse bulging over the posterior aspect of the joint on either side of the Achilles tendon, indicating a joint effusion, this is a different situation, which is described on p. 136. (Haemarthrosis associated with osteochondral injury to the talus).

Further investigations. If the patient walks into the surgery and there is minimal or very localized swelling over the lateral ligaments of the ankle, associated with no laxity on stress tests, a sprain may be confidently diagnosed and X-rays are not indicated. However, a suspicion of ligament rupture, and therefore instability, may arise from the following:

inability to bear weight;
inability to walk with a heel-toe gait;
substantial soft tissue swelling and tenderness;
laxity on ligament stress tests.

Under these circumstances AP and lateral X-rays are compulsory. Stress X-rays should be employed under local anaesthesia (at least for the inversion stress test) if facilities are available. If not, the above suspicions indicate probable ligament rupture, and the patient is treated accordingly (Jackson and Hutson 1986). To avoid undue exposure to the clinician the radiological anterior stress test may be performed with the patient comfortable in the supine position, the heel resting on a small plinth, and a sandbag of weight approximately 4.5 kg applied to the anterior distal tibia; this creates a posterior distracting force to the tibia at the ankle, and thus an anterior distracting force to the talus (Fig. 8.7). Two minutes are allowed for the patient to relax his leg, after which a lateral X-ray is taken and compared with the non-injured side. A positive *anterior drawer* sign (Fig. 8.8) is one in which the measured distance between the posterior articular surface of the tibia and the most adjacent articular surface of the talus is 6 mm or more (Lindstrand and Mortensson 1977). Local anaesthesia or peroneal nerve block with 0.25 per cent bupivacaine or 1 per cent lignocaine may be required for the inversion stress test, in which the clinician passively inverts the foot; if local anaesthesia alone is used, this remains an uncomfortable procedure, and care is required. AP X-rays are taken, and once more comparison is made with the non-injured side. Talar tilt, when present, is usually quite obvious, being at least 10° greater than on the other side (Fig. 8.9), and indicates a positive inversion stress test.

One of four situations may be found and the following conclusions drawn:

(i)   no instability = a sprain only;
(ii) positive anterior drawer sign + normal inversion stress test = rupture of the talofibular ligament;
(iii) positive anterior drawer sign + positive inversion stress test = biligamentous rupture—that is, of the anterior talofibular and calcaneofibular ligaments;
(iv) normal anterior drawer sign + positive inversion stress test = isolated rupture of calcaneofibular ligament (rare).

Confirmatory investigations have historically included ankle arthrography or peroneal tenography. The basis of either investigation is that a tear of the calcaneofibular ligament inevitably tears the capsule and adjacent peroneal tendon sheath. Dye introduced intra-articularly or into the sheath thus extravasates into the other compartment and may be determined radiologically. The author's experience is that the peroneal tenogram

FIG. 8.7 The technique used for the radiological anterior stress test is demonstrated.

FIG. 8.8 A positive anterior drawer sign is present: the distance between the posterior articular surface of the tibia and the most adjacent articular surface of the talus is over 6 mm.

does indeed confirm biligamentous tear, though the need for this definitive confirmation in the presence of firm suspicions and stress radiological evidence should be critically questioned. To reduce the incidence of false negatives on stress radiology, it is highly recommended that maximal patient relaxation is employed in the manner described.

Management

Sprain. Early mobilization is imperative for the establishment of rapid normal function. The resumption of heel-toe gait, if this has been temporarily lost, and reduction of oedema are encouraged by the therapist. The adverse effects of periarticular swelling and immobilization if this is not done may be particularly disadvantageous in soft tissue injuries around the ankle. The application of ice, ultra-sound, and effleurage are usually employed. Friction massage is useful after three or four days. Strapping, for example

FIG. 8.9 A talar tilt of 20° is present.

double Tubigrip, is frequently applied to help reduce oedema and temporarily improve proprioceptive deficit. The efficacy of its mechanical supportive role is questionable.

Acute ligamentous instability. Although biligamentous rupture is more likely to give rise to the weak ankle syndrome, comprising recurrent episodes of giving way, pain, and swelling, uniligamentous rupture alone may have the same effect. Therefore, it is imperative for functional support to be supplied. Historically, orthopaedic surgeons have favoured surgical repair followed by plaster of Paris immobilization in the young athletic patient in whom there is definite evidence of recent tear

(Freeman 1965; Brostrom 1966; Staples 1975). However, virtually all observers admit that the prolonged rehabilitation time is a major disadvantage. Ruth (1961) reviewed the results of surgical repair and found a high percentage of patients with residual symptoms. Early mobilization and strapping, on the other hand, run the risk of recurrent symptoms from ligamentous insufficiency. Brostrom (1966) found that 25 per cent of patients with primary tears treated conservatively complained of subsequent instability. If used, eversion strapping should be reapplied daily to accommodate the gradually decreasing ankle girth resulting from reduction of oedema.

Experience with a cast-brace for ankle ligament tears at the Sports Injury Clinic, General Hospital, Nottingham over several years (Jackson and Hutson 1986) has suggested a number of advantages of this form of treatment. A well-fitting Scotchcast cast is applied from below the knee to the ankle. This is followed by the application of a plastic heel cup attached to medial and lateral plastic hinges (Fig. 8.10) and held by a Velcro strap. This arrangement allows a limited amount of plantarflexion, though no eversion/inversion. It is applied for three weeks; removal is followed by proprioceptive rehabilitation. The most gratifying initial effect is that patients are immediately very comfortable and resume a normal gait spontaneously. Other than comfort the following advantages embrace the very essence of early mobilization with functional support.

1. Muscle tone is maintained, thus avoiding the muscle wasting seen after immobilization.
2. Articular cartilage nutrition is maintained, thus preventing degeneration (Salter and McNeil 1965).

3. Sound ligament healing is encouraged, thus reducing the likelihood of reduction of strength (Noyes et al. 1974).
4. Skin hygiene is improved if the brace is constructed in such a way that the hinges can be removed from the cast, thus allowing washing.
5. Early return to work is possible, as the patient is able to walk with comfort. Safe and comfortable car driving may also be possible (not so in a POP splint).
6. Early rehabilitation follows, thus allowing the earliest possible safe return to specific sports training.

The Nottingham trial suggested that the results are no worse, and may be better, than with surgery and/or immobilization. Forty-one out of forty-two patients with radiological instability returned to sport, including a number of international athletes and soccer players. One patient failed to resume sport because of pain (though her ankle became 'radiologically normal'). Nineteen per cent commented on occasional giving way, though this was not disabling, and 29 per cent complained only of occasional twinges of pain. Of significance was that no athlete required further attention as a result of the 'weak ankle syndrome'.

An Aircast inflatable stirrup brace is a commonly used alternative to a cast-brace, and avoids the need for a plaster-room setting.

Proprioceptive, strengthening and flexibility exercises are commenced after removal of a cast or cast-brace. They should also be undertaken as soon as possible after a sprain, and when an athlete presents with the weak ankle syndrome. Manual resistive (isometric) exercises are performed in all planes of movement,

Fig. 8.10 A cast-brace is a useful form of treatment for lateral ligament tears of the ankle. Views from the medial and anterior aspects are shown.

with particular emphasis on maintenance of the strength of the ankle dorsiflexors and evertors. Subsequently isokinetic exercises are employed; when testing reveals a return to at least 75 per cent of normal muscle strength, jogging may be allowed.

Limitation in joint-capsule mobility is detected by manual testing, and corrected by active and passive exercises. Active range of motion exercises are started immediately. The use of passive exercises and mobilization techniques for the ankle and foot joints are particularly important after immobilization; they will be required to a much less degree otherwise. Anterior and posterior gliding movements at the ankle joint are particularly useful, and are performed during traction of the talus from the tibia.

Deep friction massage mobilizes the affected ligament as soon as reduction of oedema allows. Proprioceptive exercises have a crucial role. They include the use of the wobble board (an invaluable piece of rehabilitative equipment) and frequent tip-toeing exercises (Fig. 8.11). Finally, weightbearing stretching exercises, particularly for the calf muscles, are demonstrated to the patient.

Complications of inversion injury. Patients who suffer from recurrent giving way, pain, and swelling (the *weak ankle syndrome*) following previous injury should be carefully examined for evidence of mechanical instability. Absence of ligament laxity indicates the need for proprioceptive rehabilitation; a short course of treatment may improve function dramatically. A significant degree of laxity, particularly inversion laxity, should be managed initially by exercises and eversion strapping should be applied during sport. It is likely that, under such a regime, sufficient function will be restored to allow further participation in sport; functional stability is present, despite demonstrable (clinical) instability. If rehabilitation does not adequately control the symptoms—that is, if functional instability persists—referral to an orthopaedic surgeon should be considered for surgical reconstruction. The results of extra-articular carbon fibre, for instance, have been encouraging. The more traditional method of functional reconstruction, using the peronei, continues to be applied successfully.

Occasionally the signs of persistent *capsulitis* are apparent. Slight restriction of passive dorsi- and plantarflexion of the ankle, often associated with synovial tenderness or thickening, are found. An intra-articular injection of steroid—for example, 20 mg of triamcinolone hexacetonide—is a worthwhile technique. A suitable approach is between the tendons of tibialis anterior and extensor hallucis longus (see Fig. 12.23, p. 220). A 2I gauge needle is introduced in a slightly cephalic direction to accommodate the dome of the talus.

Occasionally a traumatic *capsulitis of the subtalar joint* complicates an ankle injury. This is not surprising, perhaps, when it is appreciated that a considerable percentage of patients with positive tenograms are found to have contrast medium in the subtalar joint (Blanshard *et al.* 1986). Furthermore, instability of the subtalar joint as a result of inversion injury has been described (Brantigan *et al.* 1977). Detection of subtalar joint capsulitis is made with the ankle in the plantigrade position; inversion/eversion movements at the subtalar joint are assessed using the heel for leverage, and found to be restricted (comparison is made with the normal side). Injection of steroid is usually helpful; a 23 gauge needle is introduced in a slightly cephalic direction from the superior aspect of the sustentaculum tali into the joint (see Fig. 12.25, p. 221).

Other inversion injuries. Straight X-rays may reveal an avulsion fracture of the tip of the lateral malleolus. This should be

FIG. 8.11 The wobble board is an invaluable piece of equipment for use during rehabilitation of ankle injuries.

managed as a ligament tear. A common injury is a sprain of the *calcaneocuboid ligament* in which localized swelling and tenderness, and pain on passive inversion and plantarflexion of the tarsus, are found. Occasionally it is associated with a flake fracture. It usually responds well, over two or three weeks, to local anti-inflammatory measures and instep support. *Avulsion fracture* of the *base of the fifth metatarsal* gives rise to localized pain, swelling, tenderness, and pain on passive inversion. X-rays confirms its presence (see Fig. 10.7, p. 172). A lightweight below-knee walking cast for between two and four weeks is advisable for pain control, though some athletes may be sufficiently comfortable in Elastoplast strapping alone. *Subluxation* of the peroneal tendons may cause temporary localized pain; it is not always recognized as such by the patient, and therefore must be looked for specifically if there is no evidence of ligament injury. Surgical relocation is indicated if recurrently troublesome. Compression injury to the talus may be a further complication of inversion stress (see 'Osteochondral injury to the talus').

Eversion injury

The tough deltoid ligament supports the medial aspect of the ankle. It is stressed by a combination of eversion and dorsiflexion. There is a range of relatively serious injuries of the fracture-dislocation type involving the malleoli and/or metaphysis of the tibia which are associated with deltoid ligament rupture (Fig. 8.4). They require the attention of the orthopaedic surgeon. An 'isolated' oblique fracture of the distal fibula (Fig. 8.12) is associated with some degree of disruption of the distal tibiofibular interosseous ligament. If there is no involvement of the medial ankle structures, however, it usually heals well in a B/K walking plaster applied for four to six weeks. Straight X-rays are necessary to exclude a medial malleolus fracture. In the presence of

FIG. 8.13 Tomogram revealing an osteochondral injury to the anterome-dial aspect of the dome of the talus (resulting from ankle inversion)

Osteochondral injury to the talus

A jarring injury to the ankle, such as is sustained by landing heavily on the foot, may result in chondral or osteochondral injury to the dome of the talus (Fig. 8.13). Inversion of the ankle is a common cause of fracture of the posteromedial aspect of the dome (Mukherjee and Young 1973). There may be periarticular swelling, though haemarthrosis within the ankle joint is more likely to have been sustained; it is recognized by observing the diffuse bulging in the para-Achilles depressions. Passive ankle movements are restricted in the capsular pattern, though there are no signs of instability and no pain on resisted muscle contraction. Tenderness is localized to the injury site, usually the medial or lateral margins of the articular surface of the dome of the talus; on careful palpation it is differentiated from tenderness related to the ankle collateral ligaments. In the subacute stage discomfort is usually felt upon the extreme of passive dorsiflexion. Initially X-rays may not reveal a fracture, and the patient may not seek attention until a later date, complaining then of recurrent pain on attempted running or jumping. AP X-rays should be taken with the foot plantarflexed as well as in the neutral position, when the typical lesion on the dome may be seen (Thompson and Loomer 1984). Further investigations by tomogram, CT scan, or arthrography may be necessary. Haemarthrosis has also been reported after stumbling with no evidence of chondral injury, presumably due to rupture of a small synovial vessel.

In the absence of major fracture, the haemarthrosis should be aspirated using the technique described on p. 137 for intra-articular injection; immediate improvement in symptoms is to be expected. Subsequent management depends on the severity of the injury. Healing may occur over some months, though radiological evidence of separation and history of repeated impingement may indicate the need for surgical intervention.

FIG. 8.12 An oblique fracture of the distal fibula is associated with disruption of the distal tibiofibular ligament.

NBI (no bony injury) localized soft tissue swelling and tenderness should not automatically be dismissed, as they may indicate deltoid ligament tear i.e. an unstable ankle. Orthopaedic surgical referral is then indicated. A partial tear of the deltoid ligament is recognized by a mild degree of lateral talar tilt on stress films and, when unaccompanied by a fracture, may be managed by a cast-brace in a similar way to lateral ligament tear. A sprain should be mobilized without a brace, though an instep support to prevent heel eversion may be useful.

Occasionally an isolated syndesmotic sprain (involving the distal tibiofibular ligaments) is encountered, and is identified by reproduction of pain on the combination of passive dorsiflexion and eversion at the ankle. In the absence of any other structural injury it settles quickly. In collision injuries, for instance in block tackles on the soccer field, a syndesmotic sprain is often associated with a partial tear of the deltoid ligament, and with a compression injury to the articular surfaces of the ankle joint. In this situation resolution occurs much more slowly, often over several months. Subsequently, heterotopic calcification of the interosseous membrane may be visible on X-ray.

Rupture of the Achilles tendon

Achilles tendon rupture has been well documented, though cases are regularly missed, particularly in the middle-aged and elderly. The sudden onset, with no history of extrinsic trauma (though the patient often suspects that he has been struck in the back of the ankle) should make one suspicious. It should be recalled that the action of the other plantarflexors of the ankle and foot, for instance tibialis posterior, may allow the patient to maintain the upright walking posture (after a fashion). Standing or walking on tiptoe is impossible; there is often excessive dorsiflexion of the ankle, and Thompson's squeeze test (loss of plantarflexion at the ankle on squeezing the calf) is positive. Careful palpation will reveal the defect, usually felt some few centimetres above the insertion into the os calcis. If necessary, MRI confirms (see Fig. 10.20(b), p. 179).

Debate continues on the relative merits of conservative and surgical management (Gillies and Chalmers 1970; Lea and Smith 1972; Nistor 1981). If the non-operative approach is used, a prolonged period of plantarflexion of the ankle by POP immobilization is necessary. The value of surgery lies not so much in the tendon suturing as in the removal of haemorrhagic material to allow closer approximation of the frayed ends of the tendon. Subsequent cast revisions to allow graded repositioning of the ankle into the plantigrade position are necessary, followed in due course by physiotherapy. Referral for orthopaedic surgical opinion is thus indicated. Patients should be advised that full recovery will take six months at the very least.

If the initial diagnosis has been missed, *partial* recovery of function is to be expected. However, the extensive fibrous union often results in permanent weakness of the calf that is noticed by the patient when attempting vigorous weightbearing exercise.

Summary of examination procedures

Standing/walking

1. *Observation*
   - limp
2. *Weightbearing ankle dorsiflexion* (squat)
   - except in 'acute' ankle injury

Supine

1. *Observation*
   - swelling? localized
     - ? diffuse
     - ? effusion within ankle joint
   - bruising
2. *Active movements*
   - dorsiflexion of the ankle
   - plantarflexion of the ankle
3. *Passive movements*

ankle	dorsiflexion
	plantarflexion
subtalar	inversion
	eversion
midtarsal	dorsiflexion
	plantarflexion
	inversion
	eversion

- abduction
- adduction

4. *Stress tests*

ankle
   - anterior stress test (anterior talofibular ligament)
   - inversion stress test (calcaneofibular ligament)
   - eversion stress test (deltoid ligament)
   - peroneal subluxation

5. *Resisted muscle contraction*
   - ankle dorsiflexion
   - ankle plantarflexion
   - inversion
   - eversion

6. *Palpation*
   - localized tenderness

Prone

1. *Observation*
   - ankle effusion
   - Achilles swelling
2. *Palpation*
   - Thompson's squeeze test
   - Achilles defect

References

Blanshard, K. S., Finlay, D. B. L., Scott, D. J. A., Ley, C. C., *et al.* (1986). A radiological analysis of lateral ligament injuries of the ankle. *Clin. Radiol.*, **37**, 247–51.

Brantigan, J. W., Pedegana, L. R., and Lippert, F. G. (1977). Instability of the subtalar joint. *J. Bone Jt. Surg.*, **59A**, 321–4.

Brostrom, L. (1966). Sprained ankles; treatment and prognosis in recent ligament rupture. *Acta Chir. Scand.*, **132**, 537–50.

Freeman, M. A. R. (1965). Treatment of ruptures of the lateral ligament of the ankle. *J. Bone Jt. Surg.*, **47B**, 661–8.

Gillies, H. and Chalmers, J. (1970). The management of fresh ruptures of the tendoachillies. *J. Bone Jt. Surg.*, **52A**, 337–43.

Jackson, P. J. and Hutson, M. A. (1986). Cast brace treatment of ankle sprains. *Injury*, **17**, 251–5.

Lea, R. B. and Smith, L. (1972). Non-surgical treatment of tendoachilles rupture. *J. Bone Jt. Surg.*, **54A**, 1398–1407.

Lindstrand, A. and Mortensson, W. (1977). Anterior instability in the ankle joint following acute lateral sprain. *Acta Radiol. Diagn.*, **18**, 529–39.

Mukherjee, S. K. and Young, A. B. (1973). Dome fractures of the talus *J Bone Jt. Surg.*, **55B**, 319–26.

Muwanga, C. L., Quinton, D. N., Sloan, J. P., Gillies, P., *et al.* (1986). A new treatment of stable lateral ligament injuries of the ankle joint. *Injury*, **17**, 380–2.

Nistor, L. (1981). Surgical and non-surgical treatment of Achilles tendon rupture. *J. Bone Jt. Surg.*, **63A**, 394–9.

Noyes, F. R., Torvik, P. T., Hyde, W. B., *et al.* (1974). Biomechanics of ligament failure. *J. Bone Jt. Surg.*, **56A**, 1406–18.

Ruth, C. H. J. (1961). The surgical treatment of injuries of the fibular collateral ligament of the ankle. *J. Bone Jt. Surg*, **43A**, 229–39.

Salter, R. B. and McNeill, R. (1965). Pathological changes in articular cartilage secondary to persistent joint deformity. *J. Bone Jt. Surg.*, **47B**, 185–6.

Staples, O. S. (1975). Ruptures of the fibular collateral ligament of the ankle. *J. Bone Jt. Surg.*, **57A**, 101–7.

Thompson, J. P. and Loomer, R. L. (1984). Osteochondral lesions of the talus in a sports medicine clinic. *Am. J. Sports Med.*, **12**, 460–3.

9 Lower limb muscle and overuse injuries

M. A. HUTSON AND M. J. ALLEN

Muscle injury

M. A. HUTSON

Introduction

Since skeletal muscle contributes approximately 45 per cent of an average individual's body weight it is not surprising that, statistically, muscle injury is particularly common in sport. Fibre-type composition in different muscles has some relevance to patterns of injury, injury prevention, and rehabilitation (see Chapter 1).

Research has shown that athletes of national and international standard have fibre-type compositions that would seem to be advantageous for their particular sport. Sprinters have a high percentage of fast-twitch (FT) fibres, and endurance athletes a high percentage of (ST) slow-twitch fibres. Muscles such as the hamstrings, rectus femoris, and gastrocnemius, which require fast propulsive activity, span two joints, and are the most frequently injured by intrinsic trauma.

Quadriceps injury

Injury to the quadriceps femoris may be either extrinsic or intrinsic in origin. Extrinsic injury is common: the frequency of direct contusion is related to the relatively exposed nature of the anterior aspect of the thigh. Intrinsic injury is also common, as overload is frequently applied in sports involving kicking: the kicker is usually injured when unexpected resistance is met—for example, in kicking a heavy ball, the ground, or an opponent. Jumping is another activity in which excessive stresses are applied to the quadriceps.

The site of injury is usually the rectus femoris, which is the only component of the quadriceps that spans both the hip and the knee joints. A complete tear of the rectus femoris is not unusual, though subsequent loss of function is often only slight. The defect in the muscle may not be palpable initially, as swelling soon occurs. It becomes obvious after some weeks, when the swelling of the muscle belly (on contraction) adjacent to the scar may be confused by the unwary with a myosarcoma (see Fig. 1.5, p. 4).

Little difficulty is normally experienced in the diagnosis of muscle tears. Pain is localized to the anterior thigh, and dysfunction is immediate. Pain is felt and weakness is demonstrated on resisted contraction of the knee extensors; passive stretching is painfully restricted (Fig. 9.1). The basic principles of RICE (rest, ice, compression, and elevation) apply to early management. Of special importance during rehabilitation is the establishment of normal elasticity prior to resumption of training. Therapists and trainers should not allow their players to proceed to unsupervised training, particularly if joining other squad members in team sports, until the two 'Ss'—*stretch* and *strength*—have been restored.

The 'charley horse' injury is caused by direct contusion to the anterior aspect of the thigh. In its mild form it is well known to many sportsmen as a 'dead leg', which happily usually recovers inside five to seven days. In its more severe form, however, there is much swelling of the anterior thigh, and often a sympathetic effusion of the knee joint. Flexion of the knee with the hip extended is less than 90°—often 30°–45° only on day 2. Dysfunction is obvious, and the risk of myositis ossificans is very high. Subsequently, if myositis is suspected, X-rays are taken at least two weeks after injury. Acute quadriceps contusion is one of the few musculotendinous injuries which justify immobilization in a cast: a long leg cast for two weeks to rest the quadriceps appears to be effective in prophylaxis. A severely contused quadriceps may require up to six to eight weeks to settle and for restoration of the physiological parameters necessary for commencement of training. Surgical drainage is rarely indicated in the acute stage; subsequently, if an encysted intramuscular haematoma develops, a surgical approach may be necessary.

If myositis ossificans develops, immobilization is pointless and the time for resolution extends to three to six months. Although serial X-rays which reveal increasing bone maturity and contraction may be used to monitor progress, clinical appraisal is preferable. Occasionally an area of ectopic ossification may require excision if residual symptoms are still present after six months.

In the growing child the anterior inferior iliac spine (AIIS), the apophysis to which rectus femoris is attached, may sustain

FIG. 9.1 The position of the examiner and patient when assessing both contraction and stretch of the quadriceps femoris, and performing the femoral stretch test, are demonstrated.

FIG. 9.2 Avulsion of the anterior inferior iliac spine is demonstrated in a child.

avulsion fracture (Fig. 9.2). Therapy other than rest is to little avail in the first few weeks; thereafter healing occurs rapidly, and should be augmented by stretching exercises.

Tears of the quadriceps tendon and patella tendon are discussed in Chapter 7.

Hamstring injury

Injury is almost entirely by overload when the hip is flexed and the knee extended, as in hurdling and sprinting. The degree of injury varies from a strain which prevents full stretch of the muscle to a more severe tear that may cause pain on walking. The site of the injury is usually mid-belly, sometimes more proximally close to the origin from the ischial tuberosity. Pain on resisted contraction (Fig. 9.3) and restricted painful stretch are features of acute injury;

FIG. 9.3 The position of the examiner and patient when assessing contraction of the hamstrings is demonstrated.

prognosis is improved by the appearance of early bruising. The poor reputation that muscle injuries have for recurrence is epitomized by the hamstring tear. The usual cause is inadequate rehabilitation. On the question of predisposition, it is unfortunately only too common to find that either hamstring stretch or strength is poor on routine 'screening' examination of the asymptomatic athlete. As indicated previously (Chapter 1) those muscles which have explosive capacities require preloading by stretching for maximal performance and for protection from injury. Any biomechanical deficiency, such as hamstring–quadriceps imbalance, will lead to a tendency to recurrent breakdown.

Some patients complain of recurrent 'niggles' in their hamstrings, though overall function is adequate. This may be due to an increasing percentage of scar tissue resulting from previous tears; irritable foci may be satisfactorily treated by transverse friction massage.

Avulsion fracture of the ischial apophysis may occur in the child (see Fig. 1.13, p. 13): rapid healing over six weeks is to be expected. At the same site in the adult chronic traction injury, sometimes associated with an osseous erosion, may be caused by inadequate resolution of an acute tear in the muscle adjacent to the hamstring origin (see Fig. 6.13, p. 111).

Both sprinting efficiency and incidence of injury may be improved by eccentric conditioning of the hamstring muscle group. The knee flexors undergo eccentric contraction in the late recovery phase of sprinting (before foot-strike); the biceps femoris undergoes maximal stretch. The elitist sprinter generates propulsive forces earlier during the support phase, suggesting that the critical phases are late recovery and early support (when the foot descends rapidly and then moves back rapidly) (Wood 1987). Appropriate hamstring training is thus essential for sprint running.

Distally the biceps femoris tendon may be avulsed as a component of an injury that causes rupture of the posterolateral structures of the knee (see Chapter 7).

Adductor injury

This is principally an injury of the adductor longus. Rupture (partial or complete) may occur mid-belly, at the origin from the pubic ramus, or at the insertion on the linea aspera. Extensive bruising distal to the site of the lesion may be observed. Initially a boggy swelling is usually palpable when a significant tear has

FIG. 9.4 Wasting of the medial belly of the right gastrocnemius within a week of rupture is demonstrated.

occurred. Passive abduction of the thigh is restricted, and resisted adduction is virtually impossible. Although surgical management has been propounded by some authorities for distal avulsions, uneventful resolution may normally be expected following a conservative regime. Referral to an experienced therapist is advisable, as overenthusiastic mobilization may give rise to ectopic ossification (see Fig. 6.6, p. 106).

Calf muscle injury

The gastrocnemius component of the triceps surae contains a high percentage of FT fibres and spans three joints (knee, ankle, and the subtalar joint). Injury usually occurs when a sudden explosive contraction is undertaken: the patient feels a sudden 'rifle shot' in the calf. Initially the only method of ambulation is on tiptoe. The medial belly is nearly always affected, the usual site being a few centimetres proximal to the musculotendinous junction. Dysfunction is immediate, though maximal discomfort is not usually felt until the second day. Active heel raise on standing (and therefore normal ambulation) is usually impossible for ten days. Bruising and oedema tracking to the ankle are observed within a few days of injury. Wasting of the medial belly becomes obvious within a week or so (Fig. 9.4).

Initially a heel raise is required for ambulation. Various proprietary materials or pads are available. After ten days this may be dispensed with, and graded stretching exercises instituted. Unlike other muscles, non-weightbearing strengthening exercises are virtually useless. The function of the gastrocnemius is propulsion during weightbearing, and recovery takes place as ambulation gradually becomes more comfortable. It takes a month or more for the endurance capacity of the muscle to have recovered sufficiently for jogging to be resumed. At this stage weightbearing strengthening may be accomplished by overload—for example, by repeated jumps whilst holding dumbells.

A tear of the medial belly of the gastrocnemius used to be known as 'tennis leg' and was thought to be due to rupture of the plantaris muscle—this is not the case. Less severe strains also occur at the proximal attachment of gastrocnemius, masquerading as (and therefore requiring differentiation from) posterior knee or hamstring insertional strain. The diagnosis should be made by the establishment of pain on stretching the calf, either in the standing position (leaning forward) or when supine (the foot is passively dorsiflexed), with the knee extended.

At the musculotendinous junction injuries tend to take longer to resolve. (It should be recalled that the Achilles tendon is much longer than might be supposed from its colloquial appellation of 'heel cord'.) At this site, just inferior to the muscle bellies, injury may be best treated by a course of friction massage and graded stretching.

Overuse injuries of the knee

M. A. Hutson

Introduction

A wide variety of conditions resulting from overuse are responsible for those leg and foot pains which frequently occur in many athletic activities. Some are sufficiently common to have received colloquial names such as 'runner's knee', 'jumper's knee', and 'shin splints'. The signs on examination are often subtle. All require pathoanatomical identification and an understanding of the aetiological factors involved in their pathogenesis. Of these exercise risk factors biomechanical considerations, particularly involving the patellofemoral and subtalar joints, are of prime importance. Risk factors are identified and summarized at the end of the chapter.

Patellofemoral function and dysfunction

The classification and aetiology of anterior knee pain have for long been confused, though they are gradually becoming clearer with a greater understanding of patellofemoral biomechanics. One reason for the confusion is to be found in the origins of the term 'chondromalacia patellae'. In the past 'chondromalacia patellae' has been used as an all-embracing term to describe those clinical conditions giving rise to anterior knee pain which are categorized by the presence of the classical patellofemoral examination findings of compression pain, facet tenderness, etc. Since it is established that patellofemoral pain often exists in the absence of arthroscopically detectable chondromalacia, it is accepted that 'chondromalacia patellae' should be reserved for the histopathological condition that includes such features as softening and fissuring of the articular cartilage of the patella. Patellar and peripatellar pain are associated more frequently with a number of detectable abnormalities of patellofemoral function, which may be more fully understood by reference to the biomechanical function of the patella.

In extension the patella lies proximal to the trochlea. As the knee flexes the patella enters the trochlear groove from the lateral side, owing to the Q-angle that has been established by the screw-home mechanism of terminal extension (Fig. 9.5).

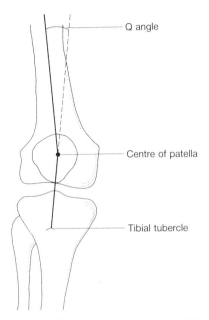

Fig. 9.5 The Q-angle is the angle between the line of the femur and the line of the patella tendon.

During flexion the patella is maintained within the trochlear groove by the combination of the relatively increased height of the lateral femoral condyle, the contraction of the oblique fibres of the vastus medialis (VMO), and the ligamentous support of the patella retinaculi. The contact areas on the articular patella facets vary as flexion proceeds to 90° (Fig. 9.6). Medial and lateral contact is equal at 90°. Thereafter, as flexion increases further, the patella describes a somewhat lateral course again—the medial facet enters the intercondylar notch and the 'odd' facet contacts the lateral margin of the medial femoral condyle (Goodfellow *et al.* 1976).

During extension the lateral shift of the patella in the later stages of the movement is accentuated by the abnormal Q-angle

Fig. 9.6 Contact areas of the patella during flexion (after Goodfellow *et al.* 1976).

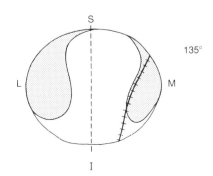

that is associated with external tibial torsion (see Patellofemoral stress syndrome). Alternatively, excessive lateral pressure upon the patella may be associated with abnormalities of the patellofemoral articulation, such as hypoplasia of the lateral femoral condyle, hypoplasia of the patella (Wiberg–Baumgartl classification III, IV, and V; see also Wiberg (1941) and Baumgartl (1964)), patella alta, and abnormalities of the supporting structures such as tightness of the lateral retinaculum, laxity of the medial retinaculum (for example, owing to previous dislocation/subluxation) and weakness/atrophy of vastus medialis. Such functional lateralization of the patella has been termed *excessive lateral pressure syndrome* (ELPS) by Ficat and Hungerford (1977).

The presence of wasting of the VMO is often secondary to prolonged patellofemoral pain. However, it may be a primary aetiological factor, and thereby play a significant role in the development of this condition in a percentage of patients, particularly adolescent girls. The specific functions of the different muscle groups within the quadiceps femoris complex are highlighted in long-distance cyclists, in whom patellofemoral pain may be exacerbated (or caused) by the fact that full knee extension rarely occurs, with the resultant relatively poor development of VMO, despite hypertrophy of vastus intermedius, vastus lateralis, and rectus femoris.

The pathological condition of *chondromalacia patellae* is characterized by the progressive features of softening, fissuring, fasciculation, and subsequently erosion to subchondral bone. It is often an incidental finding in conditions of the knee; when associated with malalignment syndromes the articular cartilage is not responsible for the symptoms of pain, which probably originate either in the sensory nerve-endings of the peripatellar soft tissues or the subchondral bone. It has been considered by some authorities that chondromalacia is found more commonly on the medial patella facet, which is not the facet that is the usual site of osteoarthritis (OA). Therefore, it is doubtful whether the one condition leads to the other: in the younger patient it is relatively unusual for chondromalacia to develop into OA.

However, *recurrent subluxation or dislocation* of the patella is very likely to give rise to patellofemoral OA. Such patellar instability may progress to a state of permanent subluxation or dislocation, in which case OA is inevitable.

Stress fractures of the patella are occasionally found. They may take the form of a transverse fracture across the patella, or occur in a vertical direction. If vertical separation occurs the condition may need to be differentiated from a painful bipartite patella, in which recurrent stress changes are found at the fibrous union (Fig. 9.7).

In summary, the known *structural abnormalities* which are associated with the development of anterior knee pain are as follows:

(i)   patella instability;
(ii)   stress fracture patella/bipartite patella;
(iii) congenital hypoplasia of patella or trochlea;
(iv)   patella alta;
(v)   VMO atrophy;
(vi)   lateral retinacular tightness;
(vii) OA patellofemoral joint;
(viii) Chondromalacia patellae.

Patellofemoral stress syndrome

Notwithstanding the possibility of structural pathology, the majority of patients who complain of exercise-related anterior knee pain do *not* have any obvious patellofemoral abnormality, and may be considered to be suffering from the patellofemoral stress syndrome. In the absence of patellofemoral pathology the most likely aetiological factors in those sports which involve running are *training errors*. James *et al.* (1978) consider that 60 per cent of all injuries to (long-distance) runners are due to training errors. When considering the possibility of inappropriate training schedules it should be borne in mind that the serious athlete, particularly the long-distance runner, may not utilize the degree of common sense that is commensurate with either his running experience or his intelligence. The inexperienced runner may have received little or no advice. In any event the motivation to continue to maintain schedules despite warning symptoms may be formidable. The 'high' that is associated with good physical conditioning in the endurance sports does not always promote a healthy detached attitude when decision-making is required in response to the needs of competition, injury, climatic conditions, illness, and a whole host of other situations. During history-taking it is often necessary to take considerable time over analysis of the training schedule for the purpose of identification of adverse aspects of training.

FIG. 9.7 A stress fracture of the patella which may need to be differentiated from a bipartite patella.

In a minority of cases there is evidence of *malalignment* that is associated with an excessive Q-angle. Genu valgus is one condition in which Q-angle is increased: 'thus runner's knee' is considered to be more common in women. The condition known colloquially as the 'miserable malalignment syndrome' is due essentially to increased femoral anteversion that effectively results in medial femoral torsion, 'squinting' patellae, compensatory external tibial torsion (otherwise 'pigeon toes' would result), and functional equinus and foot pronation (see Fig. 11.6, p. 188). When the syndrome is bilateral spurious genu varum is observed.

The cause of patellofemoral pain in cyclists may be a *technical* fault in the bicycle. Functional malalignment may result from a worn (or poorly adjusted) bottom bracket axle, excessive play on the pedal spindle bearings (or a bent spindle), or a loose connection between the crank and the bottom bracket.

Assessment

History. Irrespective of its cause, *pain* is usually located at the patella or the posterior surface of the patella. Other symptoms commonly complained of are 'clicking' or 'creaking' related to the patellofemoral joint. Although, when marked, this is a feature of patellofemoral arthritis, it is often present to a greater or less extent in the normal knee. Sharp twinges from the patellofemoral joint on weightbearing flexion—for example, on ascending or descending stairs—may give rise to a sensation of 'the knee giving way'. This should be differentiated from temporary locking, either due to a loose body or from ligamentous instability. Typically, prolonged sitting is accompanied by increasing patellofemoral discomfort.

Examination of the patient with chronic anterior knee pain should commence with the lumbar spine and pelvis. Hip disease and L4 root pressure both give rise to anterior thigh pain radiating to the knee. Knee pain only may be complained of. Examination of the patellofemoral joint often reveals varying degrees of tenderness along the medial margin of the patella and pain on posterior patella compression in anterior knee pain from whatever cause. Increased lateral mobility of the patella suggests the possibility of recurrent subluxation. Patella alta may be suspected clinically and confirmed radiologically. The Q-angle may be measured using a marker pen and goniometer. Wasting of the vastus medialis becomes obvious to the naked eye and is confirmed by palpation of the muscle undergoing isometric contraction. Further investigations include the use of radiographic techniques and occasional use of scintigraphy. The patella is viewed by AP, lateral, and skyline projections. The benefit of the skyline (tangential) views in different degrees of knee flexion—for example, 30°, 60°, and 90°—is contentious: however, it is clear that in certain patients with ELPS maltracking of the patella, as well as subluxation, may be determined by this means (Fig. 9.8). Increased patellar uptake on technetium scan is seen in a stress fracture. Arthroscopy is usually required when an effusion accompanies patellofemoral dysfunction—otherwise its usefulness is limited.

Management

The management of patellar instability should be dictated by the specialist knee surgeon. A variety of procedures are available once patellar instability has been established (Kettelkamp 1981). Medial plication and lateral release are acclaimed for their simplicity, though unfortunately they may not control the situation. The disadvantage of further procedures that adjust patellofemoral biomechanics—for example, the Elmslie–Trillat medial transfer of the tibial tubercle—is that they too may be unsuccessful, resulting in an increasingly disenchanted patient. It may be kinder in the long run to advise the patient who is disadvantaged by inadequate patellar biomechanics to resist the desire to pursue exercise that loads the patellofemoral joint excessively.

For a patient with patellofemoral pain (from whatever cause) that is not incapacitating simple advice to avoid exercises which

FIG. 9.8 Skyline views of the patella in different degrees of knee flexion may reveal lateral subluxation.

involve weightbearing flexion of the knee may be helpful. Thus hill running (or cycling) should be avoided, and exercises involving the squat position should be banned from training programmes. Reduction of stress by review and subsequent adjustment of the other aetiological factors—outlined later—is often profitable. The mainstay of any management schedule is to *redevelop the VMO*. Whether primary or secondary to the pathological process, wasting of the VMO requires reversal. A suitable isometric strengthening regime must be instituted and maintained for some time (Hungerford and Barry 1979). Abolition of symptoms in the mild case and amelioration in the more entrenched is to be expected. An understanding by the patient of the difference between isometric contraction (with the knee extended) and isotonic contraction (involving knee flexion, and thereby loading the patellofemoral joint) must be gained.

The use of patella straps to elevate the patella, and patella supports or taping to control lateral deviation, may occasionally be helpful. However, this should not be a substitute for adequate muscle control. Excessive rotation of the tibia associated with abnormal biomechanics of running may be prevented by the use of orthotics in the running or training shoe. Biomechanical readjustments in cyclists include alteration of the alignment of the cleat on the sole of the shoe, thereby affecting lower limb rotation.

Peripatellar problems

Superior to the patella

Stress fracture of the femur. Gradually disabling and poorly localized pain felt deep in the thigh and related to exercise should raise the possibility of stress fracture of the femoral shaft. Since the femur is well hidden by supporting musculature there are no abnormal signs on clinical examination. X-ray is mandatory, though it may not be positive for one to two months. Therefore, a technetium scan must be employed, and this will identify a stress fracture by localized increased uptake (Fig. 9.9). In

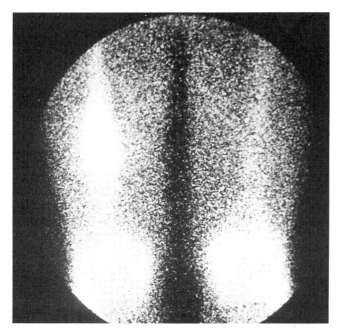

FIG. 9.9 A technetium scan reveals increased uptake in the femoral shaft due to a stress fracture.

common with the case of other lower-limb stress fractures, any form of running exercise should be discontinued, though non-weightbearing exercise, such as swimming or cycling, may be substituted as soon as the initial discomfort has settled. It is usually safe to resume running after three months provided that there is no discomfort on walking or jumping.

Quadriceps tendinitis. Discomfort is felt in the suprapatellar region, and may be reproduced on examination by stretching the quadriceps and upon resisted contraction. Crepitus may be present. Localized tenderness confirms the diagnosis, and guides the physiotherapist in the application of anti-inflammatory modalities. Ice, ultrasound, and transverse friction are complemented by quadriceps-stretching exercises.

Medial to the patella

Synovial plica syndrome (syn. synovial shelf or medial shelf syndrome). In the majority of the general population a synovial plica is palpable, running vertically alongside the medial border of the patella. It may become symptomatic, and give rise to anteromedial knee pain, when hypertrophied, either as a result of trauma or overuse. It is not uncommon in the trailing leg of hurdlers as a result of repeated trauma. Clicking may be complained of, and may need to be differentiated from retropatellar crepitus. Careful palpation reveals marked tenderness of the plica (as opposed to the medial border of the patella). Occasionally a small effusion may be present. Management by localized steroid injections may be attempted. In the refractory case arthroscopy confirms the diagnosis, and excision of the plica ('plicectomy') may be curative.

Medial retinaculitis. It is postulated that the retinaculi may be the source of pain in a considerable percentage of patients with patellofemoral pain. The medial retinaculum is torn in acute lateral dislocation of the patella, and is tender for a while afterwards. As an overuse injury, careful palpation may reveal tenderness that is felt in the soft tissues rather than the patella.

Medial coronary ligament sprain. This is a common lesion found in the middle-aged athlete engaged in sports that necessitate frequent knee rotation, such as squash or golf. It is also frequently a source of pain in the osteoarthritic knee. Alternatively it may be secondary to a torn or degenerate medial meniscus. Pain is usually present after exercise, and may subsequently prevent exercise. When unaccompanied by intra-articular pathology there is no effusion; discomfort is elicited at the extreme of flexion, and on passive external rotation of the tibia. Slight thickening and tenderness, well localized to the joint line, are found. The condition responds dramatically to one steroid injection—for example, triamcinolone hexacetonide 10 mg—followed by two weeks' rest from exercise (see Fig. 12.22, p. 220). The presence of an effusion increases the likelihood of an underlying degenerate meniscus or OA. Even in the presence of established OA, injection may give considerable relief. An alternative remedy is transverse friction massage; however, this takes significantly longer to be effective.

Chronic medial ligament sprain. Although this condition undoubtedly occurs it is often a mistaken diagnosis for coronary ligament sprain. It occurs in those sports, for instance breaststroke swimming, that involve repeated valgus/external rotation strain to the knee. In the child this is said to be the cause of 'breast-stroker's knee', though in this condition stress at the distal femoral epiphysis may be an additional factor. An inflammatory reaction at the proximal attachment of the medial collateral ligament (MCL) may be secondary to ectopic calcification (Pelligrini–Steida syndrome) (Fig. 9.10). A localized steroid

FIG. 9.10 Ectopic calcification in the femoral attachment of the MCL in the Pelligrini-Steida syndrome.

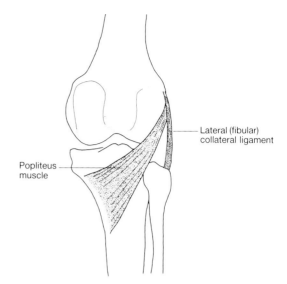

FIG. 9.11 The posterior aspect of the knee demonstrating the attachments of the popliteus.

injection is usually helpful. Orthotics for the training shoe and temporary avoidance of provocative stress may be required for the chronic MCL sprain that is secondary to excessive tibial rotation.

Anserine bursitis. A bursa usually exists deep to the pes anserinus (combined tendons of sartorius, gracilis, and semitendinosus). A bursitis secondary to overuse causes a nagging medial knee ache. Soft tissue swelling and tenderness is found several centimetres distal to the joint line, and therefore should not be confused with joint line lesions. Movements of the knee and resisted muscle-contraction tests are usually normal. Localized anti-inflammatory measures are required.

Stress fracture of the tibia. This may arise in the proximal metaphysis, particularly in the young adult, and give rise to tenderness of the tibia with overlying oedema (see Fig. 10.11, p. 174). It is said to be more common in patients with genu varum.

Tendinitis of the medial hamstrings. Both hamstring stretch and resisted contraction (knee flexion and medial rotation) may be uncomfortable, though not markedly so. Tenderness is localized to the affected tendon, and is difficult to manage other than by relative rest. If weakness of the hamstrings is found, appropriate strengthening exercises are prescribed.

Lateral to the patella

There are a number of conditions which arise in close proximity to each other (see Fig. 7.3, p. 116).

Iliotibial tract (syn. band) syndrome. This common condition, usually found in long-distance runners, is an inflammatory reaction caused by friction between the iliotibial tract and the under-lying lateral femoral condyle. It is more common when the iliotibial tract is tight, and is thus found in patients with genu varum or hyperpronation of the foot, and in runners who persistently run on heavily cambered roads or on banked bends (which causes varus stress on the lower leg) during the indoor sprinting season. When acute it is accompanied by palpable crepitus. When less severe, tenderness is well localized to the proximal margin of the lateral condyle adjacent to the tract. It usually takes several weeks to resolve, and may be helped initally by anti-inflammatory measures, including steroid injection, and subsequently by stretching the iliotibial tract (see Fig. 11.14, p. 199). Orthotics are occasionally required.

Popliteal tendinitis (tendinitis of the tendon of the popliteus). The tendon of the popliteus is attached proximally to the lateral aspect of the lateral femoral condyle, having an intimate relationship with the lateral meniscus (and its associated popliteal bursa), and for some of its course blending with the capsule of the knee joint and lined by synovium. Its distal muscle attachment is to the posteromedial aspect of the tibia (Fig. 9.11). It medially rotates the tibia, being involved in the early phase of knee flexion from the extended position. It also assists the posterior cruciate ligament in restraining anterior displacement of the femur on the tibia, for instance in downhill running. In this situation additional stress is imposed on the posterolateral aspect of the knee owing to hyperpronation of the foot. Therefore, overuse injury is often secondary to excessive hill running (Andrews 1983). In common with the medial hamstrings pain may be reproduced on resisted medial tibial rotation. Tenderness is localized to the tendon attachment, posterior and distal to the source of iliotibial tract pain, and anterior to the biceps femoris tendon. Reduction of abnormal biomechanical stress and localized steroid injections are the mainstays of treatment.

Cyst of the lateral meniscus. Although a lateral coronary ligament sprain, comparable to medial coronary ligament sprain, is relatively rare, a cyst of the lateral meniscus is more common. It is often associated with an abnormal (discoid) meniscus and may require excision. Movements of the knee may be uncomfortable at the extremes of range, though they are largely unrestricted. A palpable cyst is often approximately 1 cm in diameter, though its size varies in different positions of the joint. An inflammatory reaction appears to be involved in the causation of symptoms, as a steroid injection is often helpful and may abolish the need for surgery.

Biceps femoris tendinitis. This apparently affects certain groups of sportsmen, for instance, cyclists, though it does not appear to be very common. Diagnosis and management are similar to that for medial hamstring tendon strain. Cyclists are usually accustomed to adjusting the distance between their seat and the pedals in an attempt to resolve such problems.

Inferior to the patella

Patella tendinitis (jumper's knee). In one form or another this is an extremely common complaint. In high jumping, excessive knee extensor activity is required to translate the horizontal approach into vertical lift. In weight-training and weight-lifting regimes additional loading is applied to the patella tendon by various forms of hand-held weights. In its mild form it may be considered to be an enthesitis of the superior attachment of the patella tendon to the inferior pole of the patella (when it is sometimes referred to as 'patella apicitis'). Discomfort is well localized by the patient to the pathological site and in common with patellofemoral disorders, is felt principally under conditions of weight-bearing flexion. Histologically it affects the calcification front (the so-called 'blue line' transition of fibres) between bone and mature tendon. Discretely localized tenderness and thickening of the proximal tendon are often the only positive signs on examination, though the squat position may become uncomfortable. In common with Achilles tendinitis a spectrum of pathology is possible, so that in its more severe form partial rupture of the patella tendon may be found. Swelling is then more substantial and dysfunction more profound. Occasionally complete rupture occurs.

A self-perpetuating inflammatory response occurs, so that spontaneous resolution may be extremely slow. Physiotherapeutic modalities are often ineffective. Although intratendinous steroid injections are eschewed, localized injections around the medial or lateral aspect of the lesion are often helpful, and may need to be repeated. However, reduction of stress is necessary. Bodybuilders and weight-lifters who depend on quadriceps loading in knee flexion for good muscle definition and strength find this particularly frustrating, as they need to rely for some time on isometric contraction only. Athletes involved in jumping and racket sports must restrict their levels of activity or consider exercising on a different more resilient surface if appropriate. In common with other enthesopathies, surgical debridement is occasionally required. Cystic lesions within the patella tendon distal to the lower pole of the patella have been described by King *et al.* (1990). CT scanning, MRI, and ultrasound reveal the lesion, which may be treated effectively by excision and paratenon strip. Partial rupture usually responds to conservative measures, though complete rupture requires surgery.

Soft tissue lateral X-rays reveal thickening of the patella tendon in the more severe cases (Fig. 9.12). In the presence of infrapatellar swelling this may assist in the differential diagnosis between 'jumper's knee' and infrapatellar bursitis. Both infrapatellar and prepatellar bursitis are the result of repeated friction ('housemaid's' or 'beat' knee), and require local anti-inflammatory measures to aid resolution.

Sinding–Larsen–Johannson syndrome is the juvenile form of jumper's knee. Small fragments of bone from the inferior pole of

FIG. 9.12 Soft tissue lateral X-rays of the knee may reveal swelling of the patella tendon in partial rupture.

the patella, representing a chronic traction osteochondrosis, may appear on X-ray. Reduction (or temporary restriction) of exercise for some months is necessary.

Osgood–Schlatter's disease. This is so common that many parents of affected children have heard of the condition. It occurs mainly in active boys aged 12 to 14, and is a similar traction osteochondrosis to Sinding–Larsen–Johannson syndrome, though occurring at the distal end of the patella tendon, causing fragmented avulsion of the tibial apophysis. Commonly a talented junior athlete increases his time spent on sport by becoming involved in representative fixtures at the weekends as well as his involvement in the school sports curriculum. Eventually increasing discomfort prevents his effective contribution.

The diagnosis is usually straightforward. Localized swelling and tenderness are the principal features. X-ray is often not required; if requested the lateral film reveals fragmentation and separation of the apophysis. Rest or reduction of activity is required for periods lasting a couple of months to a year. Very occasionally, with a failed conservative approach, surgical excision of bony fragments is necessary. Immobilization is rarely required, though it is occasionally used for short periods if this is considered to be the only effective way to reduce involvement in sport.

Shin pain

M. J. ALLEN

Introduction

The name 'shin splints' is most often used by doctors, athletes, and trainers alike as an umbrella term to describe lower-limb pain during exercise. It includes such distinct conditions as:

(1) stress fracture;
(2) chronic compartment syndrome;
(3) medial tibial syndrome (periostitis);
(4) muscle hernia.

These conditions commonly occur in young fit sportsmen and sportswomen, although symptoms may appear in patients of all ages and fitness levels. During the recent fitness boom, in which more and more people took up running, often unsupervised and without proper training schedules, it became increasingly common. In addition to walkers, casual joggers, and competitive runners, it also occurs in such sports as soccer, rugby, cricket, tennis, and aerobics. It results from the running involved in each particular sport. These conditions are never seen in cyclists or swimmers.

The condition most frequently encountered is chronic compartment syndrome, particularly involving the anterior compartment, which accounts for approximately 75 per cent of all patients suffering from exercise-related pain in the lower leg. Approximately 25 per cent of patients with shin splints have a medial tibial syndrome; approximately half of these syndromes are found in conjunction with a compartment syndrome, when they are an additional irritation rather than the major problem. Both compartment syndromes and medial tibial syndromes are bilateral in 50 per cent of patients. Stress fractures account for less than 5 per cent of problems, and are usually limited to the serious runner or 'pavement pounder' (for example, postmen), often being related to repetitive exercise and hard surfaces. Muscle hernias are extremely rare, accounting for less than 1 per cent of patients.

It should be stressed that none of these conditions is mutually exclusive; any combination of two or three, or even all four together are possible. Sometimes the patient may progress through each one in turn. This is not entirely surprising, as all can be regarded as 'overuse injuries' sharing the same underlying causes.

Pathophysiology

A stress fracture, as the name implies, is a partial fracture affection only one cortex of the bone which is caused by repeated exercise, often on hard surfaces. This condition is usually self-limiting, because of the acute pain, though if the patient does not rest it is possible, although extremely rare, for the fracture line to spread across the bone, resulting in a conventional fracture.

A chronic compartment syndrome results from an elevation of pressure in the affected compartment(s). There are four major compartments in the calf (Fig. 9.13), each of which is a separate anatomical entity containing specific muscles, nerves, and blood vessels, and bounded by an osseofascial envelope. The normal compartment pressures in athletes both at rest and during exercise are between 10 and 15 mmHg. In those patients with a chronic compartment syndrome the pressures during exercise will rise to exceed 50 mmHg. On exercise the increase in blood flow and retention of fluid by muscle causes swelling which, combined with the relative inelasticity of the fascia, results in an increase in pressure. As the pressure rises the blood supply to the muscles is compromised, causing ischaemic pain. When exercise stops the pressure drops, the blood supply returns to normal, and the pain ceases. All this usually takes place within a few minutes.

The pathophysiology of medial tibial syndrome remains unclear. Some authors suggest that it may be due to inflammation of the periosteum caused by abnormal or excessive pull of the muscles. However, this has not been borne out by the author's experience, when tissue removed from the periosteum has been examined both histologically and under the electron microscope, and has always been of normal appearance.

A muscle hernia is a defect in which nerves or vessels pass through the fascia. On exercise the muscle mass protrudes through the defect, and on reaching a certain size becomes strangulated, causing pain.

The reason why some athletes are affected by these conditions and others are not is unknown, though in certain cases it is related to biomechanical factors—for example, overpronation resulting in muscle hypertrophy.

Clinical presentation

Stress fracture. Patients complain of an acute or subacute onset of lower limb pain that is well localized, normally to the lower third of the tibia or fibula. There is very well localized bony tenderness. Tapping the affected bone reveals a specific fingertip area of tenderness. Palpable callus may be present.

Chronic compartment syndrome. A gradual onset of cramp-like pain is experienced. This may increase over a period of time to such an intensity as to make running impossible. On ceasing exercise the pain usually subsides over a short period of time (usually minutes or a few hours). Occasionally it may take longer, perhaps even as long as a day. The pain may be localized to the lateral side of the calf (anterior compartment) or to the inner aspect of the calf (posterior compartment) (Fig. 9.13). This occurs in approximately 50 per cent of cases, and in the other half the pain is poorly localized and felt throughout the whole of the calf. It is extremely rare to have a chronic compartment syndrome of the lateral or superficial compartments. Occasionally pain may be accompanied by distal neurological symptoms, such as tingling in the foot during exercise.

Fig. 9.13 Compartment syndromes:
(a) anatomy of the calf compartments;
(b) site of localization of pain to the anterior
compartment; (c) site of localization of pain to
the deep posterior compartment

Examination is invariably normal, other than the possibility of some slight lower tibial border tenderness in those with deep posterior compartment involvement.

Medial tibial syndromes. The pain is described as either cramp-like or aching in character, and can occur either during or after exercise. When compared with compartment pain it usually takes much longer to disappear—periods of days, or even constant pain, are not unusual. It can vary from an irritable niggle to being totally incapacitating. The pain is always felt in the inner aspect of the leg over the inner tibial border, usually the lower third. On examination there is always an acutely tender area to palpation in the lower third of the inner aspect of the tibia.

Muscle hernia. This produces a localized intense pain around the fascial defect which is directly proportional to the amount of exercise. On ceasing exercise the pain rapidly disappears. Fascial defects may be papable. They are usually fairly small, about the size of a fingertip, and usually involve the anterior compartment fascia. On stressing the affected muscle (tibialis anterior) against resistance a noticeable lump is apparent.

Investigations

Plain radiographs are important to exclude other conditions such as bone tumour. A stress fracture will not appear on a plain X-ray until several weeks after the onset of symptoms, when either a transverse fracture line or callus formation may

be seen. Hence they are only of use for confirmation of the diagnosis. In all other conditions the radiograph is normal. Tibial cortical hypertrophy may be present, though this is not a pathological entity, and is seen equally in normal athletes and those complaining of shin splints.

Bone scans are generally unhelpful. A stress fracture will show up, earlier than on a plain radiograph, as a 'hot spot.' Often a patchy uptake is seen, which is equally prevalent in normal individuals and those suffering from medial tibial or chronic compartment syndromes (see Fig. 1.3, p. 3).

Intracompartmental pressure monitoring (ICPM) should be carried out during exercise. This is achieved by placing a slit catheter into the anterior and deep posterior compartments of both legs and measuring the pressures as the patient runs. Figure 9.14 shows the technique involved. The heparinized-saline-filled catheters are connected to pressure transducers which convert the hydrostatic pressure in the compartment into an electrical signal which can then be amplified and displayed on a chart recorder. Figure 9.15 shows a typical recording obtained from a patient with bilateral anterior compartment syndrome.

Management

A stress fracture requires rest from running. Often abstinence from sport is sufficient, though occasionally the patient requires protective weightbearing in the form of crutches or a cast.

FIG. 9.14 Intracompartmental pressure monitoring during exercise.

duration are advised to rest for a few months before any further treatment is undertaken. Physiotherapy appears to be of little help in treating this condition. Surgery, when indicated, takes the form of a subcutaneous fasciotomy of the affected compartment(s). Post-operatively the patient should be encouraged to commence light activities as soon as possible, to prevent the fascia from closing over and the condition recurring. Athletes should be back to full performance in six to eight weeks after surgery to the anterior compartment, and after a little longer if the deep posterior compartment is involved.

Treatment of the medial tibial syndrome is difficult. If the symptoms are not incapacitating, the athlete should continue activities. Rest is generally unhelpful. Physiotherapy in the form of ice or ultrasound is also unhelpful, and occasionally the ultrasound may aggravate the condition. Steroid injections may be tried, though they tend to be of temporary benefit only. Surgery takes the form of a fasciotomy of the deep posterior compartment, followed by stripping the periosteum off the inner tibial border and drilling three holes in the tibia. The patient should not undertake any strenuous exercise for twelve weeks following surgery. It usually takes approximately six months before the athlete is back to full activities, although results are by no means guaranteed.

Symptomatic hernias should be treated surgically by a subcutaneous fasciotomy of the affected compartment. Closure of the defect should never be undertaken, as it usually gives a poor result and can lead to an acute compartment syndrome.

Differential diagnosis

There are many and varied conditions that may mimic any one of the causes of shin splints.

Sciatica resulting from a prolapsed intervertebral disc or spinal stenosis due to narrowing of the spinal canal may give rise to lower-leg pain. In the spinal stenotic condition neurological features may present in the lower limbs upon exercise. Such conditions are excluded by careful examination, followed by plain radiographs and computerized tomography or MRI if indicated.

Popliteal entrapment syndrome occasionally occurs, though it is very rare. Owing to the abnormal anatomy of the popliteal artery in the popliteal fossa, temporary occlusion may occur when exercising, giving rise to pain in the lower limbs. This condition is diagnosed by palpating the dorsalis pedis pulse with the knee flexed. If it disappears it is suggestive of the entrapment syndrome. Confirmation is made by arteriography. When dealing with a population of young patients it is rare to find

Training on soft grounds can be resumed after about ten to twelve weeks for tibial fractures and a little sooner for fibular fractures, depending on symptoms and radiological appearance.

Rest should also be prescribed for the compartment syndrome, as undoubtedly some individuals respond to a period of two to three months' rest followed by gradual resumption of activities, which should begin on a soft surface. This is especially true for the so-called 'fresher's leg'—that is, those young students leaving school and going on to higher education who suddenly and dramatically increase their level of sporting activities. Hence all patients with a suspected compartment syndrome of short

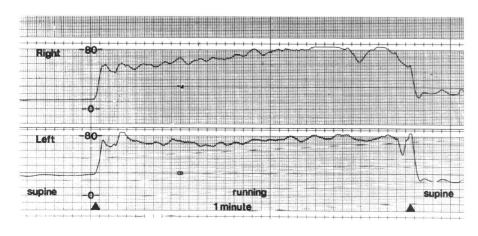

FIG. 9.15 Pressure recording of a bilateral anterior compartment syndrome (values in mmHg).

intermittent claudication, though this must be excluded by palpation of the distal pulses.

Very occasionally a bone tumour, either benign or malignant, may mimic shin splints. It should be excluded by plain radiographs of the leg.

Occasionally chronic muscle injury or tenosynovitis may be mistaken for shin splints.

Superficial peroneal nerve entrapment may mimic anterior compartment pain. This occurs when the superficial peroneal nerve becomes trapped at the level of its exit through the fascia, giving rise to symptoms in the leg. Diagnosis is often difficult, and EMGs are often not conclusive. Clinically, patients will have a positive Tinel's test. A trial injection of local anaesthetic at the site where the nerve passes through the fascia alleviates symptoms. Once a positive diagnosis has been confirmed the condition can be relieved by surgery.

Compression of the deep peroneal nerve (in the anterior compartment) may occur with an acute compartment syndrome. This is occasionally seen when a very intensive burst of activity is taken by a normally sedentary person. Alternatively it follows direct soft tissue trauma (contusion of the muscles in the anterior compartment) or a fracture, or it may occur as a complication of surgery on the tibia. The symptoms are throbbing and paraesthesia, followed by anaesthesia, in the web between the first and second toes. Icing and elevation are required. If there is doubt about the viability of the compartment tissues, particularly if motor weakness develops, referral for decompression should be undertaken.

Overuse injuries of the ankle and foot

M. A. HUTSON

Anterior to the ankle

Anterior impingement syndrome. Pain may result from repeated impingement *in ankle dorsiflexion* of the adjacent articular margins of the tibia and talus (Hontas *et al.* 1986). As the syndrome evolves osteophytic projections from the adjacent bony margins may develop. Compression of previously avulsed bony fragments from the anterior joint margins may occur, giving rise to a localized capsulitis and periostitis. Alternatively, repetitive stress to the anterior aspect of the ankle in *plantarflexion*—for example, when kicking a 'dead ball' in soccer or rugby

football—may be the initial cause of the osteophytic projections (McMurray 1950). The term 'footballer's ankle' is coined to reflect the presence of such avulsed fragments and osteophytes, which are typically seen in professional soccer players. Anterior impingement may also be seen in dancers, particularly in classical ballet, as a result of the repeated ankle dorsiflexion required by the demi-plie position. Examination findings are reproduction of pain on passive ankle dorsiflexion and localized anterior joint line tenderness. The range of dorsiflexion may become limited owing to intervening fragments. X-ray usually confirms the bony abnormalities (Fig. 9.16). However, the joint space is well

FIG. 9.16 Typical 'footballer's ankle': anterior (and posterior) osteophytes and avulsion fragments.

Fig. 9.17 Osteoarthritis of the ankle in an ex-professional soccer player: in comparison with Fig 9.16 there is additional subchondral sclerosis and joint-space narrowing.

maintained. Elastoplast adhesive strapping may control the extent of ankle dorsiflexion in footballers prior to the introduction of a suitable rest period. Occasionally surgical excision is required.

Care should be taken to differentiate the marginal osteophytosis present in 'footballer's ankle' from osteoarthritis, in which loss of joint space and subchondral sclerosis occur (Fig. 9.17). The prognosis is different, and the former condition does *not* inevitably lead to the latter.

Extensor tenosynovitis. This either results from unaccustomed intensive running—for example, in ultramarathoners—or is secondary to overtight lacing of running shoes. Localized swelling of the extensor tendons may be seen. Passive plantarflexion and resisted dorsiflexion of the foot and/or toes are painful. Local anti-inflammatory measures and reduction of stress are indicated. Surgical release is occasionally necessary in the chronic case.

Posterior to the ankle

Achilles tendon pathology and bursitis

All grades of injury to the Achilles tendon (syn. tendo-Achilles (TA)) are seen and are a common source of pain in runners. The most common type is *Achilles tendinitis* that is due to repeated microtrauma. Typically, at an early stage discomfort is felt after running and morning stiffness is a feature. Subsequently discomfort is experienced at the beginning of a run, though it improves later. However, it soon becomes increasingly difficult to 'run off' the symptoms, at which stage advice is usually sought. Precipitating factors are training errors of all kinds: inadequate footwear, the presence of a whiplash effect on the Achilles tendon due to overpronation of the foot, pressure from a shoe-heel tab, and inadequate elasticity of the musculotendinous unit. Pain is elicited on active contraction (rising on to tiptoe) and, unless the condition is mild, on stretch, either weightbearing or supine. Localized tenderness is found, commonly 4–6 cm from the TA insertion into the os calcis. In more severe cases thickening of the affected area is noted. The presence of a fusiform swelling may indicate a central (core) degenerative process.

Since the Achilles tendon is surrounded by a paratenon rather than a tendon sheath, an inflammatory reaction in this tissue is described as a *paratendinitis*. It may be secondary to underlying tendinitis, in which case a more diffuse swelling than that found in a tendinitis is observed. It may also develop as a primary response to repeated friction from a shoe or walking boot. Crepitating paratendinitis may be felt: this responds quickly to a steroid injection into the paratenon.

Partial rupture presents as a more acute injury. Pain then prevents active heel raise. A more substantial degree of swelling and tenderness are observed: however, the tendon is intact, as determined by a negative Thompson's squeeze test. With the patient lying prone the calf is squeezed—a resulting plantarflexion of the foot takes place in the presence of an intact tendon (a negative Thompson's test). A positive test indicates complete rupture (see Chapter 8).

Examination of the foot, particularly the biomechanics of subtalar function, is essential. The running or training shoes are examined. An assessment is made of the degree of stretch of the TA by reference to the normal side. Soft tissue lateral X-rays may reveal haziness of the anterior margin of the TA or the presence of tendon swelling (Fig. 9.18). Management schedules are according to the following guidelines.

1. A heel lift in the early stages. Shock-absorbing materials such as PPT are useful, both in early management and during later rehabilitation.
2. Ultrasound, ice applications/massage, and deep friction massage.
3. Subsequently, graded stretching.
4. Podiatric assessment and provision of antipronational orthoses, if appropriate.

5. Advice on footwear, with particular reference to a supportive heel counter, an effective shock-absorbing midsole, and a non-irritating (or excised) heel tab.
6. Advice on graded rehabilitation including eccentric loading.

Steroid injections are useful in paratendinitis (see Fig. 12.24, p. 221). In refractory cases of tendinitis an injection to the paratenon may be considered. In the chronic or relapsing case an adhesive paratendinitis often complicates tendon pathology; MRI is helpful, and subsequent referral to a specialist surgeon. A variety of measures, which usually include stripping of the paratenon, are often successful.

Sever's apophysitis. In juveniles repeated stress more commonly manifests itself as a traction osteochondrosis of the posterior calcaneal apophysis into which the TA is attached. Localized tenderness is felt over the posterior aspect of the os calcis: the tendon itself is apparently normal. Although X-rays are frequently taken, the normal apophysis often has a fragmented appearance and interpretation may be difficult. Therefore a clinical diagnosis should be made. Localized physio-

Achilles tendinitis
Retrocalcaneal bursitis
Postcalcaneal bursitis
Peroneal tendinitis
Stress fracture of navicular
Cuboid syndrome
Stress fracture of metatarsal
Plantar fasciitis

FIG. 9.19 Sites of overuse injury in the ankle and foot.

Normal Achilles soft-tissue shadow

Abnormal enlargement of Achilles soft-tissue shadow

Contraction of Kagar's triangle

FIG. 9.18 'Soft tissue' lateral X-rays of the ankle may reveal swelling of the Achilles tendon in the presence of Achilles tendinitis or partial rupture.

therapeutic measures are unhelpful. Reduction of stress is required, with assistance from a shock-absorbing heel cushion.

Retrocalcaneal (pre-Achilles) bursitis. Pain and swelling arise from the bursa that is situated between the Achilles tendon and the superoposterior angle of the os calcis (Fig. 9.19). Although the symptomatology is similar to that caused by tendon pathology, bursitis is characterized by a tender swelling that may be palpated both medial and lateral to the distal TA. In common with plantar fasciitis, retrocalcaneal bursitis may be a manifestation of a rheumatological condition—for instance, one of the spondyloarthritides, especially Reiter's syndrome. Bursitis is very responsive to steroid injections or non-steroidal anti-inflammatory drugs. However, blood tests should be undertaken to determine a possible rheumatological basis.

Postcalcaneal (tendo-Achilles) bursitis. A bursa exists between the TA and the skin, and may become inflamed as a result of friction from a running shoe or boot. It is also common in the non-athletic population, particularly in women who wear shoes with closefitting heel counters. Tenderness and thickening overlying the insertion of the TA is often accompanied by bossing of the os calcis, giving rise to the common 'pump bump'. Haglund described a syndrome (Torg *et al.* 1987) characterized by the combined presence of bursitis, insertional tendinitis, and bossing (Haglund deformity). Shoes should be examined, as simple measures to smooth over any roughened internal surface of the heel counter may be effective. The heel may also be protected by suitable padding around the tender area. Postcalcaneal bursitis is less responsive than retrocalcaneal bursitis to steroid injections.

Insertional tendinitis of the TA. Occasionally an isolated tendinitis is found at the insertion of the TA, where it should be differentiated from bursitis (both pre- and postcalcaneal) and stress fracture. It is an enthesitis, akin to patella tendinitis. Its management follows the guidelines already outlined for Achilles tendinitis.

Non-Achilles pathology

Stress fracture of the os calcis. Although one of the least common stress fractures associated with running, stress fracture of the os calcis does enter into the differential diagnosis of heel pain. A typical crescendo pattern of pain is usually found, so that by the time the athlete is forced to stop running he has discomfort on walking, and particularly on stamping the heel on the ground.

Fig. 9.20 A typical stress fracture of the os calcis is demonstrated by the sclerotic line parallel to the posterior margin of the os calcis on the lateral X-ray, and oblique to the inferior border of the os calcis on the AP.

In contrast with the other conditions in the heel region, the tenderness is found on compressing the os calcis between thumb and forefinger from the medial and lateral aspects. X-ray is positive after a few weeks, when a sclerotic line may be seen running parallel to the posterior margin of the os calcis (Fig. 9.20). Meantime a technetium scan reveals increased uptake. Up to three months' abstinence from all sport involving running is required; other activities such as swimming and cycling are permissible (and encouraged for maintenance of overall fitness).

Tibialis posterior tendinitis. Tendinitis of tibialis posterior and flexor hallucis longus may give rise to posteromedial heel pain, often radiating to the instep. They are more common in pronated feet. Tendinitis of tibialis posterior is characterized by discomfort felt on passive eversion and resisted supination of the foot.

Precipitating situations are those demanding prolonged and repeated inversion, as in speedskating. The condition is also seen in sprinters and long-jumpers if loss of ankle dorsiflexion—for example, owing to tightness of the Achilles tendon—is compensated by eversion of the foot. If a lesion of the flexor hallucis longus exists, discomfort is felt on passive dorsiflexion of the big toe and resisted plantarflexion of the big toe. It is common in ballet dancers. Tenderness may be felt behind the medial malleolus or more distally—for example, at the insertion of the tibialis posterior into the navicular bone or, in the case of flexor hallucis longus, along the instep. Anti-inflammatory therapy may need to be combined with reduction of pronation by the use of orthotics, or with stretching exercises for ankle equinus.

Posterior (ankle) impingement syndrome (syn. talar compression syndrome). Repeated impingement of the posterior bony margins resulting from plantarflexion of the ankle may give rise to localized pain (Brodsky and Khalil 1986). It is usually due to impingement of the posterior process of the talus against the posterior lip of the tibia. It is more likely in the presence of an os trigonum (an accessory ossicle behind the talus) which is then caught, much as a nut in a nutcracker, between the tibia and os calcis when the ankle is plantarflexed. Occasionally either the posterior process of the talus or the os trigonum is fractured.

The condition is common in ballet dancers, as a result of time spent *en pointe*. It is observed in footballers, when it is due to kicking, particularly when kicks are blocked. Javelin throwers and other field athletes are a further 'at risk' group. Passive plantarflexion of the ankle reproduces the pain. Resisted muscle contraction is painless, thus differentiating the condition from tendinitis of tibialis posterior, flexor hallucis longus, the peronei, and the Achilles tendon. Tenderness is localized to the posterior joint margin, detected by palpating from either side of the Achilles tendon. Lateral X-rays may reveal a talar posterior process or os trigonum (Fig. 9.21). Bone scan is positive if a fracture has occurred, though if negative it does not preclude the diagnosis of impingement. Conservative management is instituted initially; a steroid injection may be followed by POP immobilization for a few weeks. Surgical excision of the os trigonum may be necessary in refractory cases, and is usually successful.

Lateral to the ankle

Peroneal tendinitis. This results from overactivity of the peronei, which evert the foot. Frequent running across slopes or in the gutter of a cambered road may be responsible. Pain is felt over the peroneal tendons, and may be accompanied by swelling or crepitus. Passive inversion of the foot is uncomfortable, and pain is reproduced on resisting peronei contraction. Localized anti-inflammatory measures are useful, and recognition of training errors important. A stronger heel counter, if appropriate, may help. Occasionally tendinitis is secondary to an inversion sprain. Lateral ankle soreness is also associated with lateral instability due to previous lateral ankle ligament rupture: proprioceptive exercises are then required (see Chapter 8).

Inferior to the heel

Plantar fasciitis. This common condition arises at the proximal attachment of the plantar fascia to the medial calcaneal tubercle. It is often mistakenly ascribed to the presence of a calcaneal spur (should one exist), though it occurs irrespective of any bony irregularity. It is often associated with a heavily pronated foot when the plantar fascia is overstretched. It may also occur in the rigid cavoid foot (Doxey 1987). The history is of gradually increasing discomfort felt under the heel during running. Examination reveals tenderness that is localized to the medial calcaneal tubercle, just to the medial side of the midline.

FIG. 9.21 (a) An os trigonum is demonstrated in a patient suffering from posterior (ankle) impingement: when the ankle is plantarflexed a 'nutcracker' effect occurs between the tibia and the os calcis.(b) A positive bone scan confirms the diagnosis.

Occasionally discomfort is reproduced by stretching the plantar fascia (passively dorsiflexing the big toe with the foot also dorsiflexed). The presence of more substantial pain on this manoeuvre, particularly when accompanied by a pronounced limp, indicates the likelihood of a partial tear of the fascia in the instep (Leach *et al.* 1978). Muscle contraction tests are normal.

Management is by the combination of anti-inflammatory measures and protection of the foot by appropriate antipronational devices. Thus a localized steroid injection at the point of tenderness in fasciitis is very helpful (see Fig. 12.26, p. 221), though it may fail to prevent recurrence unless the heel is protected by a shock-absorbing pad and the fascia is supported by medial arch support. A suitable appliance is a Rose insole with the addition of a PPT heel.

Contusion of the heel pad. The heel pad has a shock-absorbing function, and is composed of fatty and fibroelastic tissue divided by septa into compartments. Repeated contusion may give rise to localized pain on heel-strike. Protection is required by additional shock-absorbing heel inserts in the athletic shoe.

Injuries to the tarsus

Stress fracture of the navicular (Fig. 9.22). This is uncommon, though it should be suspected when an athlete, often involved in a discipline in which jumping or hurdling are essential elements, complains of instep pain. The pain is worse on weightbearing on the affected foot. Localized tenderness and surrounding oedema are the only abnormal clinical signs. X-rays are often negative in the early stages, so that a technetium scan should be performed for confirmation of the diagnosis. Localized increased uptake is then clearly seen. Management is by rest from weightbearing sport for a disappointingly long period of time. It is not unusual for several months, or even a year or more, of rest to be necessary. If discomfort is felt during everyday activities, a period of non-weightbearing immobilization in a POP cast should be utilized for confirmation of the diagnosis. Further assessment and timing of the reintroduction of training should be on a basis of comfort and loss of tenderness, rather than on a change in the bone scan or X-ray.

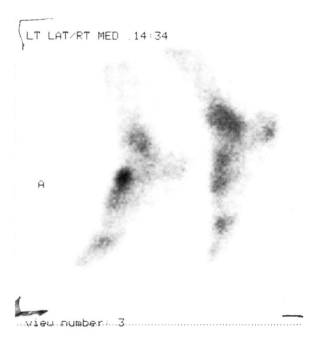

LT LAT/RT MED 14:34

A

view number 3

Fig. 9.22 (left) The typical X-ray appearance of a stress fracture of the navicular confirmed by a technetium scan (above).

An accessory ossicle, the os naviculare, may cause pain at its fibrous union with the navicular bone. If localized anti-inflammatory measures are ineffective, excision may be necessary.

Nerve entrapment. Pain felt along the instep, particularly in association with radiation to the medial aspect of the heel, may be secondary to nerve compression. The tarsal tunnel syndrome, in which the posterior tibial nerve or one of its branches is compressed just posterior to the medial malleolus, is well recognized. Medial collapse of the hindfoot is a common cause. Pain is usually sharp or electric in nature, and is often associated with paraesthesiae and/or numbness felt in the sole. There may be an associated os trigonum. Diagnostic signs are localized tenderness over the groove behind the medial malleolus and a positive Tinel sign. Nerve conduction studies may be performed for confirmation.

Other nerve entrapments occur: compression of the medial calcaneal nerve should be considered in the differential diagnosis of plantar fasciitis, as commonly pain is felt in the medio-inferior aspect of the heel. Instep pain may be due to compression of the nerve to the abductor digiti minimi that courses deep to the abductor hallucis muscle (Murphy and Baxter 1985). Entrapment of the medial plantar nerve close to the calcaneonavicular ligament has also been described. Localized steroid injections may be helpful: otherwise, surgical release is indicated in refractory cases.

Cuboid syndrome. This relatively rare condition behaves as a stress injury to the cuboid, though without the progress to stress fracture that is seen with the navicular. Localized discomfort, tenderness, and soft tissue swelling resolve over a period of a few weeks' rest. The condition does not appear to be related to overactivity of the peronei.

Arch strain. This may be secondary to muscle weakness or fatigue, ligamentous inadequacy, or overstrain of the plantar fascia (when it is felt particularly on toe-off). Inadequate support of the instep from the running shoe is often observed. The pronated foot is at most risk. Although there is minimal muscle activity in the standing position, when aching may predominantly be felt, both extrinsic and intrinsic muscle-strengthening exercises are prescribed to correct any imbalance during running or walking.

Degenerative changes in the tarsus. This may be secondary to previous injury, and gives rise to a loss of mobility of the tarsus. Superior osteophytic projections may cause localized discomfort in a shoe that is too tightly laced or inadequate in size. Generalized discomfort is felt during or after exercise, and should be controlled by an adequate instep support.

Metatarsalgia and forefoot pain

Stress fracture (see Fig. 10.10, p. 170). One of the commonest stress fractures in the lower limb is the metatarsal (MT) stress fracture, usually occurring at the distal metaphysis of MT2 or MT3, although fracture at the base of MT5 is also recorded. Usually it results from increased walking or running activities in the relatively untrained—for instance, in military recruits or inexperienced joggers. Localized tenderness and swelling are found over the distal shaft of the relevant MT. Diagnosis is made on clinical grounds: X-rays may not become positive for two or three weeks. A suitable metatarsal pad (on elastic or on insole) is effective for comfort when combined with four weeks' reduction in activity.

Inadequacy of the transverse arch. This is usually found in the more mature runner, and may be combined with other struc-

tural abnormalities, for instance, hallux valgus. Reversal of the superior convexity of the arch is associated with the formation of callosities under the second and third metatarsophalangeal (MTP) joints. In its more severe form it is commonly found in rheumatoid arthritis, when dorsal subluxation of the proximal digits occurs. Localized tenderness under the MTP joints is found. Although the introduction of intrinsic muscle exercises does not influence the structural configuration found on examination, it may help dynamically. An appropriately applied metatarsal pad—that is, one proximal to the MTP joints—is usually helpful.

Freiberg's disease is an osteochondritis affecting the head of MT2 or MT3 in the skeletally immature. Discomfort may be felt at this time; metatarsalgia is a secondary manifestation in adulthood. A metatarsal pad is required.

Hallux rigidus. Degenerative changes in the first MTP joint give rise to restriction of mobility of the joint—hallux rigidus. This common condition may be secondary to a previous osteochondritis; at least, there is often a history of synovitis that subsequently settles, only to lead to a more chronic condition in which repeated stress results in pain and increasing restriction of mobility. Pain is felt when the joint is forcibly dorsiflexed—for example, in toe-off on running and in gymnastics or ballet. Examination confirms restricted dorsiflexion and plantarflexion. Osteophytes may be palpated around the joint. Tenderness is felt over the dorsal joint margin. It is a problem which may be difficult to overcome, though the use of a metatarsal 'rocker' in the running shoe may help. In a ballet dancer it may herald a premature end to a career.

Trauma, as in stubbing the toe, may cause a haemarthrosis of the first MTP joint. Aspiration allows earlier resolution than would otherwise be the case, and thus an earlier return to activity. If an assistant delivers an axial distracting force to the joint, dorsal needle entry is facilitated.

Sesamoiditis. Stress may give rise to pain from the sesamoid bones that are associated with the insertion of flexor hallucis brevis along the plantar aspect of the first MTP joint. This is particularly common in ballet dancers. An inflammatory reaction, chondromalacia, or a stress fracture may develop (see Fig. 10.15, p. 176), occasionally necessitating excision of the affected sesamoid.

Bunions. Bunions (adventitious bursae) may be troublesome over the first and fifth MTP joints. The former is often associated with *hallux valgus*, caused by tight-fitting shoes. There may be a primary metatarsus primus varus and subsequent development of hammer and overriding toes. The choice of adequate shoe-width is essential. Advice from a podiatrist or chiropodist may be required.

Morton's interdigital neuroma. Pain that radiates between the second and third or third and fourth toes may be due to a neuroma of a plantar digital nerve. There are accompanying paraesthesiae, and numbness radiating along the adjacent toes. Tenderness may be elicited on pressure applied to the web at the point of division of the nerve to the adjacent digits. Injections of the associated intermetatarsal bursa, accompanied by restriction of activities, may help, though excision is usually required.

Aetiological factors

Identification of the aetiological factors involved in the development of overuse injury in the lower limb is of paramount importance. Following the establishment of the patho-anatomical nature of the injury and recovery therefrom, relapse may be expected unless adverse aetiological factors are corrected. These factors may be considered by reference to the following groups:

    training errors;

    terrain characteristics;

    inadequate flexibility and muscle imbalance;

    pathology elsewhere;

    biomechanical abnormalities;

    inadequate footwear;

    growth characteristics.

Although reference is made particularly to running injuries, the same principles may be applied to all sports that involve weight-bearing activity.

Training errors. Training errors probably account for the majority of running injuries. Although it is understandable that the inexperienced jogger/runner may indulge in an inappropriate training programme, often with too rapid an increase in mileage, the experienced or elitist athlete is by no means exempt. On the one hand risk may be taken with new or innovative programmes; on the other a lack of common sense may prevail. The body's adaptive process may be compromised by excessive mileage, overfrequent (for instance, daily with no rest-day) or infrequent activity, addition of extra loading (for example, frequent hill work or fartleking), and excessive incremental increases in training distances. Although it may be a question of being wise after the event in individual cases, the most extraordinary circumstances are reported. The author has interviewed one runner with multiple stress fractures who increased his mileage from 0 to 110 miles per week in three weeks!

Information on suitable schedules for beginners are readily available in other texts, and particularly in the various running magazines. Having overcome the initial phase of muscle soreness, further progression should be at a comfortable pace. Adaptive responses are compromised by the inappropriate targeting of a future race meeting that allows an inadequate amount of training time, thereby imposing excessive musculoskeletal strain.

Terrain. It is clear that the transmission of shock on foot-strike is affected by the nature of the running surface. Exaggeration of shock waves is found on concrete; a marginal improvement may be expected on asphalt. Although it is usually stated that running on grass is desirable, particularly when recovering from injury, there are obvious drawbacks. Wet grass may be too slippery, and dry grass may cover a bumpy surface; in any event, apart from well-prepared recreational surfaces, potholes may be a problem. The best surfaces are perhaps a level dirt track or a prepared bark surface, though in Britain these are rarely available. Sand should normally be avoided, as it imposes a considerable strain on the Achilles tendons. Banked surfaces, such as heavily cambered roads, impose an excessive pronational strain on the higher foot and a varus strain on the lower knee. Competitive athletes often experience problems in the spring and autumn—that is, between running seasons—when adjustments are required from road or cross-country running to running on tartan tracks, and vice versa. Tartan surfaces vary in their shock-absorbing quality, depending to some degree on their thickness. Transitional programmes should be as graded as possible.

Flexibility/Muscle balance. Sprinters, who often have the benefit of advice on training programmes from qualified coaches at club level, are usually diligent in performing stretching exercises. However, both their longer-distance club colleagues and 'fun-runners' have in the past been notoriously negligent in this

Fig. 9.23 Biomechanical abnormalities of the foot: (i) forefoot varus (inversion deformity of the head of the talus and the forefoot in relation to the calcaneus); (ii) subtalar varus (inversion deformity of the calcaneus in the neutral position); (iii) forefoot valgus (eversion deformity of the head of the talus and the forefoot in relation to the calcaneus).

(i) Forefoot varus   (ii) Subtalar varus   (iii) Forefoot valgus respect. Yet loss of musculotendinous flexibility contributes to the development of many injuries, such as Achilles tendinitis and iliotibial tract bursitis. Elsewhere in the text it has been suggested that restricted flexibility around the hip joint, often due to tight soft tissues, contributes to chronic pelvic and back strains.

Not enough data are available on muscle imbalance to be certain how significant this is in the development of injury. It appears to be a logical concept, however, so that clinical appraisal should always be made of the strength of the major muscle groups in the legs.

Pathology elsewhere. The presence of (a) ligamentous instability, for example at the ankle, (b) structural deformity, for example after previous tibial fracture, and (c) joint stiffness, for example as a result of degenerative change, increases the stress applied to the leg during running. This increased loading may cause stress symptoms some distance away from the affected site. Examination of the lumbar spine, pelvis, hips, and knees, as well as the lower legs, should be carried out routinely.

Biomechanical abnormalities. Traditionally, convention has dictated that foot shape be described by reference to the longitudinal arch on standing. Thus the 'flat foot' or pes planus is easily recognizable, as is the rigid cavoid (supinated) foot. Of these the most common abnormality is the pronated *pes planus*, which may be either congenitally or developmentally determined. Usually, however, such a foot will be capable of revealing a substantial longitudinal arch when standing on tiptoe.

Dynamic biomechanical studies have demonstrated that during the foot contact (stance) phase of running the foot has the ability to change from a rigid lever in the supinated state to a mobile adaptor in the pronated state (Subotnik 1985). Incorrect timing of this biomechanical change, leading to the application of abnormal forces to the leg, may result from either excessive or prolonged pronation (Donatelli 1987). Problems may also arise when the foot remains on the running surface for too long—that is, dorsiflexing too much as a result of plantarflexor weakness or of the nature of the terrain (e.g. sand or ice). The centre of gravity then extends too far anteriorly at toe-off, creating hyperextension of the knee. Within the gait cycle (just prior to toe-off), as the heel leaves the ground, the foot should be in the neutral position. In this position the heel is perpendicular to the ground, the subtalar joint is neither supinated nor pronated, and the plane of the metatarsal heads is at right angles to the heel. This normal position may be demonstrated in the static standing position by externally rotating the leg with the foot on the ground. When a patient is examined in this position and the articulation of the talar head with the navicular is palpated, abnormalities between the rearfoot and the forefoot, and their relationships with the leg and the ground, may be detected. Such abnormalities may be the cause of overuse injury.

A number of variations from the norm of both forefoot and hindfoot are seen (Fig. 9.23). *Abnormal compensatory pronation* at the subtalar joint (STJ) is usually secondary to forefoot varus (Brown and Yavorsky 1987) or to ankle equinus, which is often due to tightness of the Achilles tendon. The uncompensated and compensated positions of the foot with forefoot varus are shown in Figs 9.24 and 9.25. The excessive STJ motion is necessary for the forefoot to reach the ground. The resultant excessive internal rotation of the tibia is accompanied by transmission of similar forces to the femur. Injury patterns include Achilles tendinitis, posterior tibialis tendinitis, plantar fasciitis, medial periostitis of the tibia, and the patellofemoral stress syndrome (McKenzie *et al.* 1985).

The *cavoid foot* is quite different: the dissipation of forces on heel strike is inadequate, as unlocking of the foot does not take place owing to the relative rigidity of the subtalar and midtarsal joints. Rearfoot varus (an inverted heel) may be substantial. Supination persists through the stance phase, resulting in loss of the normal internal rotation of the lower leg: the knee retains a slight varus position, contributing to tightening of the lateral knee structures. Injury patterns include a predisposition to iliotibial tract bursitis, stress fractures, Achilles tendinitis, and lateral ankle sprains.

The positions of the STJ in neutral and of the forefoot relative to the hindfoot may be observed when the patient lies prone on the couch with his feet hanging over the edge. A weightbearing assessment is required to appreciate fully the degree of excessive pronation (in the relaxed compensated position) that is associated with a 'weak' foot due to ligamentous laxity or hypermobile first ray (MT1 and medial cuneiform). On the other hand, abnormal pronation may be due to biomechanical abnormalities associated with malalignment—for example, femoral anteversion, increased Q-angle, genu varum and valgum, and leg-length inequality. Video recordings and clinical observations on a treadmill often give valuable information on the prevailing biomechanical forces, and may be augmented by a study of the distortion and wear pattern of the running shoe.

Therapeutically, simple mechanical measures may effect adequate control. An extra insole of a few millimetres thickness

Fig. 9.24 Forefoot varus: (i) uncompensated; (ii) compensated (by subtalar pronation); (iii) orthotic posting under first ray (MT 1 and medial cuneiform).

Forefoot varus   (i) Uncompensated   (ii) Compensated   (iii) Orthotic posting under first ray

FIG 9.25 Clinical appearance of everted heel (subtalar pronation) as a compensatory mechanism for forefoot varus.

inside the running shoe of a short leg may adjust the running biomechanics so as to reduce incidence of injury, even when the leg-length inequality is of the order of 1 cm or more. If the insole forces the foot too far out of the shoe, a responsible shoe manufacturer may be prevailed upon to increase the depth of the sole. An athlete may attempt to control pronation by the substitution for the running-shoe insole provided by the manufacturer of a soft arch-support purchased 'off the shelf'. If this measure fails, podiatric assessment is desirable in order to determine the cause, whether from within the foot or from the lower limb as a whole, of any abnormal subtalar biomechanics. A soft insole or temporary posting of the hind- or forefoot may be employed. Subsequently a hard orthotic is used if necessary. The long-term use of orthotics to control biomechanical abnormalities appears to reduce the likelihood of further injury. Orthotics are considered further in Chapter 11, p. 187.

Training characteristics may need to be examined further. Counter-clockwise sprint training around athletic tracks leads to different supinating and pronating forces on the left and right feet. For example, excessive torque on the right knee due to external rotation of the right leg during 'push off' may lead to medial symptoms. Care should be taken to achieve a well balanced training schedule.

Inadequate footwear. The modern training shoe incorporates a number of features that assist in shock absorption and support for the foot (see Fig. 11.3, p. 186). The midsole (often made from the polyurethane compound ethylene vinyl acetate (EVA) in varying densities) and the wedge assist in shock absorption. This may be further assisted by other materials that can be incorporated into the manufacture of a running shoe in the form of an insole. The wedge also contributes to heel lift. A firm heel counter and 'arch cookie' help to control subtalar joint motion, though regrettably the flimsy arch support (cookie) is often ineffective. Pronation may be controlled by a firm heel counter, medial arch support, and a board-lasted shoe (in which the upper part of the shoe is connected to a firm fibrous innersole board). Shoes with lateral rearfoot flares should be avoided; varus wedges may help (Anthony 1987). The cavoid foot requires a board-lasted rearfoot, a lateral flare, and a firm heel

counter, combined with a decent wedge and slip-lasted forefoot (in which the upper has been brought beneath the foot and stitched as a moccasin to provide greater flexibility).

It is essential for the patient with a running injury to bring in his training shoes for inspection. Inappropriate shoes (for example, casuals sold as trainers) may have been used, and it is not unusual to find over-worn footwear. Simple advice on the purchase of a suitable shoe may be all that is required for some patients. For further information on the running shoe the reader is referred to Cavanagh (1980).

Growth characteritics. Carefully graded intensification of training schedules is obviously necessary for young athletes. It is important to recognize that, during growth spurts, increased bone-length may not always be accompanied by corresponding musculo-tendinous elasticity. Hence there is a particular need for an adequate long slow stretch programme. Youngsters are prone to heel pain if insufficient support is available from footwear. All too often children are expected to participate in physical education programmes of all kinds, including running, in flimsy plimsolls. Physical education should include advice on warm-up, stretching, and footwear to all age groups.

References

Andrews, J. R. (1983). Overuse syndrome of the lower extremity. *Clin. Sports Med.*, **6**, 291–320.

Anthony, R. J. (1987). The functional anatomy of the running training shoe. *Chiropodist*, **42**(12), 451–9.

Baumgartl, F. (1964). *Das Kniegelenk*, p. 452. Springer Verlag, Berlin.

Brodsky, A. E. and Khalil, M. A. (1986). Talar compression syndrome. *Am. J. Sports Med.*, **14**,(16), 472–6.

Brown, L. P. and Yavorsky, P. (1987). Locomotor biomechanics and pathomechanics: a review. *J. Orthop. Sports Phys. Ther.*, **9**, 3–10.

Cavanagh, P. R. (1980). *The running shoe book*. Anderson World, Mountain View, CA.

Donatelli, R. (1987). Abnormal biomechanics of the foot and ankle. *J. Orthop. Sports Phys. Ther.*, **9**, 11–16.

Doxey, G. E. (1987). Calcaneal pain: a review of various disorders. *J. Orthop. and Sports Phys. Ther.*, **9**, 25–32.

Ficat, R. P. and Hungerford, D. S. (1977). *Disorders of the patello-femoral joint*. Williams and Wilkins, Baltimore, MD.

Goodfellow, J., Hungerford, D. S., and Zindel. M. (1976). Patello-femoral joint mechanics and pathology. *J. Bone Jt. Surg.*, **58B**, 287–90.

Hontas, M. J., Haddad, R. J., and Schlesinger, L. C. (1986). Conditions of the talus in the runner. *Am. J. Sports Med.*, **14**(6), 486–90.

Hungerford, D. S. and Barry, M. (1979). Biomechanics of the patellofemoral joint. *Clin. Orthop. Relat. Res.*, **144**, 9–15.

James, S. L., Bates, B. T., and Ostering, L. R. (1978). Injuries to runners. *Am J. Sports Med.*, **6**(2), 40–50.

Kettelkamp, D. B. (1981). Current concepts review: management of patella malalignment. *J. Bone Jt Surg.*, **63A**, 1344–8.

King, J. B., Perry, D. J., Mourad, K., and Kumar, S. J. (1990). Lesions of the patellar ligament. *J. Bone Jt. Surg.*, **72B**, 46–8.

Leach, R., Jones, R., and Silva, T. (1978). Rupture of the plantar fascia in athletes. *J. Bone Jt. Surg.*, **60A**, 537–9.

McKenzie, D. C., Clement, D. B., and Taunton, J. E. (1985). Running shoes, orthotics and injuries. *Sports Med.*, **2**, 334–7.

McMurray, T. P. (1950). Footballer's ankle. *J. Bone Jt. Surg.*, **32B**, 68–9.

Murphy, P. C. and Baxter, D. E. (1985). Nerve entrapment of the foot and ankle in runners. *Clin. Sports Med.*, **4**(4), 753–63.

Subotnick, S. I. (1985). The biomechanics of running: implications for the prevention of foot injures. *Sports Med.*, **2**, 144–53.

Torg, J. S., Pavlov, H., and Torg, E. (1987). Overuse injuries in sport: the foot. *Clin. Sports Med.*, **6**, 291–320.

Wiberg, G. (1941). Roentgenographic and anatomic studies on the femoropatellar joint. *Acta Orthop. Scand.*, **12**, 319–410.

Wood, G. A. (1987). Biomechanical limitations to sprint running. *Med. Sport Sci.*, **25**, 58–71.

10 Investigations

M. A. Hutson and D. B. L. Finlay

Non-radiological investigation

M. A. Hutson

Clinical assessment of patients suffering from sports-related injuries combines a thorough history and a detailed musculoskeletal examination. This alone is often sufficient to establish a diagnosis. For full assessment, however, further investigative procedures may be needed. Since rheumatological conditions sometimes masquerade as sports trauma, rheumatological screening may be required. Additional information on those tissues which are deep-lying and therefore not easily inspected or palpated—for example, intervertebral discs and (intra-articular) menisci—may be gained by radiological or pathological investigation. Thus CT scans, MRI scans, and scintigraphy may complement straight radiological techniques. Biopsy of muscle or synovium may occasionally be useful.

Certain procedures—for instance, joint aspiration and epidural injection of procaine—may have both diagnostic and therapeutic applications. However, the employment of local anaesthesia as a diagnostic tool should usually be unnecessary if a satisfactory clinical examination has been conducted.

Tests for muscle function may be performed on an isokinetic dynamometer, and the results computerized in a tabulated or graphical form: they are considered further in Chapters 11 and 12.

Joint aspiration

This may be performed in either a mono- or polyarthropathy for the following reasons.

1. Detection (and therapeutic aspiration) of a haemarthrosis. The additional presence of fat globules indicates an intra-articular fracture.

2. Detection of *inflammatory cells*. Other than a haemarthrosis, an effusion may be either clear (serous) or turbid. Turbidity indicates the presence of a large number of inflammatory cells which are secondary to infection or inflammatory joint disease. High white cell counts (for example, up to 50 000 per cubic millimetre) are found in infection, and also in rheumatoid and psoriatic arthropathy.

3. Detection of *organisms*. Gram-staining identifies the presence of gonococcal, staphylococcal, and streptococcal bacteria. A Ziehl-Neelsen stain is used if the presence of *Mycobacterium tuberculosis* is suspected.

4. Detection of *crystals*. The use of a polarizing microscope is necessary to detect the presence of needle-like urate crystals in gout: strongly negative birefringence is found. Weakly positive birefringence indicates pseudogout (rhomboid or rectangular-shaped pyrophosphate crystals). Spectrophotometry is required to identify hydroxyapatite crystals, which are thought to be responsible for low-grade joint inflammation (and are present in 'calcific' tendinitis).

Haematological and serological tests

Hb, WBC and differential, and ESR. Anaemia is found in chronic inflammatory disease. White cell count is elevated in the presence of infection. ESR may of course be elevated in the presence of active disease, though it is an unreliable indicator of the presence or the progress of the various polyarthritides.

Latex and Rheumatoid factor, ANF and DNA binding. The latex and rheumatoid factor tests are positive in rheumatoid arthritis and negative in osteoarthritis. ANF and DNA binding are positive in systemic lupus erythematosus.

Uric acid. Hyperuricaemia indicates a gouty tendency. Positive clinical findings or crystals are necessary to confirm the diagnosis of gout.

Tissue typing. The HLA B27 antigen test is most useful if one of the spondyloarthritides is suspected: 96 per cent of cases of ankylosing spondylitis and 50 per cent of Reiter's syndrome are positive.

Plasma proteins, calcium, phosphate, and alkaline phosphatase. These investigations are necessary to exclude metabolic and bone disease as a cause of back pain.

Creatine phosphokinase (CPK or CK). The level of this enzyme is often substantially raised in the presence of muscle damage resulting from overtraining. It is also high in polymyositis.

Biopsy

Virtually any tissue may be biopsied, should the need arise. In practice synovial biopsy is occasionally used, though its application is limited because of the non-specificity of the observed inflammatory changes. Muscle biopsy may reveal mitochondrial abnormalities, an uncommon cause of recurrent muscle dysfunction. Fibre-typing is largely a research procedure.

Urinalysis

Other than its general use in screening and in detection of certain specific diseases, there are few other indications for urinalysis in sports trauma. Haemoglobin or myoglobin may be detected in the urine after endurance activities or after gross muscle trauma.

Radiological investigations

D. B. L. FINLAY

Plain film radiography

The principal imaging technique for the diagnosis of fractures is plain film radiography. A fracture is most commonly seen on the radiograph as a line of lucency—the greater the displacement of the component parts of the fracture the wider and more obvious is the fracture line. The visibility of this line also depends on its alignment with the X-ray beam, and if it is oblique it becomes less visible. There is a degree of obliquity at which each individual fracture line will not be seen. However, it is unusual for the fracture line not to be visible on a further radiograph obtained at right angles to the first (Fig. 10.1). These

(a)

(b)

FIG. 10.1 (a) AP and (b) lateral radiographs of the ankle of a child. Fracture of the lower tibia is only visible on the lateral radiograph (arrowed). There is separation of the lower tibial epiphysis (curved arrow) (Salter II epiphyseal injury) observations apply to fractures involving most of the circumference of a bone. However, for identification of fractures which involve only part of the circumference, in particular fractures of the end of a bone within a joint or avulsion fractures by tendons or ligaments, further radiographs may need to be obtained. To a lesser extent this is also true of fractures involving the proximal or distal shaft of a bone. *Therefore it is important that information be given by the requesting physician about the precise location of the injury and the suspected nature.* This helps to ensure that adequate radiographs are obtained for diagnosis.

The sports physician is particularly interested in fractures inside a joint and in ligament or tendon avulsions. It is important to note abnormal alignment of one bone with another. Even if no fracture is visible malalignment suggests the presence of ligamentous damage, which is of particular importance in the fingers (Fig. 10.2). It is necessary to verify the articulation of individual bones in areas in which multiple joints exist in the wrist and foot.

(a)

(b)

FIG. 10.2 Lateral radiograph of finger. The proximal interphalangeal joint is hyperextended due to acute volar plate disruption.

FIG. 10.3 (a) PA and (b) lateral radiographs of the ulna and radius of a child. A greenstick fracture is demonstrated. Bulging of the posterior cortex is seen (arrowed).

FIG. 10.4 Lateral radiograph of the knee of a child. There is anterior tilting of the lower femoral ephiphysis and a large effusion in the knee joint (arrowed).

FIG. 10.5 Patellar tendon avulsion. Lateral radiograph of the knee shows that the patella lies high. (The distance from the lower pole of the patella to the tibial tuberosity should equal the longest oblique diameter of the patella). There are fragments avulsed from the inferior pole of the patella and the anterior tibial tubercle (arrowed). Soft tissue swelling is seen in the area of the patellar tendon (curved arrow).

Fractures can be seen as areas of increased density due to impaction. This is common in fractures of the femoral neck, in depressed fractures of the skull vault, and in some stress fractures (see Fig. 10.11., p. 174). In comminuted and other fractures where the alignment of fragments of bone with the X-ray beam is altered, there may be increased density. This also occurs when bones overlap, as in a dislocation.

It is important that the same rule of two radiographs, usually obtained at right angles, is remembered in examining joints. It is easy to miss a dislocation when only one view is obtained. When a long bone is fractured, the joints above and below should be included on the radiograph.

Two additional types of fracture occur in children. Incomplete fractures are commonly classed as *greenstick* fractures. One cortex may be fractured and the other bent or bowed but intact, as commonly occurs in the mid-shaft of the radius and the ulna (Fig. 10.3); alternatively they may be compression fractures, causing bulging of one or both cortices, as commonly occurs at the end of the long bones, particularly the radius and the ulna. The second group of fractures are *epiphyseal separations*. These occur with or without an accompanying metaphyseal fragment, and are the childhood equivalent of a dislocation or ligamentous injury (Fig. 10.4).

For further information on fractures the reader is referred to the book by Rogers (1982).

Soft tissue signs

Unfortunately, radiographs do not image soft tissues well. Soft tissue swelling is a useful marker of damage and possible underlying fracture (Fig. 10.5). Although some injuries, for instance complete tears of the Achilles tendon, may be identified on the radiograph, this is of little primary value. A complete tear will be seen as a disruption of the normal convex curve of the tendon. There is normally a lucent triangle bounded by the Achilles tendon posteriorly, the deep layer of posterior tibial muscles anteriorly, and the superior margin of the tuberosity of the calcaneum inferiorly. This is obliterated when there is damage— either incomplete or complete rupture of the Achilles tendon (see Fig. 9.18, p. 157).

At the knee, infrapatellar tendon ruptures are demonstrated by superior displacement of the patella (Fig. 10.5) associated

Fig. 10.6 Lateral radiograph of the elbow. Elevation of the anterior fat pad which is sail-shaped (arrow) and the posterior fat pad (curved arrow) are demonstrated. The radial head is fractured (thick arrow).

Fig. 10.7 AP radiograph of the foot. Avulsion of the base of the fifth metatarsal by the peroneus brevis has occurred (see also Fig. 9.2, p. 142).

with a soft tissue mass in the region of the infrapatellar tendon. There may be avulsion fractures from the inferior pole of the patella or from the tibial tubercle. In the normal knee the length of the infrapatellar tendon is approximately the same as the longest diameter of the patella.

When there is an effusion in the knee joint swelling of the suprapatellar pouch above the knee can be seen (Fig. 10.4). In the normal knee this is visible only as a stripe, the width of the thickness of two layers of synovial membrane surrounded by extra-synovial fat. If there has been a fracture in the joint which has released fat, this lipohaemarthrosis may be seen on a horizontal lateral radiograph as a fat fluid level within the joint.

At the elbow a joint effusion may be identified by elevation of the anterior fat pad, as a sail-shape, away from the anterior cortex of the distal humerus (Fig. 10.6). The posterior fat pad, which is not normally in evidence behind the lower humerus, becomes visible.

Avulsion fractures

Fragments of bone are avulsed by ligaments or tendons. They may vary in size from small slivers to quite large fragments, as occurs, for instance, at the base of the fifth metatarsal owing to avulsion by the peroneus brevis (Fig. 10.7). They indicate serious damage to the soft tissues, rather than just fractures of the bone. They occur in many characteristic sites, but are particularly common at the ankle and foot (see Fig. 9.16, p. 155). From the malleoli of the ankle avulsion fractures are caused by the medial and the lateral collateral ligaments; in the foot they occur from the navicular and talus. In the pelvis the anterior superior iliac spine is avulsed by the sartorius, the anterior inferior iliac spine by the rectus femoris, and the ischial tuberosity by the hamstrings (see Fig. 1.13, p. 13). It is important to note that avulsion of the ischial tuberosity commonly produces a large mass of bone in the healing phase, which may be misdiagnosed as a tumour. Avulsion fractures also commonly occur in the fingers—for example, avulsion of the extensor tendon at the base of the distal phalanx, of the profundus tendon on the volar surface of the base of the distal phalanx, and of the volar plate

FIG. 10.8 Lateral radiograph of the knee. There is a transverse fracture of the lower pole of the patella.

(ai)   (aii)   (b)

FIG. 10.9 (a) (i) and (ii) Dorsiplantar radiographs of the foot. An os tibialis externa is seen. Its margins are corticated and rounded, seen particularly laterally where its margin is seen in profile without the overlying navicular bone (arrowed). Importantly, this is the characteristic site of this os. (b) Lateral radiograph of the foot. An os supranaviculare with rounded margins is seen at its characteristic site.

at the base of the middle phalanx. In the knee, damage to the extensor mechanism may cause avulsion of the superior and inferior patellar tendon attachments, avulsion of the tibial tubercle, or complete fractures of the patella (Fig. 10.8).

In the foot avulsion fractures must be distinguished from accessory ossicles and a normal apophysis. The ossicles occur in characteristic sites. Examples are the os tibialis externa (Fig. 10.9(a)), which lies proximal to the medial tuberosity of the navicular, the os supranaviculare, which is related to the dorsal aspect of the navicular (Fig. 10.9(b)), and the apophysis of the base of the fifth metatarsal. These do not 'fit' the adjacent bone and have rounded corticated margins. In these sites avulsed fragments which are larger than slivers should fit with the underlying bone, should have sharp well-defined margins, and may be associated with soft tissue swelling.

Stress fractures

Stress fractures occur in normal bone in response to the stress of repeated activity. Their sites are characteristic. They commonly occur in the distal part of the second and third metatarsal shafts (Fig. 10.10), the proximal and distal shaft of the tibia and fibula, the neck of the femur, and the pubic rami. A radiograph of the area involved is normal at the time of injury. No evidence of a fracture will be seen for between ten days and three weeks. The

FIG. 10.10 Oblique radiograph of the foot. A stress fracture of the third metatarsal neck is identified by the presence of callus formation, without a fracture line being evident.

FIG. 10.11 AP radiograph of the upper tibia of a child. Sclerosis (arrowed) and periosteal elevation (curved arrow) are due to a stress fracture.

Fig. 10.12 Lateral radiograph of the tibia. Marked thickening of the anterior cortex is seen. The wavy appearance is due to multiple old stress fractures.

Fig. 10.13 (a) AP and (b) lateral radiographs of the tibia. Initially, an osteosarcoma may be visualized predominantly as periosteal elevation.

fracture may first be seen as a thin translucent line, or periosteal callus may be visualized without evidence of the fracture line. Occasionally the fracture may be seen as sclerosis due to impaction, for example, in the tibia or calcaneum (Fig. 10.11).

In the tibia, multiple stress fractures in the anterior cortex may produce marked thickening, with a wavy outline that is sometimes associated with multiple horizontal radiolucent defects (Fig. 10.12). This appearance represents multiple stress fractures at different stages in healing. Occasionally periosteal and endosteal thickening of the cortex may be observed without a fracture line. If not seen in profile, a stress fracture may appear as a rounded lucency within thickened cortical bone.

There is often concern that these radiological abnormalities may be due to bone tumours. This is particularly so in lesions in the tibia, especially near the knee joint. An osteosarcoma may initially be visualized predominantly as periosteal elevation (Fig. 10.13); an osteoid osteoma normally causes sclerosis and cortical thickening. In the latter case a well-defined area of rarefaction is commonly seen in the bone (Fig. 10.14); in an osteosarcoma rarefaction is indiscrete. The osteoid osteoma gives a history of pain, predominantly at night, which is relieved by aspirin. Other tumours and infection do not usually cause great problems in differential diagnosis, provided that the history and the characteristic sites of stress fractures are remembered. Very occasionally the diagnosis can only be determined by biopsy.

Fig. 10.15 Oblique radiograph of the big toe. A fragment is seen distally which fits 'with the rest of the sesamoid'. Its margins are not rounded—a fracture of the medial sesamoid.

muscle, and produces an area of calcification which is orientated longitudinally along the limb (see Fig. 1.8(b), p. 7). Initially the appearances are of a cloud of calcification within the tissues, but, with time, this becomes organized and actual bony trabeculae can be identified.

Calcification is occasionally seen in certain areas of the body after chronic trauma, for instance in the medial collateral ligament of the knee (see Fig. 9.10, p. 149), the Pellegrini-Steida lesion, and in the adductors of the thigh, as seen in horse-riders. Bands of calcification, indicative of chondrocalcinosis, may be seen in fibrocartilage such as the knee menisci.

Osteochondral and chondral fractures

Abnormal joint movements associated with subluxation or dislocation may produce fractures of one or both joint surfaces. The resulting fragment may be cartilage alone, which will not be visible on plain radiographs, or may consist of a fragment of bone and cartilage. These fractures occur in characteristic sites, and close examination of the radiograph is often necessary to detect them. They are found after dislocation of the patella, and arise from the medial facet of the patella (Fig. 10.16) or the lateral femoral condyle. They are often best seen on the skyline view. Osteochondral fractures of the dome of the talus occur on both the medial and lateral aspects, and result from inversion injuries. They are usually best seen on the mortise view of the ankle joint (see Fig. 8.13, p. 138). Osteochondral fractures are also commonly observed in the capitellum and radial head.

Fig. 10.14 AP radiograph of the tibia. Marked thickening of the cortex with a central lucency (arrowed) is due to an osteoid osteoma.

Sesamoid fractures

In common with avulsion fractures, the opposing surfaces of a fractured sesamoid should appear to fit together and seem sharp and possibly jagged (Fig. 10.15). In practice it is probably impossible to make the diagnosis in the absence of suitable clinical findings. Sesamoid fractures, when they occur, are most commonly seen in the medial and fibular sesamoids related to the big toe.

Myositis ossificans

This results from calcification arising in a post-traumatic haematoma. It occurs characteristically in the quadriceps

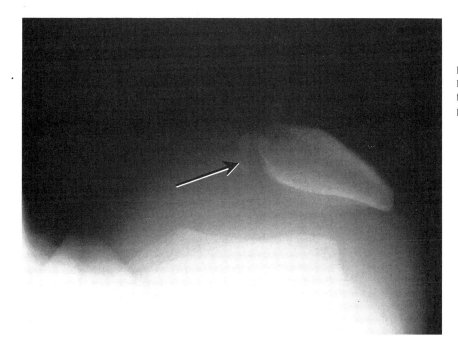

FIG. 10.16 Skyline view of patella. Fragments of bone (arrowed) have fractured from the medial surface of the patella after dislocation.

Osteochondritis dissecans

In osteochondritis dissecans a fragment of bone which is concave away from the joint becomes separate from contiguous bone, although the overlying articular cartilage may be intact. At its most minimal it may be identified only by a line of lucency around it (Fig. 10.17); at its most maximal a fragment of bone and its overlying cartilage may become free within the joint. These lesions are seen particularly in the femoral condyles, and may be demonstrated also in the talus and hip joint.

Dislocations

The need for suitable clinical information upon which the correct radiological views are taken is highlighted at the shoul-

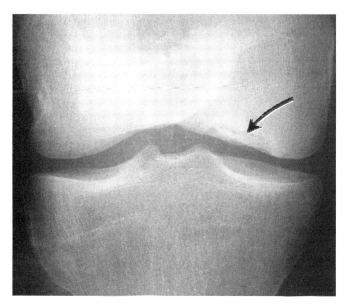

FIG. 10.17 AP radiograph of the knee. An area of osteochondritis dissecans with a line of lucency around it (curved arrow) is demonstrated.

der. Posterior dislocation of the shoulder joint is easily missed on the AP radiograph, as the radiographic features are subtle. The most reliable sign is that the head looks unusually oval because the upper arm is in forced internal rotation. It is important that when a posterior dislocation of the shoulder joint is considered a second view is obtained, preferably an axillary view.

Recurrent dislocations

These commonly occur in two sites—the patellofemoral and the glenohumeral joints. At the knee, the patella is dislocated in a lateral direction: this is associated with a low lateral femoral condyle seen on the skyline view of the patella, and a long infra-patellar tendon (patella alta). Recurrent anterior dislocation of the shoulder is associated with damage to the anterior glenoid labrum with or without the separation of a bony fragment (Bankart lesion).

Radioisotope bone imaging

In the diagnosis of sports injuries, radioisotope bone imaging is most commonly used to detect stress fractures. The images are obtained by a gamma camera after the intravenous injection of technetium-99m-labelled phosphate or diphosphonate. The amount of local radioactivity seen on the isotope scan correlates with the rate of mineralization of the bone; increased tracer localization or so-called 'hot spots' are seen in stress fractures. Hot spots can be seen at fracture sites as early as twenty-four hours after injury. This is well before evidence will be available on a radiograph.

Radioisotopic bone imaging is also of use in a patient in whom there is a history of pain, but in whom no fracture or abnormality can be detected radiologically even after a delayed period. This occurs particularly in the foot, where fractures of the navicular and cuneiforms may be difficult to see on a radiograph (see Fig. 9.22, p. 160). The detection of a hot spot on the radioisotopic scan allows a more localized search of the radiographs for a fracture; further views or CT scanning may be indicated.

Investigation of the joints

Magnetic resonance imaging (MRI) is now becoming the investigation of choice for the examination of many joints. Relying for its effect on the excitation of protons by magnetic fields and not requiring ionizing radiation, it has no known side-effects. It is extremely sensitive and has a higher diagnostic accuracy than arthrography in joint investigation.

Arthrography allows the surface of the joint to be examined, and is comprehensively described elsewhere (Freiberger and Kaye 1979). The aim is to coat the articular surfaces with a thin

(a)

(b)

FIG. 10.18 MRI investigation of the knee. (a) T1-weighted sagittal image through the intercondylar fossa of the knee. The anterior cruciate ligament is torn; its inferior part only is seen (arrowed). (b) Coronal T1-weighted image through the knee. A line of reduced density (arrowed) is seen surrounding a minimally depressed fracture of the lateral tibial plateau. This injury occurred in a skier; the clinical diagnosis was a lateral meniscal tear. Plain films were normal.

layer of radiological contrast medium, with air being introduced into the rest of the joint space. This is the so-called double-contrast arthrogram (Fig. 10.19(a)).

The knee

The advent of MRI has revolutionized the investigation of traumatic knee disorders. In addition to lesions of the articular cartilage, tears of the menisci can be diagnosed with high accuracy (Fig. 10.19(b)). Stress fractures of the tibial plateau, which are not unusual in athletes presenting with meniscal pain, are also well visualized (Fig. 10.18(b)). Furthermore, the severity of injuries to both the cruciate and collateral ligaments, as well as the patellar tendon, can be readily evaluated by this technique (Fig. 10.18(a)).

Knee arthrography is used principally to diagnose tears of the menisci. In Britain the usual approach into the joint is medial–at the junction of the upper third and lower two-thirds of the patella. About 6 ml of radiological contrast medium, for instance Hexobrix or Niopam, is introduced into the joint, followed by room air through the same needle—a volume of 30 ml is satisfactory. The patient is then asked to walk, or the leg is moved passively, before the radiographs are obtained. If fluid is obtained on puncture of the joint, it should be aspirated before the introduction of air and contrast.

The menisci are examined individually under radiographic screening with the leg positioned in appropriate degrees of rotation to obtain sequential radiographs from anterior to posterior, or vice versa. The number of these spot radiographs will vary from department to department, but about eight is satisfactory. An AP radiograph and a lateral radiograph with the anterior draw are obtained to demonstrate the integrity of the collateral ligaments and the cruciate ligaments respectively. The lateral is obtained with the leg hung over the table, with a pillow or foam pad behind the upper tibia, so that the foot is vertically ahead of the knee. A weight is placed on the foot to produce anterior draw at the knee. When the examination is completed, as much air and contrast as possible are removed from the knee through a needle introduced into a site similar to that used before.

The appearance of meniscal tears varies from case to case. They may be seen as lines of contrast crossing the menisci (Fig. 10.19(a)), as cleaves in the menisci, with contrast coating both lips, or as areas of increased density in the medial portion of the meniscus. The latter occurs with the so-called bucket-handle tears. The direction of the abnormality is commonly vertical, horizontal, or oblique, although more complex patterns may arise. It must be remembered that it is easier to be confident about the absence or presence of tears in the medial meniscus than in the lateral meniscus. This is because the anatomical features of the lateral meniscus are more complex, particularly its relationship to the popliteus tendon.

Post-meniscectomy arthrograms may present problems in interpretation. Often it is difficult to be certain whether abnormalities present are due to the remaining meniscus or to a new tear.

The ankle

Ankle arthrography is used to demonstrate tears of the calcaneo-fibular ligament. When this ligament is torn, contrast is seen to fill the peroneal tendon sheath, which lies in immediate proximity to the calcaneofibular ligament. Ankle arthrography can also be used to confirm that loose bodies lie within the joint.

(a)

(b)

Fig. 10.19 (a) Vertical tear of the posterior horn of the medial meniscus (arrowed) demonstrated by an arthrogram. (b) Oblique tear (arrowed) of the posterior horn of the medial meniscus demonstrated by MRI on a T1 weighted sagittal slice through the medial aspect of the knee.

The arthrogram is performed by the introduction of a needle under radiographic screening into the anterior tibiotalar joint space on its anteromedial aspect. One to two millilitres of radio-opaque contrast are introduced, and the joint is then distended by the introduction of approximately 6 ml of room air. Antero-posterior and lateral and both oblique radiographs are obtained. Tomography may be necessary to confirm the presence of fragments of bone within the joint.

Peroneal tenography is occasionally used after acute ankle injury, when rupture of the calcaneofibular ligament is suspected. After peroneal and sural nerve block, a needle is introduced into the peroneal tendon sheath behind the lateral malleolus under radiological screening control. Contrast is introduced into the tendon sheath in a volume of about 5 ml. If the investigation is positive, signifying a rupture of the underlying calcaneofibular ligament (and commonly rupture of the anterior talofibular ligament in addition), contrast will be seen in the ankle joint.

The shoulder

MRI is particularly useful in the evaluation of tears of the rotator cuff. Disruption of the elements of the cuff, commonly the supraspinatus tendon, may be visualized. Fluid in the sub-acromial bursa is also well demonstrated. The ability of MRI to evaluate the soft tissues and the availability of images in any plane required provide valuable assistance to the clinician in dealing with the impingement syndrome (Fig. 10.20(a)).

(a)

(b)

Fig. 10.20 MRI investigation of tendon injuries. (a) Coronal oblique T1 weighted image of the shoulder showing an osteophyte arising from the acromion (arrow) impinging on the supraspinatus tendon; there is also an osteophyte arising from the acromioclavicular joint (curved arrow) impinging on the supraspinatus muscle. (b) T2 weighted sagittal image of the ankle showing haemorrhage (arrow) at the site of a tear in the Achilles tendon; haemorrhage is also seen in the soleus muscle (curved arrow).

Although defects of the glenoid labrum are readily seen on MRI, shoulder arthrography is more commonly performed as part of the investigation of recurrent dislocation of the shoulder. In the case of an anterior dislocation, deformity of the anterior inferior rim of the glenoid and its overlying articular cartilage may be seen (Bankart lesion). In the case of a posterior dislocation, a defect of the posterior aspect of the labrum may be seen. These appearances are often difficult to diagnose with certainty on the radiographs, and CT scanning is of great value.

In the diagnosis of tears of the rotator cuff contrast may be seen extending into the subacromial and subdeltoid bursae. When a frozen shoulder is present, the joint capsule is shown to be contracted; this is particularly evident in the small size of the axillary recess.

The arthrogram is performed by the introduction of a needle, most commonly anteriorly, between the humeral head and the glenoid. Under radiographic screening approximately 4 ml of radio-opaque contrast is introduced followed by 10 ml of room air. In the case of a frozen shoulder, it is often useful to introduce local anaesthetic and steroid into the joint, and distend it until rupture and leakage of air from the joint capsule occurs. Active physiotherapy with maximum movement of the joint is then encouraged.

The spine

When available, MRI has almost completely replaced the use of myelography in the evaluation of disc disease. Images in both the axial and sagittal planes demonstrate the patho-anatomy of the disc prolapse and its relationship to the central neural tissue and the emerging nerve roots—loss of epidural fat signal is an important observation. The diagnosis of disc sequestration is assisted by the evaluation of the integrity of the posterior longitudinal ligament.

Radiculography may be used in the assessment of disc prolapse. A radiographic contrast is introduced into the spinal theca by a lumbar puncture. In the UK it is customary to keep patients in bed for twenty-four hours after this investigation. With newer contrast agents there few side-effects, the only one of any note being headache. Disc prolapses are demonstrated as filling defects in the contrast column, accompanied by poor filling or obliteration of the relevant nerve roots.

Muscle and tendon

MRI is the technique of choice for the assessment of injuries to the musculotendinous unit. In difficult or complicated cases MRI helps in the clinical grading of muscle injuries by the identification of haematoma, ossification, fibrosis, and muscle herniation. In tendinopathies the extent of intratendinous degeneration of fibre disruption can be gauged (Fig. 10.20(b)). This is particularly helpful in the Achilles tendon, but also applies to injuries to the patellar tendon when surgery may be contemplated.

Computerized tomography

Computerized tomography (CT) is at present the principal diagnostic tool in the evaluation of trauma in the brain. Both

Fig. 10.21 CT slice through the skull. A dense extradural haematoma is revealed.

extradural and subdural haematoma (Fig. 10.21) are well visualized. An extradural haematoma produces a biconvex abnormality in relation to the skull vault. A subdural haematoma is seen as a layer outlining the surface of the brain. Both types of haematoma appear dense in the first two weeks, after which time they reduce in density, eventually becoming less dense than the underlying brain. There is a stage at which they show the same density on the CT scan as the underlying brain tissue Both these collections of blood cause displacement of the midline of the brain away from the haematoma and tend to obliterate the ventricular system.

Evidence of concussion to the brain may be seen either as an area of increased density due to oedema, or as increased density due to blood lying within the brain tissues. The number and size of areas of haemorrhage may vary greatly. CT scanning may occasionally reveal an increase in brain volume recognizable by obliteration of the ventricles, basal cisterns, and cerebral sulci.

CT is the primary modality in the diagnosis of subarachnoid haemorrhage. Increased density due to blood may be found in the sylvian fissures and the basal cisterns, and in the ventricular system. In approximately 25 per cent of cases of subarachnoid haemorrhage, however, the CT scan is normal.

CT scanning is now used in the assessment of brain damage in boxers. This may reveal the presence of a cavum pellucidum, which is formed in the septum pellucidum, or frontal atrophy (Fig. 10.22).

CT is also of use in injury to the skeleton. It is of particular benefit in the spine, where it allows the production of images in the transverse plane. This is particularly helpful to the surgeon prior to consideration of operative intervention. CT is also capable of showing fractures at levels which appear normal on

Fig. 10.22 CT scan of the head of a boxer. A cavum pellucidum is illustrated (arrowed).

plain radiographs. In the pelvis, CT assists in the assessment of traumatic conditions which require surgery, and in the identification of loose bodies present within the hip joint.

Diagnostic ultrasound

This investigative modality uses sound with frequencies ranging from 3 to 10 MHz. The sound is transmitted into the patient by a transducer coupled to the skin with oil. The transducer receives reflected sound and demonstrates it as a two-dimensional picture. The picture is in 'real time', i.e. it is an image of what the transducer sees at the time.

Intramuscular haematoma may be demonstrated by ultrasound (Vincent 1988). Damage to tendons, particularly the Achilles tendon, can be demonstrated by a defect or thickening (Mack 1988; Fornage and Rifkin 1988).

The place of ultrasound in the management of these conditions is at present unclear.

References

Fornage, B. D. (1988). Ultrasound examination of the tendons. In: *Ultrasonography of the musculoskeletal system*. Radiologic Clinics of North America, W. B. Saunders, Philadelphia, PA.

Freiberger, R. H. and Kaye, J. J. (1979). *Arthrography*. Appleton-Century-Crofts, New York.

Mack, L. A. (1988). *Sonographic evaluation of the rotator cuff. In: Ultrasonography of the musculoskeletal system*. Radiologic Clinics of North America, W. B. Saunders, Philadelphia, PA.

Rogers, L. F. (1982). *Radiology of skeletal trauma*. Churchill Livingstone, New York.

Vincent, L. W. (1988). Ultrasound of soft tissue abnormalities of the extremities. In: *Ultrasonography of the musculoskeletal system*. Radiologic Clinics of North America, W. B. Saunders, Philadelphia, PA.

11 Prevention of injury

M. A. Hutson

Responsibility of the medical profession in sports injury prevention

Members of the medical profession, in particular those involved with sports injuries (and in the broader context with sports medicine), have a responsibility to advise both sports groups and individuals on aspects of prevention of injury resulting from sport. Such advice may be offered at all levels, with the recipients ranging from sports governing bodies on the one hand to local sports clubs and individual sports participants on the other. Major strides in injury prevention have been made in certain directions, though progress is slow in others, particularly where there are financial implications and where there are possibilities of infringement of personal freedom. This advisory function should be the responsibility not only of the various associations of sports physicians on behalf of their membership, but also of individual practitioners, acting in concert with administrators, managers, and coaches in their own localities.

Protective equipment

Reduction in the incidence of injury due to direct trauma is influenced by the design of protective equipment and the obligation upon the wearer to comply with the regulations of sports associations. An obvious example is the wearing of suitable helmets by horse-riders. In horse-racing the wearing of a skull cap of acceptable design is mandatory. In competitions under the control of the British Horse Society or the Pony Club it is also compulsory for the riders to wear a protective helmet that conforms to British Standards Institute regulations BS 4472 or BS 6473 (Fig. 11.1). However, many competitions are not held under such control, with inevitable consequences. Even when a helmet is worn, it is important to stress the need for attachment of the chinstrap. Of course, fashion plays a part. Not long ago Mike Brearley (an outstanding captain of English cricket in recent times) was advocating the use of head and facial protection while batting at cricket. At first, the reaction from the 'macho' element was of disbelief, but the application of protection in specific risk situations, for example batting or fielding close to the wicket, is now commonplace. In some sports, such as American football, motorcycling, cricket, and hockey (goal-minders), the helmet has a visor or grille extension to reduce the incidence of maxillofacial injury (Fig. 11.1). Standards and statutory requirements vary in different sports: in some it is also necessary to comply with international regulations.

In American football body protection has become so extensive that the sceptic is inclined to the view that the game is effectively a licence to injure. However, the incidence of head, neck, and shoulder injuries appears to be on the decline. In cricket batsmen often protect the forearms and thighs as well as the genitals. In karate the use of fist pads has been shown to reduce the severity of head injuries, which account for the majority of injuries sustained in tournaments (Johannsen and Noerregaard 1988).

Goggles are worn in a number of sports in which high speeds are encountered (see Fig. 2.7, p. 28). Special goggles made from

(a) (b) (c)

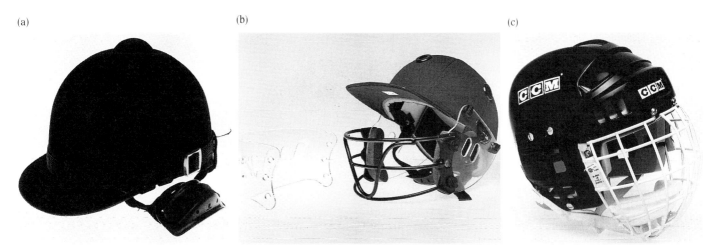

FIG. 11.1 Protective equipment: (a) equestrian helmet to BSI standards; (b) an example of a cricketer's helmet (alternative forms of visor are demonstrated); (c) ice hockey goal-minder's helmet.

tough polycarbonate material are available for squash, though to date none are approved by the Squash Rackets Association (see Chapter 2, Ocular injuries). However, one should not assume that the mere replacement of spectacles by contact lenses protects the eye. Increased damage to the eye may result from direct trauma to a contact lens; soft lenses are safest.

Mouth guards are compulsory in some sports, for example boxing, and their use is encouraged though not mandatory in others, such as rugby football. All contact sports participants are at risk; the highest incidences of injury to the mouth and teeth are in rugby football in the UK and American football in the USA. 'Non-contact' sports participants are not exempt, as direct trauma in these sports is not uncommon (for example, in squash and field hockey). It has been mandatory for some time for all high school and college footballers in the USA to wear mouth protectors: in the UK progress has been somewhat slower. A suitable protector acts against trauma to the teeth, fillings, bridges, and crowns. Additionally, the likelihood of laceration of lips, mouth, and tongue from the teeth is drastically reduced, as are mandibular fractures and concussion injury which may result from the teeth being forcefully clenched together by an impact from below (Chapman 1988).

A number of different mouth guards are available. 'Off the shelf' guards are the least adequate, as they may fit badly and easily be displaced. An inexpensive guard made from a thermoplastic material, for instance a polyvinyl acetate-polyethylene polymer, and moulded by the patient usually fits better, though it may not be sufficiently extensive or resilient at points of maximal stress. A custom-made mouth guard constructed from a cast impression taken by a dental surgeon is the most satisfactory (Fig. 11.2). A number of different materials are available; however, the cost is considerably higher than in the non-custom-made types.

The design of ski boots has helped to reduce certain types of injury such as ankle fractures, though to some extent these have been replaced by boot-top tibial fractures. 'Modern two-mode ski-release bindings have allowed earlier release of the ski under excessive rotational stress, and thereby reduced the incidence of grade I medial collateral ligament (MCL) knee injuries, though not the more severe knee ligament disruptions (Johnson and Ettlinger 1982). Proper care of bindings helps to reduce incidence of injury. It is also possible that further sophistication in the release system, for example from the present-day sensitivity to forward lean at the posterior attachment and twist at the toe, to a multimode system, might lower the incidence of lower-extremity injury still further.

Attention to specific clothing is important in certain sports—for example, the use of fireproof material for racing drivers, and the utilization of neoprene, reinforced by nylon, in the manufacture of water-skiing pants to prevent vaginal or rectal douches. Light-weight emergency anti-exposure clothing should be carried by hill-walkers and mountain-climbers to protect against sudden changes in the weather.

Sports arenas

Safety designs of arenas and training and competition surfaces, including pole-vaulting, high jump, and gymnastic landing areas, are important considerations. In gymnastics the basic basemat requirement of $1\frac{1}{2}$ inches of padding should be augmented by mats of 4 inch thickness around the various pieces of equipment. Suitable padding of essential props (for example, the goalposts in rugby football and ski-lift pylons) reduces the incidence of direct traumatic injury. Spring-back flagposts of non-breakable material should be used. Injuries to the thumb on dry-ski slopes may result from a fall in which the thumb is caught in the diamond-shaped gaps between the links. It seems likely that the incidence of this type of injury will be reduced when skiing on other recently introduced artificial surfaces. Indoor arenas should be designed to exclude obstacles such as radiators, which are potential sources of injury.

Rules of the game

Although body protection of different kinds may be custom-designed and, if necessary, made obligatory for sports which involve risk from extrinsic trauma, the enforcement of safety measures by the participants' adherence to rules is not always so easy. Illegal play is often dangerous. Prime examples are to be seen in rugby (union) football: both illegal collapsing of the scrum and the deliberate ploy of 'popping' the opponent upwards out of the scrum impart excessive strain on the cervical spine of front-row forwards (Burry and Calcinai 1988). A similar danger exists in the head-high short-arm tackle. Silver (1984) emphasized the risks to the cervical spine, and encouraged the Rugby Football Union to change certain interpretations of the laws for schools to make the game safer. The New Zealand Rugby Football Union has insisted on matching boys by weight,

FIG. 11.2 A variety of mouth guards are available. On the left an 'over the counter' gum-shaped shield is moulded by the player's teeth. On the right a 'custom made' guard is constructed from a disc of plastic (demonstrated) following a plaster impression taken by a dentist.

a sensible approach that appears to have been more difficult to enforce in the UK. Both Silver (1984) and Davies and Gibson (1978) related a percentage of rugby injuries to foul play; the collation of statistical medical information of this kind provides an example of the way in which the medical profession can be of considerable assistance to the governing bodies of sports.

Regulations regarding physical contact vary from one martial art to another; injury may result from the novice's inexperience or clumsiness, or from the expert's manipulation of the rules. Of course, lack of skill is to be expected in the beginner in any sport. In downhill snow-skiing, for instance, statistics often reveal a higher incidence of injury in the novice (Johnson *et al.* 1980; Davis *et al.* 1977). The pattern of injury may be different at the elitist level. Expert skiers tend to have a relatively higher incidence of shoulder injuries and the more severe type of knee injury. Professional soccer players accept a relatively high incidence of injury, which is more often due to the intensity of physical commitment than to dangerous play.

The control of dangerous play is in the hands of referees, umpires, and sports administrators; nevertheless it is incumbent upon the sports physician to advise on the medical implications of unnecessary violence. Regrettably, criminal proceedings have been necessary on occasions for assault on the field of play, and it seems likely that prosecutions will become more common.

Pre-participation screening

Guidelines on individuals' fitness to compete should be established in co-operation with the relevant sports bodies. The practice of medical screening (or 'profiling') prior to participation in sport varies enormously from country to country. On the basis of prevention of illness and injury, screening makes sense. As an example, the existence of hyperextension of the knees or hypermobility in general should result in a ban from contact sports because of the risk of ligament and/or joint injury. In the UK, however, the provision of such screening services within the framework of a National Health Service that is already stretched in other directions is debatable. Nevertheless a healthy debate should include the advocacy of a changing emphasis in health care towards prophylaxis against injury.

Participation in certain sports or recreational activities such as subaqua diving requires a medical examination and certification of fitness. Other sports require medical certification if the participant has reached a certain age—for example, is over 40 in parachuting. It is of some interest that people with certain medical conditions (which include giddiness and fainting) are prevented from parachuting, whereas there is no proscribed level of lower-limb musculoskeletal incompetence. Participation in the majority of sports in the UK does not require any statutory examination procedure.

A suitable pre-participation medical examination which encompasses the techniques described in individual chapters is summarized as follows.

History

Sports
Illnesses
Injuries
Surgery
Orthotics

Physical examination

Somatotype
General (body systems)

Musculoskeletal:

Spine
- Scoliosis
  Kyphosis
  Lordosis
  Pelvic tilt/leg length
  Cervical ROM ⎫ flexion, extension,
  Thoracic ROM ⎬ side flexions, rotations
  Lumbar ROM ⎭
  SLR
  Reflexes : upper limb
              lower limb

Shoulders
- Symmetry/Deformity
  ROM : abduction
      : external rotation
      : internal rotation
      : adduction
      : flexion
- Impingement/apprehension signs
- Muscle power: abductors
          :external rotators
          :internal rotators

Elbows
- Cubitus valgus
- ROM : flexion
      : extension/hyperextension
- Forearm ROM : supination
          : pronation
- Muscle power : flexors
        : extensors
        : supinators
        : pronators

Wrist/hands
- ROM   : wrist dorsiflexion
          : wrist palmarflexion
          : finger/thumb mobility
- Muscle power : wrist dorsiflexors
          : wrist palmarflexors
          : hand intrinsics

Hips
- Femoral anteversion (squinting patellae)
- ROM: flexion
      : extension
      : abduction
      : adduction
      : medial rotation
      : lateral rotation
- Muscle power: flexors
        : extensors
        : abductors
        : adductors
        : medial rotators
        : lateral rotators
- Flexibility: hamstrings
        : quadriceps
        : iliotibial tract

Knees
- Genu varum/valgum
- Effusion
- Q-angles
- Patella mobility/apprehension/alta
- Patella compression
- ROM : flexion/squat
       : extension/recurvatum
- Laxity : medial
       : lateral
       : anterior drawer (10˚ / 90˚)
       : posterior drawer
       : jerk test/pivot shift
- Muscle power : flexors
               : extensors

Lower legs
- tibia vara
- Achilles stretch
- Heel deformity
- Muscle power : triceps surae (tip-toe)

Ankles
- ROM : dorsiflexion
       : plantarflexion
       : squat
- Laxity: anterior drawer
       : talar tilt
- Muscle power : foot dorsiflexors
               : foot plantarflexors
               : invertors
               : evertors

Feet
- Pes cavus/planus
- Forefoot/toe deformity
- ROM : subtalar
       : midtarsal
       : first MTP

Technical factors in overuse injury

Introduction

Reduction in incidence of overuse injury is dependent upon the prior identification of the relevant aetiological factors responsible for overload. Thus excessive or abnormal biomechanical stress, caused by poor sports technique or associated with anatomical malalignment, needs modification by appropriate means. Further stress reduction should be achieved by the choice of suitable sports shoes and equipment (such as squash and tennis rackets). Training schedules should be critically assessed in conjunction with coaches and trainers—excessive training may improve some physiological parameters, but often leads to biomechanical injury.

Flexibility

Lack of flexibility in one or more joints may be found during medical examination or noted by the trainer/coach. It may be congenital—for example, the cavoid foot. Alternatively it may be due either to intrinsic joint pathology (for instance, capsular contracture or early degenerative disease) or to a lack of elasticity of the surrounding musculotendinous structures. Athletes generally may not receive appropriate advice on the relevance of stretching exercises, or may become non-compliant as a result of boredom, shortage of time, or for other reasons. It is of the utmost importance that exercise is preceded and followed by a flexibility programme for all major muscle groups to help prevent injury. Using dance as an example, considerable hip extension is required for arabesque; restriction of extension results in pelvic sway and excessive lumbar lordosis. Hamstring muscle tears (particularly in sprinters) and tendinitis are common if the hamstrings are not regularly stretched. Cyclists may also develop hamstring tendinitis, and therefore should utilize a stretching routine. Long-distance runners who have a 'shuffling' gait tend to develop limited hip movement as a result of soft tissue contracture, and are prone to pelvic stress injuries. Squash players are liable to back injury due to the combination of flexion and rotational stresses on the thoraco-lumbar spine; inadequate spinal flexibility compounds this risk. To help prevent subacromial problems in swimmers and tennis players (in whom external rotation of the shoulder may become restricted) an adequate warm up should include a comprehensive stretching routine for the shoulders.

Sports shoes

There has been a consistent improvement in design of running shoes over the last decade (Fig. 11.3). Excellent texts describing the construction of shoes are available (Anthony 1987; Cavanagh 1980; James *et al.* 1978), and a detailed account will not be reproduced here. However, one or two relevant general points should be made. An unsatisfactory level of support or shock absorption may be associated with the following:

(1) an inadequate shoe, for example a casual 'trainer' or squash shoe, being chosen instead of a running trainer;

FIG. 11.3 The construction of the modern running (training) shoe incorporates a number of features designed for support and shock absorption.

Padded tongue
Padded collar
Padded (cutaway) Achilles protector
Firm heel counter
External stabilizer
Toe box
Ridged outersole
Midsole
Wedge

(2) distortion occurring in the worn shoe;
(3) inadequate heel counter;
(4) inadequate arch support;
(5) early deterioration of the shock-absorbing properties of the midsole;
(6) disruption between the upper and the sole.

Pressure effects, giving rise to bursitis or tendinitis, may be due to the following:

(1) laces that are too tight;
(2) insufficient breadth of shoe;
(3) irritation from the heel tab;
(4) anatomical foot deformities;
(5) biomechanical abnormalities.

The overall level of medial arch support is often inadequate. The flimsy insole that is so often provided in a running shoe may be replaced by a more substantial commercially available arch support. An orthotic may be required for correction of excessive biomechanical stresses. Orthotic appliances ('orthoses') are used to realign an abnormally balanced foot by controlling either the subtalar joint or the forefoot (Fig. 11.4). A temporary 'soft' orthotic may be constructed in the surgery by the use of small pads of chiropody felt positioned on to a flexible insole: support under the medial arch and under the medial aspect of the heel is useful for overpronators. For greater sophistication, and for a long-term approach, a more rigid orthotic should be manufactured from a cast of the patient's foot made by an orthotist or podiatrist. The foot is cast in subtalar neutral; a positive mould is formed from this plaster cast by pouring in moulding plaster. (Alternatively, a foam cast may be used to replace the traditional casting method.) Suitable posting may be added to correct deformities. The orthotic is then constructed using one of a number of materials, according to the orthotist's or the manufacturer's inclination.

The most common reason for the use of orthotics is correction of compensatory overpronation of the foot associated with conditions such as forefoot varus (Subotnick 1985). Less satisfactory results are obtained with the supinated foot. Orthoses may be used to prevent injury or the recurrence of injury, or be part of the therapeutic armamentarium that is used for established conditions, such as metatarsalgia, plantar fasciitis, 'runner's knee', and iliotibial tract bursitis, when there are identifiable biomechanical foot abnormalities.

In comparison with running shoes, which have thick soles to reduce impact (and thus are unstable on change of direction), squash shoes provide greater stability, as they allow the foot to be closer to the ground.

Bicycle maintenance

Bicycles should be regularly overhauled, not only to prevent accidents resulting from major structural faults, but also to reduce the likelihood of the insidious onset of overuse injury due to abnormal biomechanical stress. In particular, emphasis should be given to the pedal–crank–bottom-bracket axle interconnections. Excessive wear or poor adjustment may result in patellofemoral pain. Further information may be gained from manuals such as *Richard's Bicycle Book* (Ballantine 1976).

Racket construction

Over the last few years artificial materials such as graphite and boron have been used increasingly in racket construction. Although unsubstantiated at present, it may be demonstrated later that the incidence of forearm and elbow overuse injury has been altered for the worse by this trend (despite some manufacturers' claims to the contrary). Sports physicians should monitor the incidence of injury so as to be able to advise on future construction patterns in the manufacture of sports equipment.

Technique

It is apparent that inadequate technique throws abnormal biomechanical strains upon the athlete's musculoskeletal system: examples are given throughout the text in individual chapters. Vigilance is required by teachers and coaches in order to prevent injury from poor technique. The incidence of low back problems, including spondylolysis, in young dancers should be kept to a minimum by attention to posture in certain exercises. Thus care should be taken to avoid an excessive lordosis at the barre and in floor exercises (Fig. 11.5). For the older (male) dancer a correct lifting technique is necessary to reduce lordotic stress. The foundation of proper dance technique is a strong well-balanced lumbar spine and pelvis. Excessive pelvic flexion or extension will undermine technique and increase the likelihood of injury.

The pivotal area of the spine, the lumbosacral junction, is also at particular risk in other sports if technique is faulty. Too much forward swing prior to powerful leg action in rowers should be corrected. Hyperflexion and hyperextension, both in the air and on water-entry, is a cause of low back injury in highboard divers. Overuse of the butterfly stroke is a further cause of low back pain in swimmers. In weight-training, injury risk may be lessened by preventing spinal flexion on attempting heavier loads.

Technique is particularly important in the various field athletics disciplines. In javelin throwing, for instance, power is maximized by rotation of the chest and body. During the throw, the

FIG. 11.4 Orthoses for the running shoe help to realign an abnormally balanced foot by controlling the subtalar joint and the forefoot.

FIG. 11.5 Excessive lordosis in gymnasts and dancers may cause low back problems: (a) a stylish finish; (b) poor posture at the barre.

(a)   (b)

knee ipsilateral to the throwing arm is brought through quickly to block forward momentum and 'square off' the body, thereby reducing the likelihood of a side-arm throw, which is more likely to incur shoulder strain. Varying degrees of upper body rotation are utilized in the different throwing styles.

In other sports, such as Alpine skiing, it is clear that technical guidance from qualified instructors may reduce the incidence of certain types of injury—for example, reduction of likelihood of injury to the first MCP joint by excluding the thumb from the leather wrist strap.

Malalignment

Femoral anteversion in young dancers increases the likelihood of lower limb injury (Fig. 11.6). Excessive internal rotation of the hips, detected most easily when a patient is examined in the prone position, is suggestive of femoral anteversion. The additional features of squinting patellae and excessive Q-angle are poor prognostic indicators for athletes contemplating long-distance running. Both pes cavus and pes planus are associated with increased incidence of foot and lower limb injury. Performance targets should be adjusted accordingly.

Biomechanics

A basic knowledge of sports mechanics is required to appreciate the factors involved in prevention of injury, aetiology of injury, and management of injury. Consideration should be given to such concepts as force, torque (force around an axis of rotation), centre of gravity, and lever arms. The axis of rotation itself has great relevance in certain joints such as the subtalar joint. In other joints the resultant force in different positions of the surrounding levers is of greater relevance—for example, in the patellofemoral joint. Of course, muscle function depends on its physiological state of training. Its force of contraction depends

FIG. 11.6 An abnormally large Q-angle due to femoral anteversion is demonstrated in the right leg of this patient.

on its cross-section, and its effectiveness on its position in relation to a joint. The ground-reactive forces—that is, those forces which are applied to the body by contact with the ground—depend on the magnitude of the force with which the athlete presses on the ground. Such external vertical forces amount to two and a half to three times the body-weight in running, and may increase to three or four times the bodyweight in jumping, and to even higher levels on bouncing (Nigg 1988). Therefore, activities such as the more aggressive forms of 'aerobics' impose considerable repetitive strains on the legs, commonly resulting in injuries such as Achilles tendinitis and shin splints. The suitability of shock absorption, either in the training shoe or the training surface, is an important consideration in the prevention of these injuries.

The mechanics involved in locomotion in its various forms, and the technical requirements of various sports, may not be obvious in a particular individual without more refined study. Video recordings that allow slow-motion playback of running style on a treadmill, EMG tests, stress plate analysis, high-speed motion photography, and discussions with the trainer or coach are all ways of identifying faults. Some of the instrumentation is available principally as a research tool, though increasing use is now made of video analysis in the clinical setting. The qualified coach or trainer is familiar with kinetics (analysis of movement) and dynamics (the muscle forces required for movement), so that under his guidance suitable flexibility and strengthening regimes are included in the athlete's training programme. The sports physician should also develop a suitable baseline of knowledge of kinesiology and be able to relate this to clinical

problems. For example, in sprinting, high knee action is coupled with early elevation of the heel towards the buttock as soon as the foot leaves the ground—rapid leg movement is achieved by the use of a small swing radius. Strong hip flexors and knee flexors are required. Training should concentrate on strengthening these muscles (principally the iliopsoas and the hamstrings), and creating a balance with the gluteals and the quadriceps. Routine stretching of all these muscle groups is equally important, and in hurdlers is particularly necessary for the hamstrings (Fig. 11.7).

The running style of long-distance runners (when compared with sprinters) is quite different: muscle economy is required. The running style is more of a shuffle, with little hip movement. Although powerful hamstrings are not required, nevertheless the athlete is at risk of developing hamstring contracture unless flexibility exercises are performed regularly. Poor elasticity of the hamstrings creates a risk of muscle 'pull' during bursts of activity—for example, in downhill running—that invoke greater stretch.

Further biomechanical considerations are identified by reference to the following examples, which are particularly relevant to a number of sports.

Abdominal muscle exercise

Well-developed abdominal muscles are required to stabilize the spine, acting as antagonists to the paraspinal extensors. They also reduce shear strain by their action on the dorsilumbar fascia, and unload pressure on the intervertebral discs during lifting. The extensors are rarely weak, either in athletes or in the general population, as they are postural muscles. However, the abdominals are often relatively weak: abdominal strengthening exercises are thus useful for all. A critical study of exercises which are commonly prescribed for abdominal strengthening reveals a need for differentiation between abdominal muscle contraction and hip flexor (iliopsoas) contraction. When hanging from a bar and raising the legs to the horizontal, or lying supine and raising both legs in the air, the iliopsoas contracts powerfully. There is a considerable transmission of force to the lumbar spine, increasing intradiscal pressure and increasing lordosis, thereby incurring risk of injury to the lumbar spine in those individuals who do not have established strong abdominal musculature. To offload the spine and yet exercise the abdominals instead of the hip flexors, trunk curl exercises should be performed in a specific way (Fig. 11.8(a)). In the supine position the hips and knees are flexed as far as possible and the feet placed flat on the floor. Alternatively both hips and knees are flexed to 90° as shown in Fig. 11.8(b). In this way the hip flexors are disengaged. Curled trunk sit-ups ('half' sit-ups only are possible) strengthen the rectus abdominae, and angulations to each side strengthen the external and internal obliques. Commonly, exercises are performed in less hip flexion with the ankles/feet supported under a wall bar for example. Although the lumbar lordosis has been abolished to a considerable degree in this position, the iliopsoas is able to assist the abdominals (Norris 1993). The earlier part of the sit-up is by concentric abdominal contraction, and the latter half is by concentric iliopsoas contraction.

Although elitist athletes are able to perform multiple hip flexor repetitions, the relatively less fit or those recovering from injury, particularly back strain, require expert guidance in the first instance on the correct way to exercise the abdominals in isolation.

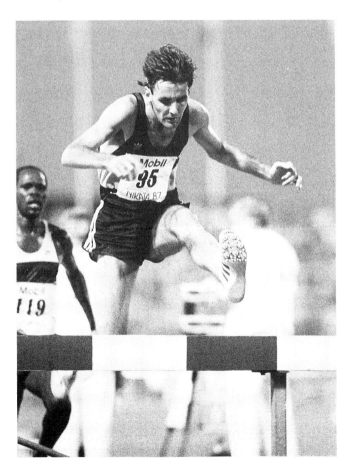

FIG. 11.7 Regular stretching of the hamstrings is especially important in hurdlers.

FIG. 11.8 Abdominal strengthening exercises are demonstrated (the hip flexors are disengaged and the trunk is curled).

Quadriceps femoris exercises

The rectus femoris flexes the hip and extends the knee. The vastus lateralis and intermedius extend the knee only. The vastus medialis obliquus (VMO) stabilizes the patella by pulling it medially. Examples of exercises which strengthen the knee extensor components of the quadriceps femoris are as follows:

(a) 'sitting' against a wall with both hips and knees flexed to 90° (isometric contraction);
(b) step-ups, particularly when extra load is applied by carrying free weights;
(c) squat jumps.

The muscle force increases as knee flexion increases (the lever arm extends significantly). Patellofemoral compression also increases alarmingly at the extreme of flexion—up to as much as eight times the bodyweight. Thus it may be seen that zero force is required to maintain the extended knee, i.e. in the upright position, and the VMO is not exercised significantly in these regimes.

Following injury, however, it is necessary to develop the VMO at the onset: the likelihood of patellofemoral pain is high if isotonic exercises are performed too early. Thus therapists take patients through a carefully graded sequence of straight leg raises—that is, isometric contractions in full knee extension (see Fig. 12.3, p. 208). Subsequently, progressive resistance training is performed using weights from flexion through to extension. Many gymnasia contain items of equipment which load the knee concentrically in this way. However, when this type of exercise is undertaken the patellofemoral joint is increasingly loaded, and the quadriceps work increasingly hard *in extension*, not flexion (see Fig. 7.8, p. 121). This is an unnatural situation for most everyday activities and sports. When 'unnatural' stress is applied, for instance when the relatively untrained or the skeletally immature engage in unsupervised exercise using gymnasium equipment that utilizes a weight-stack resistance principle, particularly the leg-press station, the risk of injury is significantly raised.

Biomechanics of running

The terms 'overpronation', 'podiatric assessment', and provision of 'orthosis' have become familiar to many competitive athletes,

who may assume (not unreasonably) that functional support in the running shoe is an important factor in prevention of injury. It behoves the physician to understand the basic principles involved in a biomechanical assessment, to eschew a too theoretical approach to mechanics, and to search for the practical applications. An understanding of the biomechanics of running facilitates this strategy.

The subtalar joint (STJ) is a linchpin of the system of stress distribution. Its axis is triplanar, passing from posterior, lateral, and inferior to anterior, medial, and dorsal (see Fig. 8.1, p. 130). It is also described as being a mitred hinge joint, reflecting its association with pronation/supination in the foot and internal/external rotation in the lower leg. Rearfoot *valgus* (calcaneo-valgus) is the hindfoot position when the subtalar joint is everted. When combined with abduction and dorsiflexion in the foot pronation takes place. On the other hand, rearfoot *varus* indicates inversion of the subtalar joint that, when com-

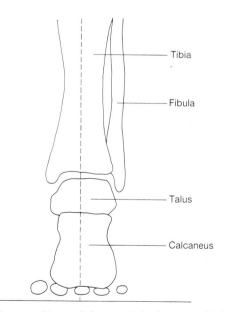

FIG. 11.9 The normal (neutral) foot (vertical calcaneus, subtalar neutral, and horizontal forefoot) observed in the midstance phase of the gait cycle.

Heel-strike   Midstance   Toe–off

F𝚒𝚐. 11.10 The running gait cycle: the phases for the right leg are shown.

bined with adduction and plantarflexion, contributes to supination of the foot.

The neutral position of the STJ (Fig. 11.9) is achieved when one-third of the movement from eversion to inversion has taken place, and is found at midstance in the gait cycle. The midtarsal (or transverse tarsal) joint comprises the talonavicular and calcaneocuboid joints, with motion occurring in all planes around longitudinal and oblique axes (see Fig. 8.2, p. 132). A full range of motion at the midtarsal joint is dependent upon the 'unlocking' of the subtalar joint in pronation. Assessment of the position of the forefoot relative to the hindfoot (with the STJ in neutral) determines any degree or forefoot varus or valgus.

The running-gait cycle includes phases of stance (heel-strike through to toe-off), float (double-limb unsupported phase), swing, and further float (Fig. 11.10). During the early stance phase the centre of gravity passes forward over the hindfoot, requiring a relative leg shortening. The STJ everts and the foot pronates. Transmission of force and motion to the midtarsal joints, and thence to the forefoot, allows the plantar surface of the forefoot to accommodate to the ground surface. Pronation is largely a passive event without muscular control. From midstance to toe-off supination takes place, during which both intrinsic and extrinsic foot muscles are active prior to the provision of heel-lift by the triceps surae. The limb then extends as the foot comes off the ground during acceleration.

Although the majority of long-distance runners use an initial heel-strike pattern, a small percentage (increasing as faster speeds are gained) have a midfoot strike. Sprinters usually have a forefoot strike pattern. The magnitude of the ground-reaction forces which occur during running may be measured by a force platform. Peak forces (in a biphasic fashion for rearfoot strikers, and uniphasic for midfoot strikers) of three times bodyweight are seen.

Abnormal biomechanics are discussed in Chapter 9.

Training schedules

Since inappropriate training schedules are a common source of overuse injury, it is clear that this is a subject with which the physician should be familiar. Naturally, a well-balanced training schedule is sought at all times, though the athlete recovering from injury is particularly at risk of relapse or further complications, unless muscle rehabilitation has been adequate and training is undertaken at the correct pace—that is, without abnormally large incremental increases in loading. His frustration during a period of disability and subsequently impatience to increase the intensity of training combine to cause further irritation if breakdown occurs. The physician may then be criticized for his 'mis-management' of the condition: indeed this may be a valid criticism if a suitable 'review' policy is not arranged on starting training. Particular care is required by the athlete at the beginning of a season (when he is relatively 'unfit') and towards the close of the season (when he may be 'stale'). Overtraining may led to generalized fatigue and poor competitive performance. Serum creatine phosphokinase may be significantly raised both in over-training and in sports such as some martial arts, in which there is repetitive direct trauma.

The risk of injury may be lessened by increasing muscle strength. Studies of American university footballers, for instance, have demonstrated that the frequency and severity of knee injuries are reduced by preseason total-body conditioning (Cahill and Griffith 1978). The importance of appropriate agonist–antagonist balance for a particular sport, in addition to muscle power and endurance, cannot be overemphasized. Loss of shock-absorbing capacity may occur in fatigued muscles, thus leading to increased stress and microfractures in the area of bone adjacent to their attachments. Recurrent stress (repetitive microtrauma) in musculotendinous units which are fatigued from repetitive eccentric contraction may result in tendinitis.

Regular strengthening of muscles which are not primarily involved in posture, such as the abdominals, should be performed by those who wish to undertake physical conditioning. Stretching exercises also contribute to muscle warm-up, thus helping to prevent the well recognized association of injury with 'cold' muscles. They also counteract the adaptive shortening of muscles that occurs with strength-training.

Common sense

Athletes who have achieved the feeling of well-being or 'high' from the endorphin release associated with endurance exercise are not always able to adopt an analytical or sensible approach when setting themselves targets or goals. The type of exercise that is chosen in the pursuit of physical fitness or conditioning may be inappropriate. It is not always appreciated by the 'prospective athlete' that endurance (aerobic) exercise is required to attain the level of 'cardiorespiratory' fitness necessary for a healthy life-style. A schedule of thirty minutes of jogging, brisk walking, cycling, or swimming three or four times a week should be the goal for those seeking recreational rather than competitive activity. For those who expand their exercise programmes, the risk is the linear association between the intensity of endurance exercise and the incidence of musculoskeletal injury.

Training characteristics
Strength training

During strength training, or recovery from disuse atrophy (for example, after immobilization), there is an increase in the number of muscle capillaries, an increase in myofibril size per cell, and an increase in mitochondria. It is possible that inter-conversion between fibre types II-A and II-B is a response to training techniques (see Chapter 1, Tissue injury—muscle, p. 6). No such interconversion appears to occur between types I and II: selective recruitment of the different type II fibres appears to be the more logical response. Generation of new fibrils occurs, and must be given time between training sessions to compensate for fibril destruction. Thus it is important to allow at least twenty-four to forty-eight hours between sessions of intensive strength training. Application of heavy workloads is necessary in strength training (for example, 80–95 per cent of the load that may be maximally managed)—and high-intensity low-repetition regimes are used. Increases in strength of up to 70 per cent are reported as typical training effects (Thorstensson 1976). However, endurance work requires repetitive stress with loads that correspond to 20–25 per cent of maximal capacity—that is, low-intensity high-repetition regimes.

Dynamic muscle activity is often a combination of *isotonic* (dynamic or concentric) contraction when muscle shortens, and *isometric* (static) contraction when there is no change in length. Muscle may also contract *eccentrically* while lengthening. Visco-elastic energy is stored by muscle when prestretched or pre-loaded by eccentric contraction prior to concentric contraction. This principle is employed during a type of training known as plyometrics when various drills are used to develop power for running, jumping, and rowing. Such drills include hops, power bounds, depth jumps, and jumping with weights. Free weights, or throwing and catching a medicine ball, may be used for the upper body.

Progressive resistance training is the mainstay of the develop-ment of strength, power, and local muscle endurance. Gradually increasing overload must be applied to the musculoskeletal system as adaptation occurs. Relatively inexpensive equipment, in the form of barbells, dumb-bells, and ankle and wrist weights, relies on gravity for resistance. At no extra expense an athlete may utilize his own bodyweight for resistance, for instance in bench-stepping and press-ups, in a conventional 'circuit'. Multi-gyms usually rely on the gravity effects of stacked weights, though at somewhat greater cost. Sets of repetitions are used, with the workload depending upon both the maximal capacity and the capability of the joint over which the muscle acts. Variation is required, as it has been observed that training by concentric contraction alone will not necessarily increase the ability to contract eccentrically.

Many health clubs and gymnasia now employ *variable resist-ance*, provided by equipment such as Nautilus or Atlanta. A series of cams and levers modifies the loading on a muscle (and therefore on a joint) at different angles of contraction. Although weight is selected in a similar way to the multi-gym, the engi-neering is such that ballistic movements are eliminated and heavier weights are capable of being handled. In distinction from the situation found using conventional weights, the athlete is not limited to using a weight that can be moved through the mechanically 'weakest' part of the muscle's range. The variable-resistance systems include a large number of pieces of equipment for exercising specific muscles or muscle-groups.

Isokinetic training employs a more specific 'accommodating resistance' by the use of hydraulics (Fig. 11.11). A dynamome-ter offers an equal resistance as soon as the preset speed is reached, thus matching the muscle contraction (Hislop and Perrine 1967). Increased muscular output produces increased resistance rather than the increased acceleration that would occur in gravity-loaded systems. Systems such as Cybex, Orthotron, and Lido include a computer linkage, so that torque in foot pounds and other measurements may be made (see Fig. 11.11(d), p. 189). Peak torque is defined as the highest point on the generated torque curve in foot pounds (1 foot pound = 1.356 newton metres). The joint angle at which peak torque occurs may be measured. A change in angular velocity affects this value: for instance, quadriceps peak torque occurs later in the range of motion with increasing speeds. Work, which is a reflection of the movement of force through an angular displace-ment, may be measured, and is represented by the area under the torque curve (Fig. 11.11(c)). There is substantial evidence that isokinetic exercise increases the work that a muscle can do more rapidly than isometric or isotonic exercise (Moffroid *et al.* 1969).

In comparing the mechanics of an isokinetic contraction with a dynamic one using weights as a resistance, the difference in the torque curve over the range of motion is striking (Grimby 1982). In an isokinetic exercise programme at the knee maximal resis-tance may be achieved throughout a complete range of motion. However, on examination of the torque values at 0° it may be seen that, if resistance work is required at or close to full knee extension, isometric training also should be employed.

Different sports require different muscle capabilities in respect of strength, power, and endurance. Eventually the establishment of a data base from testing protocols using isokinetic dynamome-ters should help to determine the function of specific muscle groups in each sport (Watkins and Harris 1993). Many sports, for instance soccer, demand a background of constant running interspersed with frequent demands for explosive power in the form of short sprints. Weight-lifters also require power—that is, strong fast contraction. Therefore training should be appropriate (sport-specific), and include a full complement of exercise, not solely that designed for endurance. Pure endurance training reduces the strength and power of muscles. Any athlete who has experienced the difficulty in coping with the bursts of activity demanded in a game such as squash rackets after a period of long-distance running training will recognize this.

Flexibility training

Adequate flexibility is essential for normal biomechanical func-tion in sport. Performance may be compromised if flexibility is inadequate.

(i) Sports techniques are difficult, if not impossible, to achieve.
(ii) Other training characteristics—for example, strength-training—may be impeded.
(iii) Excessive muscle activity is required, leading to prema-ture fatigue.

Of the factors affecting flexibility there are some which impose unyielding limitations—for instance, bone to bone, or bone to soft tissue impingement. But other factors, such as the following, may be influenced by flexibility exercises:

(i) the contractile (musculotendinous) structures that span joints;
(ii) the non-contractile (capsular/ligamentous) structures that are an integral part of joints.

Fig. 11.11 Isokinetic training (for example, with Lido isokinetic dynamometer) utilizes the principle of 'accommodating resistance' by the use of hydraulics. Muscle function may be assessed by computer linkage. (a) Knee flexors/extensors. (b) Shoulder abductors/adductors. (c) Typical torque curves are displayed for repetitions of knee flexion/extension at 90°/sec (the curves are emphasized for clarity). The positions of the joint ('joint angle') are also illustrated. (d) A typical print-out of Lido isokinetic results: bar graphs indicate average peak torque (if an injury is present this side is shaded); the remaining parameters are expressed digitally.

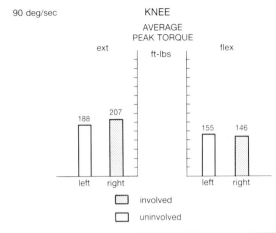

90 deg/sec

KNEE
AVERAGE PEAK TORQUE

ext · ft-lbs · flex

188 · 207 · 155 · 146

left · right · left · right

▨ involved

☐ uninvolved

(a)

(b)

STRENGTH

	Repetitions	5 LEFT	5 RIGHT	INV/UNIV %
PEAK TORQUE (ft-lbs)				
ext		198	210	106 %
flex		161	149	93 %
WORK PER REPETITION (ft-lbs)				
ext		162	153	94 %
flex		146	114	78 %
TORQUE RATIO (%)				
flex/ext		81 %	71 %	
PEAK TORQUE TO BODY WEIGHT RATIO (%)				
ext		104 %	111 %	
flex		85 %	78 %	
JOINT ANGLE AT PEAK TORQUE (degrees)				
ext		60	60	
flex		58	45	
RANGE OF MOTION (degrees)				
ext		98	86	
flex		99	86	

ENDURANCE

	LEFT	RIGHT	INV/UNIV %
TOTAL WORK DONE (ft-lbs)			
ext	811	765	94 %
flex	732	571	78 %

	LEFT	RIGHT	INV/UNIV %
FATIGUE INDEX (%)			
ext	90 %	92 %	102 %
flex	92 %	104 %	113 %

(d)

LIDO ISOKINETIC TEST RESULT

200 ft/lb 90 deg/sec   9–25–1986 9.4 seconds

Work (extension)   Peak torque

Work (flexion)   Joint angle

Torque ———
Position ———

KNEE - left	ext	flex
average peak torque (ft-lbs)	188	155
peak torque (ft-lbs)	198	161
joint angle at peak torque (degrees)	60°	58°
range of motion (degrees)	98°	99°
fatigue index (%)	90%	92%
total work done (ft-lbs)	811	732

(c)

Fig. 11.12 To maximize the force required to kick a football, the hip is extended, thereby creating viscoelastic energy in the rectus femoris which is subsequently required as a powerful knee extensor.

The term *laxity* refers to the degree of passive distraction or shear of a joint in a specific direction: it results from ligamentous insufficiency, for instance medial laxity at the knee after MCL rupture. If mobility in a wide spectrum of joints is excessive, the term *hypermobility* is applied (see Chapter 1). Neither situation is desirable.

Muscles which are used repetitively and remain unstretched, or muscles which are trained for strength only, become shorter. However, viscoelastic forces allow muscles to achieve maximum force when initially stretched to approximately 120 per cent of their resting length. Thus to maximize the force required to kick a football the hip is initially extended, thereby stretching the rectus femoris, which is subsequently required as a power knee extensor (Fig. 11.12). In throwing the javelin or discus the trunk is rotated maximally, thereby stretching the pectoralis major (among other muscle groups), which contracts powerfully in the forward acceleration phase.

Flexibility training develops this capacity for viscoelastic energy storage by overload. *Long slow (passive) stretching* is required. Passive stretching is often reinforced with the aid of external forces, thereby creating passive 'assisted' stretching—for example, resting the heel of the outstretched leg on a plinth to stretch the hamstrings. *Ballistic* stretching, on the other hand, should not be considered to be anything other than a form of 'toning up' for muscles. It stimulates the stretch reflex and, if performed too vigorously when the athlete has warmed up inadequately, may provoke muscle pulls. De Vries (1962) found that flexibility may be improved significantly (and equally) by both static and ballistic methods. *Post-contraction relaxation* is another

technique that is utilized in both training and therapeutic contexts. Muscle may lengthen further after isometric contraction at the extreme of range—therapists use this principle in the technique of PNF (proprioceptive neuromuscular facilitation).

In summary, flexibility exercises are used:

(i)   in rehabilitation to re-establish normal joint function;
(ii) prophylactically to prevent injury;
(iii) in training to achieve a maximally efficient biomechanical framework for specific sports techniques.

Examples of flexibility exercises are demonstrated in Fig. 11.14, pp. 198–201.

Fitness assessment

A number of identifiable factors are involved in the preparation of an individual or a collection of players in team sports to a level of maximal effectiveness. Some factors, such as motor skills, tactics, and team selection are clearly the responsibility of coaches, trainers, and managers. In other areas, such as the development of improved materials used in the manufacture of running shoes, and the reduction of drag in speed sports such as yacht-racing, car-racing, sprinting, and sprint cycling by streamlining including the use of wind suits, the bio-engineer plays his part. Other factors which are within the domain of the sports physician, psychologist, and physiologist are the provision of sports medical services, psychological training, and fitness assessment. A large contribution to fitness assessment may be made by the physiologist, although a 'team approach' in which the physician plays a leading role is desirable. A thorough medical examination (see previous section on 'Pre-participation screening') should precede the more dynamic (physiological) aspects of fitness evaluation.

Physiological assessment

The physiological components which may contribute to athletic performance may be outlined as follows.

1. *Physique.* Whilst somatotyping individuals into ecto-morphs, endomorphs, and the typically athletic mesomorph is interesting, it is of little practical benefit. In sports such as American football it is quite clear that size is as important as explosive power. On the other hand, the variation in body size of 800 metre runners is quite extensive. The determination of body-fat per unit bodyweight is of more relevance, and may be calculated by the use of skin-calipers. Reference is made to conversion tables once average values are determined from the four skin-sites, i.e. those overlying triceps and biceps in the upper arm, at the inferior angle of the scapula, and finally over the iliac crest. Alternatively, lean body-weight may be determined by electrical impedance.

2. *Flexibility.* Although an initial evaluation should be made during medical examination, the physiologist performs his own tests. The assessment of flexibility should not be confined to an isolated test for combined trunk flexion and hamstring elasticity (touching the toes), despite its relative importance. All the major joints are examined. Specific stretch tests for muscles which span two joints are performed. At very mobile joints range of motion in the position of function is recorded—for example, external rotation in 90° abduction of the shoulder in tennis

FIG. 11.13 Max. VO_2 may be measured using a recording of heart rate and expired air analysis (this test is being performed at the Sports and Fitness Assessment unit at the London Bridge Clinic). Cardiac function may be assessed simultaneously using a Marquette ECG.

players. Hypermobility should be recorded if present: it should be looked for routinely in dancers and gymnasts (see Chapter 1).

3. *Aerobic fitness*. The capacity of the cardiovascular system to deliver appropriate quantities of oxygen to working muscle is conventionally measured by determination of maximal O_2 intake (max. VO_2). The Astrand method, depending on the use of conversion factors from a knowledge of heart rate and work performed, has been used for some time. A more accurate method requires expired air analysis (Fig. 11.13), though increased costs may be restrictive. A sport-specific ergometer should be chosen if available—for example, bicycle, treadmill, rowing ergometer, or swimming flume. Gradually increasing effort to exhaustion is required of the athlete.

Max. VO_2 should be measured in athletes whose sports involve over two minutes of continuous vigorous activity. Aerobic capacity depends on the ability of muscles to cope with the available oxygen.Muscular endurance as well as cardiovascular efficiency is improved by training. Max. VO_2 in the relatively unfit may improve by up to 25 per cent following suitable training. Typical figures in athletes who depend on high aerobic capacity are 65–80 ml per kg bodyweight.

4. *Anaerobic threshold (AT)*. At a given submaximal exercise intensity muscle relies largely on anaerobic metabolism to deliver energy. Much greater amounts are available, although for limited periods of time; the accumulation of chemicals such as lactic acid causes increasing discomfort. The anaerobic threshold depends on the body's capacity to metabolize lactic acid. Therefore determination of the AT yields information on the capacity to *sustain* high levels of aerobic work. When used to test endurance capacity it correlates better than max. VO_2.

Its physiological basis has not been universally agreed. The onset of blood lactate accumulation (OBLA) is often measured; other parameters are associated with the sudden relative reduction of VO_2. Endurance training causes the AT to increase significantly compared with max. VO_2. The running speed at the AT correlates well with the maximal running speed over middle and long distances.

5. *Anaerobic fitness*. Explosive bursts of energy are required in a number of sports, and are provided by the creatine phosphate energy store and anaerobic glycolysis. An anaerobic test measures the quantities of work that a muscle group can produce maximally, in addition to its ability to recover. A typical example is the Wingate test using a cycle ergometer. Calculated values for the total work done and mean power output are measured for short bursts of maximal exercise, and reflect the subject's work capacity. A *recovery index* may be determined by noting the relevant recorded data on repeated tests after short rest intervals. Alternatively, an isokinetic dynamometer may be used: the time taken for torque to drop to 50 per cent of its initial value, or the torque level after 30 contractions at a high angular velocity, for example, 300° per second, are recorded. A *fatigue index* is determined by this means.

6. *Muscle strength and power*. Sheer 'strength' (which may be measured in a number of ways because it has no inherent definition) plays its part in a number of sports. It is usually required for limited periods—for example, in rugby scrummaging. The fast delivery of force—that is, of *power* which is measured in foot pounds or newton metres per second—is often much more relevant. Conventionally, when measured by an isokinetic dynamometer, the faster speeds—for example, 240° or 300° per second—are used, as it is thought that these more accurately reflect function. However, Rothstein *et al.* (1987) point out that no evidence exists to suggest that different speeds of movement test different muscular characteristics. Field tests such as sergeant jumps, short sprints, and throwing the shot in different ways offer a cruder indication of power in different muscle groups.

The Lido isokinetic dynamometer (Fig. 11.11) in use at the Sports and Fitness Assessment Unit at the London Bridge Clinic has a number of practical applications in assessment and rehabilitation, summarized as follows:

(1) determination of fatigue index—an anaerobic test of local muscle endurance;

(2) establishment of a data base of muscle function for fit individuals or team members;

(3) detection of muscle imbalance—as an assessment procedure or in established injury, for example, comparison of torque ratios of agonists and antagonists;

(4) rehabilitation after injury;

(5) isokinetic training.

Psychological assessment

Psychological factors have a significant effect on an athlete's capacity for (or perseverance in) training, and motivation for competition or increased intensity of effort (Yaffé, 1983). Factors which are generally believed to influence sports performance include anxiety, aggression, motivation, concentration, self-confidence, pain tolerance, and emotional state. Psychometric evaluation of abilities, aptitudes, and skills by objective measurement and techniques may be performed by the sports psychologist.

Yaffé (personal communication 1988) used Nideffer's Test of Attention and Interpersonal Style (Nideffer 1981) to determine the capacity of talented young tennis players to cope with stress, and Eysenck's Personality Questionnaire to gauge sociability, impulsiveness, emotionality, and toughmindedness. Response to specific training and competitive situations is assessed by a structured interview.

Community fitness

The need for an increased emphasis upon disease prevention within the framework of the National Health Service in the UK has been appreciated for some time. Various arguments, not least those involving financial implications, have apparently prevented its more extensive development. Debate still continues over the relative importance of the aetiological factors implicated in the health scourge of affluent Western civilization—coronary artery atherosclerosis. There is general agreement over the adverse effects of smoking and hypertension, though the subsidiary roles of obesity, stress, and a sedentary existence seem less clear. Hypercholesterolaemia appears to be involved, with the result that fat-reducing diets are widely available.

Studies (e.g. Kavanagh *et al.* 1979) have purported to show the usefulness of regular exercise in the prevention of progressive coronary artery disease after a first myocardial infarct. A logical extension of this argument is that exercise may prevent the initial onset of coronary artery disease in the asymptomatic subject, possibly by assisting in maintenance of serum cholesterol and weight within accepted norms. Although studies such as that by Morris *et al.* (1953) on London busmen and Paffenbarger and Hale (1975) on San Franciscan longshoremen have shown an association between active jobs and reduction in ischaemic heart disease, a causal relationship is not established. Furthermore, comparison of the apparent beneficial effects of work activity and leisure pursuits is difficult. Nevertheless it is generally accepted that exercise reduces the likelihood of developing coronary heart disease. Morris *et al.* (1980) have shown that the important aspect of this cardio-protective effect is repeated bouts of vigorous exercise, rather than overall energy expenditure. Other benefits to health from exercise are as follows:

(i)   prevention of osteoporosis;

(ii) facilitation of management of chronic disease such as diabetes;

(iii) increase in physical working capacity;

(iv) improvement of mood.

Evaluation of risk factors is available at screening centres within the private medical sphere in the UK. The more dynamic aspects of health and fitness, with particular reference to the role of exercise, are determined by appropriate tests at the Sports and Fitness Assessment Unit at the London Bridge Clinic. The testing protocol conforms to as sophisticated a system of dynamic assessment as is currently available.

1. Medical examination identifies abnormalities of the musculoskeletal system as well as other physiological systems. Flexibility is assessed. The resting blood pressure is measured.

2. Anthropometric measurements include height and weight.

3. Body fat percentage is calculated from skin caliper measurements.

4. Lung function is determined by spirometry.

5. Cardiac function is assessed by a stress ECG using a 12-channel 12-lead Marquette machine while the subject exercises on a treadmill or bicycle.

6. Aerobic fitness is measured by expired air analysis. Maximal exercise testing (to exhaustion) using one of several protocols on a treadmill or bicycle ergometer is performed on subjects who take regular vigorous exercise. Max. Vo_2 and anaerobic thresholds are calculated, where possible, and assessment made by comparison with age-related tables. Submaximal tests are used for subjects who do not take regular exercise or who are recovering from cardiac disorders or bypass surgery: nevertheless max. Vo_2 may be computed from tabulated oxygen consumption. The test is concluded when the subject's heart rate rises to the target heart rate adjusted for age.

7. Muscle power and endurance (in the quadriceps and hamstrings) are assessed on a Lido isokinetic dynamometer.

8. Urinalysis and haematological screening, including cholesterol and triglycerides, are undertaken.

9. Finally a 'prescription' is issued with suggestions for a healthier life-style, including a suitable exercise regime. The subject's inclinations, musculoskeletal capabilities, and cardiovascular tolerance are taken into account in the formulation of the prescription.

Exercise prescription

Three components should be included.

1. Warm-up. During this five-minute phase exercises to stretch large muscle-groups are performed, preparing them for sustained activity. The combination of long slow stretch and muscle-toning in the form of jogging on the spot or hopping increases muscle blood-flow.

2. Endurance or aerobic. During this phase, lasting fifteen to thirty minutes, intensity should be tailored, depending upon the baseline of fitness, to increase aerobic capacity. Although different formulae are used, a rule of thumb guide is for a target heart rate of approximately 75 per cent of maximal safe heart rate to be achieved and maintained. Maximal heart rate is usually considered to be 220 minus age. For example, for a forty-year-old $220 - 40 = 180$ beats per minute; thus target heart rate in this case would be 135 beats per minute. Clearly the type of aerobic activity will depend upon a number of factors already outlined:

fast walking, swimming, cycling, and jogging are commonly prescribed.

3. Cool down. During this phase body metabolism is allowed to return to normal gradually by the inclusion of a reduced level of muscle activity. Callisthenic exercises, which have the added desirable effect of improving anaerobic fitness, may be added to walking or a slow jog.

Injury prevention in children

An understanding of the pattern of musculoskeletal injury in children is required prior to a consideration of injury prevention. The different patterns of injury are dependent on the difference in the relative strength of the various components (bone, tendon, muscle, and ligament) in the child compared with the adult. Thus indirect stress applied to the articular framework in children is more likely to result in epiphyseal fracture than in ligament disruption. Salter and Harris (1963) classified fractures involving the epiphysis into grades I–V depending upon the extent of the involvement of the metaphysis or diaphysis. When faced with apparent joint injury in the child radiological investigation of the epiphysis should be undertaken, and orthopaedic surgical opinion should be sought if disturbance is detected. Joint instability tends to be caused by avulsion of a bony fragment attached to a ligament, rather than to an intraligamentous tear. The equivalent of the anterior cruciate ligament (ACL) tear in the adult is avulsion fracture of the inferior attachment of the ACL at the intercondylar area of the tibia. Surgical management by re-attachment of the bony fragment is advisable. In general a satisfactory outcome may be expected following such fracture management.

Traction forces which result in muscle tear or tendon rupture in the adult tend to cause fracture separation of the apophysis in the child. Examples of acute avulsion fractures are found in the pelvic girdle (see Fig. 6.14, p. 111). The affected apophyses are located at:

- iliac crest—origin of gluteus medius and insertion of external oblique
- anterior superior iliac spine—origin of sartorius
- anterior inferior iliac spine—origin of rectus femoris
- ischial tuberosity—origin of hamstrings
- lesser trochanter—insertion of iliopsoas.

Fragmentation of an apophysis that results from chronic repetitive stress is referred to as a traction osteochondrosis. Examples of stress injuries to the apophyses in the upper limb are found at the coracoid process (origin of coracobrachialis and the short head of biceps brachii) and in the lower limb at the tibial tubercle (Osgood-Schlatter's disease) and the posterior calcaneal tubercle (Sever's apophysitis). The acute injuries should be treated in the same way as muscle tears—that is, with a full stretching and strengthening programme during rehabilitation. The stress injuries require reduction of load; relative rest for two to three months may be sufficient.

Overuse injury patterns are similar to those in the adult. Stress fractures are common, though they may occur at the epiphyseal growth plate as well as the diaphysis. In the upper limb stress fractures of the proximal humeral epiphysis in Little Leaguers (baseball pitchers) and of the distal radial epiphysis in gymnasts (see Fig. 4.7, p. 57) have been recorded. X-rays often show widening of the epiphysis; bone scans may confirm the diagnosis, though interpretation is sometimes difficult as there is

increased uptake in the normal epiphysis. Stress fractures in the lower limbs conform to a similar pattern to those found in adults. Stress fractures in the partes interarticulares of the lower lumbar vertebrae (spondylolyses) are largely confined to children under twelve, when they are often relatively (or completely) painless, and to adolescents (aged thirteen to seventeen), when they are usually painful (see Fig. 5.7, p. 85). Repetitive micro-trauma may lead to compression fracture of the anterior margins of the vertebral bodies in the thoracic and thoracolumbar regions, giving rise to the clinical syndrome of Scheuermann's disease (see Fig. 5.5, p. 83). A tight lumbodorsal fascia associated with an increased lordosis are thought to be contributory factors (Micheli 1983).

Disorders of the articular cartilage may also occur during growth spurts. Osteochondritis dissecans of the capitellum is seen in gymnasts (see Fig. 4.4, p. 54). Osteochondritis dissecans of the knee occurs in juniors as well as in adolescents (see Fig. 10.17, p. 177). Although the aetiological factors remain unproven, recurrent microtrauma is suspected.

In the determination of the aetiological factors involved in overuse injury a full range of possible abnormalities of technique, malalignment, and abnormal biomechanics should be studied as for the adult. In some sports, such as swimming, the peak of potential may be realized while the child is still in the mid-teens. Miles of swimming training may be performed each day, resulting in injury to the shoulder, in particular, and to other areas, of which the most notorious is breast-stroker's knee (see p. 146). Other sports, including gymnastics and dance in its various forms, require training from an early age. Extreme flexibility is required in many joints. Injury patterns may be associated with lack of flexibility in crucial areas—for instance, inadequate hip mobility leading to low back injury in ballet dancers.

In some youngsters in their early teens recurrent injury may be associated with relative tightness of the musculotendinous structures. Growth spurts involve axial lengthening of the long bones. Unless flexibility exercises (Fig. 11.14) for the contractile tissues are undertaken at this time recurrent muscle pulls may be sustained. Usually the child is no more inclined than the average adult to perform regular stretching exercises, and therefore must be suitably encouraged.

The possibility of long-term skeletal problems resulting from repetitive intensive exercise from an early age is conjectural. Since it is accepted that a delay in sexual maturity associated with delayed puberty may occur in girls as a result of intensive and prolonged sporting activity, it is of some concern that skeletal maturation may also be affected. Murray and Duncan (1971) and Stulberg et al. (1975) have suggested that repetitive stress to the capital femoral epiphysis in childhood could be an aetiological factor in the causation of adult osteoarthritis of the hip. It is possible that a reactive hypertrophy of the humeral head, secondary to the repeated stress of throwing in childhood, may cause impingement syndromes in the adult (F. Jobe in a personal communication to L. Micheli). Further research is required in these directions before definite conclusions may be drawn.

In the protection of children from inappropriate levels of stress, responsibility should be shouldered by the relevant contact groups: parents, teachers, coaches, trainers, sports clubs, and sports associations. Parents, in particular, may need suitable counselling when their child has considerable athletic potential. Sports associations have a special responsibility for grouping children by weight, as well as height and age, in contact sports

Fɪɢ. 11.14 Flexibility exercises demonstrated by Jack Buckner.

(a) External rotation of the (right) shoulder using a stick

(b) Internal rotation of the (left) shoulder using a stick

(c) Extension of the shoulders using a stick

d) Backward roll for trunk flexion

e) Trunk rotation

(f) Side flexion of the trunk

(g) Flexion of the hip

(i) Abduction of the (right) hip, standing (adductor stretch)

(h) Extention of the right hip (psoas stretch)

(j) Abduction of the hips, sitting (adductor stretch)

(k) Adduction of the right hip (iliotibial tract stretch)

(l) External rotation of the flexed adducted hip (glutei stretch)

(m) Internal rotation of the (right) hip combined with contralateral hamstring stretch

(n), (o) Hamstring stretching

such as rugby football. In New Zealand children have been graded by weight for some time; as yet there is no statutory requirement in the United Kingdom. By definition children are immature, and therefore need advice. Very often, however, a child, if left alone to decide for himself how much sport he wishes to play, will formulate an appropriate judgement. In this respect he may be more mature than his advisers.

References

Anthony, R. J. (1987). The functional anatomy of the running training shoe. *Chiropodist*, **42** (12), 451–9.

Ballantine, R. (1976). *Richard's bicycle book* (revised edn). Pan Books, London.

Barry, H. C. and Calcinai, C. J. (1988). The need to make rugby safer. *Br. Med. J.*, **296** (6616), 149–50.

(p) Quadriceps stretching

(q) Soleus stretching

(r) Gastrocnemius stretching

Cahill, B. R. and Griffith, E. H. (1987). Effect of preseason conditioning on the incidence and severity of high school football knee injuries. *Am. J. Sports Med.*, **6**, 180–84.

Cavanagh, P. R. (1980). *The running shoe book.* Anderson World, Mountain View, CA.

Chapman, P. J. (1988). The pattern of use of mouthguards in rugby league (a study of the 1986 Australian rugby league touring team). *Br. J. Sports Med.*, **22** (3), 98–100.

Davies, J. E. and Gibson, T. (1978). Injuries in rugby union football. *Br. Med. J.*, **6154**, 1759–61.

Davis, M. W., Litman, T., Drill, E., and Mueller, J. K. (1977). Ski injuries. *J. Trauma*, **17**, 802–8.

De Vries, H. A. (1962). Evaluation of static stretching procedures for improvement of flexibility. *Res. Q.*, **33**, 222–9.

Grimby, G. (1982). Isokinetic training. *Int. J. Sports Med.*, **3**, 61–4.

Hislop, H. J. and Perrine, J. J. (1967). The isokinetic concept of exercise. *J. Am. Phys. Ther. Assoc.*, **47**, 114–7.

James, S. L., Bates, B. T., and Osternig, L. R. (1978). Injuries to runners. *Am. J. Sports Med.*, **6** (2), 40–50.

Johannsen, H. V. and Noerregaard, F. O. H. (1988). Prevention of injury in karate. *Br. J. Sports Med.*, **22** (3), 113–15.

Johnson, R. J. and Ettlinger, C. F. (1982). Alpine ski injuries: changes through the years. *Clin. Sport Med.*, **1** (2), 181–97.

Johnson, R. J., Ettlinger, C. F., Campbell, R. J., and Pope, M. H. (1980). Trends in skiing injuries. *Am. J. Sports Med.*, **8** (2), 106–13.

Kavanagh, T., Shephard, R. J., Chisholm, A. W., Qureshi, S., and Kennedy, J. (1979). Prognostic indices for patients with ischaemic heart disease enrolled in an exercise-centered rehabilitation program. *Am. J. Cardiol.*, **44**, 1230–40.

Micheli, L. J. (1983). Overuse injuries in children's sports: the growth factor. *Orthop. Clin. North Am.*, **14** (2), 337–60.

Moffroid, M., Whipple, R., Hofkosh, J., *et al.* (1969). A study of isokinetic exercise. *Phys Ther.*, **49**, 735–47.

Morris, J. N. *et al.* (1953). Coronary heart disease and physical activity at work. *Lancet*, **2**, 1053–7, 1111–20.

Morris, J. N. *et al.* (1980). Vigorous exercise in leisure time: protection against coronary heart disease. *Lancet*, **2**, 1207–10.

Murray, R. O. and Duncan, C. (1971). Athletic activity in adolescence as an aetiological factor in degenerative hip disease. *J. Bone Jt. Surg.*, **53B**, 406–19.

Nideffer, R. (1981). *The ethics and practice of applied sport psychology.* Mouvement Publications, Ithaca, NY.

Nigg, B. M. (1988). The assessment of loads acting on the locomotor system in running and other sport activities. *Seminars in Orthopaedics*, **4** (3), 197–206.

Norris, C. M. (1993). Abdominal muscle training in sport. *Br. J. Sports Med.*, **27** (1), 19–27.

Paffenbarger, R. S. and Hale, W. E. (1975). Work activity and coronary heart mortality. *New Eng. J. Med.*, **292**, 545–50.

Rothstein, J. M., Lamb, R. L., and Mayhew, T. P. (1987). Clinical uses of isokinetic measurements. *Phys. Ther.*, **67** (12), 1840–44.

Salter, R. B. and Harris, R. (1963). Injuries involving the epiphyseal plate. *J. Bone Jt. Surg.*, **45A**, 587–622.

Silver, J. R. (1984). Injuries of the spine sustained in rugby. *Br. Med. J.*, **288**, 37–43.

Stulberg, S. D., Cordell, L. D., Harris, W. H., *et al.* (1975). Unrecognised childhood hip disease: a main cause of idiopathic osteoarthritis of the hip. In *The Hip: Proceedings of the Third Open Scientific Meeting of the Hip Society*, Vol. 3, pp. 212–18. Mosby, St Louis, MO.

Subotnick, S. I. (1985). The biomechanics of running: implications for the prevention of foot injuries. *Sports Med.*, **2**, 144–53.

Thorstensson, A. (1976). Muscle strength, fibre types and enzyme activities in man. *Acta Phys. Scand. Suppl.* **443**, 1–45.

Watkins, M. P. and Harris, B. A. (1983). Evaluation of isokinetic muscle performance, *Clin. Sports Med.*, **2** (1), 37–53.

Yaffé, M. (1983). Sports injuries: psychological aspects. *Br. J. Hosp. Med.*, **29** (3), 224–33.

12 Treatment and rehabilitation

M. A. HUTSON

General concepts

It is useful at the outset to define terminology; that this is more than pure semantics should become obvious in the text. 'Treatment' usually refers to those therapeutic measures that are used in healing injured tissue. 'Rehabilitation', on the other hand, literally means restoration of a normal state of health or well-being, and is a more all-embracing term. Total rehabilitation transcends the anti-inflammatory phase (involving treatment by specific modalities, physical or otherwise) by incorporating recovery of musculoskeletal functions that existed before the injury. Furthermore, it may involve realignment of any pre-existing weakness or imbalance that precipitated the breakdown process. In many instances the psychological aspect of rehabilitation is just as or more important than the physiological. Therefore rehabilitation may be instituted from the first day of injury, and should invoke in the clinician's mind the need for maintenance of general body fitness, as well as the more specific aspect of tissue healing.

The extent of rehabilitation depends on a number of factors, including the severity and type of injury sustained, and the requirements of the specific sport. A cricketer with a fractured finger will be more severely handicapped than a long-distance runner with the same injury, though he will be able to maintain general body fitness to a large degree. Conversely, a runner with shin splints may need to modify his training substantially compared with the cricketer, who might continue to practise technical skills such as batting even though he may not be able to bowl. The timing of the re-introduction of specific training schedules is dependent upon the exact demands made by each sport. It is erroneous to pursue a narrow-minded approach of first 'treatment', then 'rehabilitation'. Muscle-strengthening and flexibility exercises may be performed concurrently with anti-inflammatory therapy, albeit in a restricted fashion.

Rehabilitation programmes should include the following stages:

(i) healing of injured tissue such as muscle, tendon, joint capsule, and ligament;
(ii) a pain-free active range of movement;
(iii) restoration of full flexibility of joints and contractile structures;
(iv) recovery of muscle strength and endurance;
(v) recovery of skill and cardiovascular fitness.

Although the final determinants of recovery (factor (v)) are often pursued by the patient after discharge to his own training schedules or to his coach, advice on timing and appropriate amendments to his schedule are required of the clinician.

Expansion of the principles of rehabilitation

Rest

The normal tissue response to injury, namely inflammation, takes at least five days, and may last for two or three weeks. During this time some degree of reduction of applied stress is necessary. Many conditions require relative rather than absolute rest of the injured part, and numerous instances have been cited in the relevant chapters. Absolute rest by immobilization may be prescribed for complicated or unstable fractures, grade III medial collateral ligament tears of the knee, Achilles tendon ruptures, and severe muscle contusions (when the development of myositis ossificans is to be avoided). Alternatively, surgical management may be undertaken for some fractures and ligament and tendon ruptures. Following surgery, a period of immobilization is usually indicated, though cast-bracing rather than casting may be appropriate.

For most soft tissue problems, however, the period of complete rest should be as short as possible—of the order of a few days only—and immobilization by external splintage should be eschewed whenever possible. Immobilization affects the proprioceptive mechanism adversely, as well as causing capsular stiffness by contracture, muscle-wasting, loss of tensile strength of all connective tissues (Akeson et al. 1967; Viidik 1967; Laros et al. 1971), and impaired nutrition of articular cartilage (Finsterbush and Friedman 1973).

Cast-bracing

The use of cast-bracing techniques for lower limb fractures has been accepted by orthopaedic surgeons for some time. Mooney (1974) summarized his own practice as follows:

> The ambulatory care of lower extremity fractures is based on two concepts: 1) Progressive weight-bearing, with its associated muscle and joint function, improved fracture-site fluid-flow, and gradually increasing skeletal stresses—these are positive factors to achieve efficient fracture healing and early limb rehabilitation; 2) prolonged recumbency is a negative factor. The improved general body metabolism associated with ambulatory activity is good for primate organ function, including the 'psyche'.

Experience with a cast-brace for patients with knee trauma, utilizing a modified single-axis joint in which the arc of motion was restricted to 30° 90°, was described by Bassett et al. (1980). Both non-operative and post-operative management were included. Rehabilitation times were considerably shortened and stability was not compromised, even with moderately severe ligamentous injuries.

The author has subsequently utilized a cast-brace for management of both acute ankle ligament injuries (Hutson and Jackson 1982) and acute knee ligament injuries to good effect. At the ankle the usual requirement is for lateral support due to inversion injury: the provision of a plastic heel-cup and stirrups allows a limited amount of plantarflexion in addition to dorsiflexion (see Fig. 8.10, p. 136). At the knee protected motion in the sagittal plane is limited to 10°–90°: valgus and varus stresses are controlled by the medial and lateral (adjustable) knee hinges, and rotational strain may be reduced by the application of an additional ankle brace (Fig. 12.1).

The protection afforded by such a brace invites an alternative strategy to the surgical management of substantial tears of the collateral and anterior cruciate ligaments, and of peripheral meniscal tears.

Haggmark and Eriksson (1979) have also reported the satisfactory use of a similar cast-brace (which included an ankle attachment) for control of rotation in the post-operative period after anterior cruciate ligament reconstruction. By comparison with the use of a standard cylinder cast the rehabilitation time was much reduced. Alternatively, a knee brace, such as the Masterhinge rehabilitation brace, may be used during the rehabilitative phase after surgical ligamentous reconstruction (Fig. 12.2(a)). For established instability the Lenox Hill derotation brace offers resistance to rotatory, A.P., and medial-lateral stresses (Fig. 12.2(b)).

Therapeutic modalities

Non-steroidal anti-inflammatory drugs (NSAIDs)

The increased interest in sports and fitness in recent years, allied to the development of sports medicine, has been paralleled by the introduction of NSAIDs for the management of musculoskeletal disorders. Although the emphasis in this text is on the application of physical modes of treatment to sports injuries, a few comments on the use of NSAIDs are of relevance.

NSAIDs and salicylates have analgesic, anti-inflammatory, and antipyretic properties. Low doses produce analgesic effects, while higher doses reduce inflammation (Calabrese and Rooney 1986). The mechanism of their action appears, in part, to be due to reduction of prostaglandins by inhibition of prostaglandin synthetase. Nevertheless, the inflammatory phase of healing is essential, and the role of the prostaglandins is important (see p. 4).

Several studies have demonstrated the usefulness of NSAIDs in the management of acute sports injuries, for example in knee ligament sprains (Hutson 1986). There is less agreement on their efficacy in overuse injuries; in the author's experience their ability to hasten recovery in these conditions is disappointing. In the presence of degenerative joint disease the prescribing physician has an ethical problem to consider in respect of the possible masking of further joint deterioration resulting from exercise. A further consideration of their use is the significant incidence of gastro-intestinal toxicity which may give rise to faecal blood loss.

Cryotherapy

The use of ice, or at least cold applications, has been established for many years (Sloan *et al.* 1989). Its vasoconstrictive activity, leading to decreased blood flow and decreased capillary permeability, has a useful effect on the control of bleeding and oedema. Of equal, or greater, importance in the immediate management of acute injury is the reduction of tissue metabolism by cooling. Often this anti-inflammatory action is combined with elevation and compression (ICE) in the early stages of tissue healing. Subsequently it may be used throughout the subacute

Fig. 12.1 An ambulatory cast-brace for management of knee ligament injuries includes both knee and ankle hinges to control varus, valgus, and rotational stress: (a) using a polycentric hinge; (b) using a Masterhinge (InCare Orthopaedics).

Fig. 12.2 (a) A knee brace may be used during rehabilitation after surgical ligamentous reconstruction: a Masterhinge rehabilitative knee brace is demonstrated. (b) The Lenox Hill derotation brace offers resistance to rotary, AP, and medial-lateral stresses for established instability.

stage during the institution of a graded exercise programme. Muscle spasm and pain are minimized, thus allowing earlier resumption of mobilizing exercises.

Cold applications or ice may be applied in a number of ways. Crushed ice wrapped inside a suitable bag or wet towel has the advantage of being moulded around the affected area to some extent. Ice that has been produced inside a polystyrene container in a freezer may be used by snipping off the top of the container, thus facilitating the technique of ice massage. The extremities may be immersed in iced water, though this does not allow the concomitant use of elevation. Finally, numerous commercial cold packs which are re-usable are available. Ice applications or cold packs should be used for ten to twenty minutes, and reapplied every two hours or so from the time of the injury for forty-eight hours.

Although cryotherapy is used almost universally, it is not without its dangers. Ice itself should not be allowed to stay in direct contact with the skin, as iceburns may result: motion or massage should be employed. Frostbite has been reported. Nerve palsy has also been documented (Drez *et al.* 1981) when ice is applied over areas in which an underlying nerve lies superficially.

Heat

Heat may be employed in a variety of ways, and is dependent upon the following therapeutic properties:

increased metabolism;

increased blood flow (vasodilatation);

increased threshold of sensory nerve endings.

Shortwave diathermy. A high-frequency current (frequency 27.12 MHz) generated in a machine circuit and coupled to a patient's circuit is used to treat the patient with as deep a form

of heat as any available to the therapist. The method of application is either via electrodes or by insulated cable. It is particularly valuable for deep-seated conditions—for example, at the hip joint—and for relief of muscle spasm prior to active exercises. Like other forms of heat, it is not used immediately after injury, particularly after haemorrhage.

Ultrasound therapy

Ultrasound therapy employs frequencies well beyond the range of hearing: 1 MHz (for deep-seated lesions such as joint capsules) to 3 MHz (for more superficial lesions). A high-frequency current is converted via a crystal into an ultrasound beam transmitted through a treatment head. Intensity is variable, though most therapeutic ultrasound is used in the range 0.25–1.0 watts/cm². Continuous wave and pulsed wave outputs are available—pulsing lowers the overall intensity. A coupling medium is required to transmit the waves. Physiological, psychological, and physical mechanisms are involved in the therapeutic effect on tissues (Dyson 1987). The principal effects are acceleration of repair and reduction of pain.

A *physiological* response within twenty-four hours of injury may be due to stimulation of the release of histamine and chemotactic agents by mast cells, thereby attracting polymorphs and monocytes to the injured site. This process involves a change in permeability of the cell membrane, thereby increasing the transport of calcium ions into the mast cells. As the inflammatory phase proceeds to the proliferative phase, fibroblasts may also be stimulated by diffusion of calcium ions, facilitated by ultrasound, resulting in increased collagen synthesis. Increased endothelial activity occurs with the formation of new capillaries. Therefore the overall physiological effect of ultrasound is to accelerate both the inflammatory phase and the proliferative phases of tissue repair (Dyson and Pond 1970). During the subsequent remodelling the strength of the scar is greater if ultrasound has been used early on.

One of the *physical* properties of ultrasound is the production of heat, which may be minimized by the use of pulsed waves; it is not usually desired immediately after acute injury. At a later stage the thermal effect may be used to increase the extensibility of collagen, and to reduce pain and muscle spasm. Among the non-thermal physical effects is a micromassage that occurs at cellular level, facilitating the reduction of oedema that is associated with both acute and chronic conditions. Acoustic streaming, a unidirectional flow of tissue fluid, affects cellular permeability, thereby increasing protein synthesis and reducing pain (possibly by stimulation of mechanoreceptors, or by a direct effect on nerves). A potential hazard is transient ('unstable') cavitation, in which cells may be damaged by the implosion of small gas bubbles: the risk is reduced by continued mobility of the transducer, and the use of a low intensity (0.1–0.2 watts/cm^2).

The *psychological* (placebo) effect is associated with alteration of plasma endorphin levels: patients often find therapy to be soothing.

A major advantage of ultrasound lies in the fact that it may be used in acute traumatic conditions, when reduction of oedema and adhesions are required. Although there is controversy over dosage schedules, perhaps the most practical guide is to rely on the personal experience of the therapist. Absorption of hydrocortisone cream is facilitated by ultrasound energy (phonophoresis). A further therapeutic use of ultrasound depends on its softening effect on established scar tissue at both an early and a later stage following injury.

Interferential therapy

Interferential therapy is so called as a result of the use of the 'interference' between two medium-frequency currents to produce the desired low-frequency current. The resultant frequency of between 0 and 250 Hz is produced in the crossover area between two applied circuits. Interferential stimulation is a form of transcutaneous electrical nerve stimulation (the classical pain-relieving form of which is better known as TENS). The electrodes are applied diagonally across the treatment site. Claimed clinical benefits are as follows:

(1) reduction of inflammation—for example, in shoulder-joint synovitis;
(2) muscle re-education—for example, foot muscle exercises, pelvic floor exercises;
(3) pain relief (150–250 Hz).

Lasers (light amplification by stimulated emission of radiation)

Cold or soft lasers produce a flow of photons in a specific wavelength. For treatment of soft tissue lesions the energy is released in a pulsed mode, which reduces the average intensity to safe levels. This energy 'helps reinstate normal conditions by overcoming tissue resistance that occurs with trauma. Healing is enhanced in this manner by the resumption of normal cellular metabolism ... Various researchers have disclosed the following results from studies involving cold lasers; (1) elevated ATP production; (2) enhanced DNA replication; (3) reduction of prostaglandin production; (4) oedema reduction, especially in the acute phase of injury; (5) increased collagen production and vascularization; and (6) increased tensile strength of collagen.' (Gieck and Saliba 1987).

Early experience is encouraging in its use in various overuse conditions.

Massage

Massage may take many forms, and may be used for a multitude of soft tissue problems. Although at one time it fell into some disrepute, as a result of its association with 'massage parlours', therapeutic massage is now being employed to its rightful extent. Undoubtedly it has physiological effects. Depending upon the type used, these effects include relaxation, neural stimulation, increased lymphatic drainage, increased local blood flow, and possibly an effect on muscles whereby recovery from post-exercise muscle soreness is accelerated. However, the indications should be clear to the clinician and therapist, and it is important that the correct type of massage is used. Types of massage which may be of therapeutic value are detailed below.

Effleurage helps to relieve congestion, particularly the unwanted presence of oedema around joints and in traumatic periostitis. Repeated upward stroking movements are employed, and the massage is repeated daily and followed by application of a double tubigrip support.

Deep friction. This technique, developed by Cyriax, helps to maintain or restore mobility to those (often deeply seated) lesions that are prone to develop adhesions or scarring. Its application is principally to muscles, tendons, and ligaments. Accurate localization of the lesion is imperative; thus the technique may not be employed until oedema has been reduced by *effleurage*. Its action is to promote mobility of the healing or scarred area and create hyperaemia, which results in analgesia, and to increase mechanoreceptor stimulation, which further reduces pain by blocking afferent sensory stimuli. It is imperative that it is used properly by transverse movements across the line of the fibres in their relaxed position, and by the abolition of any movement between the therapist's finger and the patient's skin, so that finger and skin move as one across the underlying tissues. Although it is painful initially, subsequently there is a numbing effect.

When used for muscle lesions its effect is to reduce adhesions between individual fibres, and to allow natural broadening upon contraction. For ligamentous lesions the purpose is to reproduce the normal mobility of the ligament over the underlying bone and to reduce fibrotic attachments, thereby improving joint mobility. Examples of its use are in lesions of the femoral attachment of the medial collateral ligament of the knee, of the coronary ligaments of the knee, and of the dorsal ligaments of the wrist. In tendinous lesions it may help to reduce intratendinous scarring and thus facilitate stretching. It may have an excellent effect on tenosynovitis (though steroid injections have an even quicker effect) by mobilizing the sheath around the tendon.

Other types of massage include kneading and vibration massage using commercially available vibrators; probably these assist by their pleasurable effects and by increased local blood flow.

Mobilization exercises

The benefits of mobilization are the reverse of the adverse effects of immobilization: the primary considerations are the maintenance and subsequent improvement of muscle tone, reduction of joint stiffness, and increased tensile strength of connective tissue, particularly ligaments. Although conventional orthopaedic teaching in the past has suggested that six weeks is required for healing of a ligament tear by immobilization (for example, in a POP cast) it is probable that this healing time is less when a joint is mobilized, if necessary with an appropriate degree of functional support. It seems likely that collagen deposition is more 'orderly' in respect of the laying down of fibres in parallel during this phase when under the influence of controlled exercise. The constraints to early mobilization of connective tissues should be the presence of oedema or effusion, the patient's complaint of discomfort or pain, and the minimum amount of time taken for tissues to progress to the repair stage of healing. However, such constraints should not result in an all-or-nothing situation. Sound healing of a muscle tear may take three or four weeks (and indeed many months for full maturity of the scar), though graded stretching exercises should take place well before then. The diagnosis of 'microscopic' rather than 'macroscopic' damage in ligament injury—that is, a stable joint—should lead to commencement of both active and passive mobilization exercises as soon as pain and oedema allow. The use of a cast-brace for ligament rupture allows earlier introduction of a restricted range of joint mobility.

Prolonged tissue oedema may have devastating effects on local musculoskeletal function, and is influenced considerably by the judicious use of graded mobilization. In the lower limb a distinction should be made between the adverse effects of prolonged standing and abnormal gait on the one hand (in the mistaken belief that any form of ambulation is correct), and the usefulness of deliberate careful, though biomechanically correct, gait on the other.

The acute phase. Both active and passive range of motion exercises may begin early after joint injury. They have a similar effect on joint mobility, though only active exercises maintain some degree of muscle tone. The therapist may need to encourage joint motion initially, to a point at which slight discomfort is appreciated by the patient, followed by active exercises within the same range. A skilled therapist is able to gain the patient's cooperation, and proceed through a gradually increasing range of movements on a daily basis. In many instances the patient may be taught to perform these exercises himself.

When treating muscle injury, movement of the affected muscle should be maintained passively within the limit of pain. Passive stretching should not be instituted too early, for fear of disrupting healing scar tissue, though it will begin gently after a week or so. Faradic stimulation may be considered in the early stages, when little active contraction is possible otherwise. Dynamic muscle exercise may be instituted in the recovery phase.

Recovery phase. Forced passive movements are sometimes necessary to break down adhesions or to stretch capsules. Adhesions form at the knee and ankle joints, particularly after immobilization or surgery. Capsular contracture is a common accompaniment to immobilization of any joint, whatever the pathology of the preceding injury. It is often profound at the shoulder in post-traumatic capsulitis (and in the second phase of adhesive capsulitis), and may require stretching exercises for several months (see Fig. 11.14, p. 198). The elbow joint warrants special mention, as it often responds adversely to passive mobilization or stretching. Whether secondary to dislocation, fracture, or severe contusion, stiffness of the elbow may be profound, resolving slowly over many months. Attempts at forceful extension exercises create further loss of mobility. Overvigorous exercises may cause myositis ossificans in the surrounding muscles.

Flexibility exercises should be undertaken, gently at first and more vigorously later, to restore full mobility at the affected joint and full elasticity of an affected muscle or tendon. The principle of the two Ss—full *stretch* and *strength* — cannot be overemphasized in muscle rehabilitation, as so often they are overlooked. Strengthening exercises are considered further, while the reader is referred to Chapter 11 for an account of flexibility exercises.

Strengthening exercises
Whatever the nature of the injury sustained, a well-designed management plan includes rehabilitation of weakened muscle. Muscle function may be stimulated in a number of different ways.

Isometric exercise. The phenomenon of active muscle contraction with constant length is utilized during the early stages of recovery from joint injury. In some situations, for instance disorders of the patellofemoral mechanism, it may be the only effective way of maintaining or developing muscle tone during the early stages of rehabilitation. The therapist may need to demonstrate and subsequently monitor contractions, and in certain circumstances be required to provide manual resistance. However, most isometric exercise may be performed by the patient without assistance. Examples have been provided throughout the text. Further consideration is now given to two regions that require careful monitoring: the knee and the shoulder.

Early loss of quadriceps tone and bulk are easily measured (by a tape measure) and demonstrated to the patient. During recovery from either ligament or meniscus injury it is usually possible to proceed rapidly to dynamic isotonic or isokinetic exercise once the ability to straight leg raise has been demonstrated (see Fig. 7.8, p. 121). However, recovery from injury to the extensor mechanism, particularly the variety of problems associated with the patellofemoral syndrome, is hindered by the risk of exacerbation of symptoms if muscle conditioning is attempted from a significant degree of knee flexion.

Isometric contraction drills in extension are prescribed to build up the vastus medialis and thereby maintain patellar stability (Fig. 12.3). Isometric exercise is undertaken initially in a supine or sitting position, though subsequently it may be performed on standing. A maximal contraction is maintained for as long as possible (that is, up to ten seconds), followed by two to three seconds relaxation, and then by a further similar contraction. This sequence is continued to muscle exhaustion, usually involving up to ten repetitions. The set of contractions is repeated several times a day.

Just as the vastus medialis contributes largely to patellar stability, so the rotator cuff is primarily responsible for stability of the mobile glenohumeral joint. Once tendinitis resolves, a schedule of isometric exercise for each of the elements of the cuff in turn should be instituted. Initially the therapist manually resists movement, subsequently instructing the patient in other forms of isometric exercise which may be performed at home. Particular attention is paid to contraction of the abductors (with the arm in the dependent position) and the external and internal rotators. Graded introduction of isotonic exercise follows, using surgical tubing or hand-held weights (see Figs. 3.25 and 3.26, pp. 46 and 47).

Isotonic exercise. Concentric contraction occurs when muscle shortens during contraction. Resistance may be provided by a variety of methods that are available to the therapist and patient. Exercise with climband, surgical tubing, weighted boots,

FIG.12.3 Isometric exercise in extension for the knee extensors may be augmented by loading—for example, with a weight attached to the ankle.

(a)

(b)

FIG.12.4 (a) Cliniband (made from pure latex) is a suitable material for use in remedial exercise. (b) The patient's own body weight is often utilized in circuit training exercises.

and free weights may be undertaken in the treatment room (Fig. 12.4(a)). More sophisticated equipment—for example, multi-gym stations—may be available in a gymnasium. The patient's own body weight is often utilized in circuit-training exercise.

Strict monitoring is required to establish and expand a suitable programme of exercises.

Eccentric exercise. Eccentric contraction takes place when muscle contracts during lengthening—for example, triceps contraction during controlled elbow flexion using body weight as a resistance (Fig. 12.4(b)). Mennell (1960) emphasizes the importance of this aspect of management by stating that 'when a long muscle becomes weakened by shortening through any cause it can only be strengthened once more by the use of lengthening, eccentric decelerating exercises rather than by concentric, shortening accelerating exercises which are more commonly used in a routine manner by most therapists.' The author considers that a sensible balance is advisable.

Isokinetic exercise. Isokinetic contraction is dynamic muscle activity performed at a constant angular velocity. The speed of motion is preselected and controlled by an isokinetic dynamometer, in which internal resistance is created to accommodate to the force applied. As soon as the preset angular velocity is reached (which takes a few degrees of movement) the resistance offered by the machine is determined by the effort of the patient, and may be measured as torque (in foot-pounds). Grimby *et al.* (1980) have described the usefulness of isokinetic rehabilitation after knee ligament surgery. There are now numerous reports on rehabilitative isokinetic exercise involving the quadriceps and hamstrings. Most recorded work has been performed on the Cybex, originally developed by Perrini in 1969, although there are other machines such as the Orthotron and the Lido (see Fig. 11.11, p. 193).

Isokinetic exercise differs from dynamic exercise using externally applied weights by allowing muscle to work maximally throughout the full arc of motion. In addition, an athlete's training or rehabilitation programme may be adapted by selection of

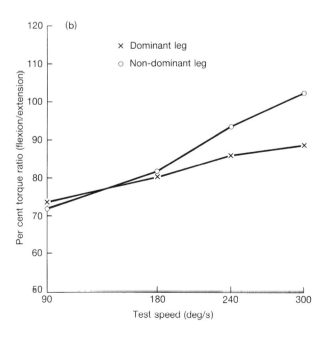

FIG. 12.5 (a) Comparison of power output of the combined knee flexors and extensors per pound body weight (i) shortly after injury to the knee and (ii) after three weeks' rehabilitation on a Lido isokinetic dynamometer. (b) % Torque ratio (knee flexion/extension) vs. test speed in tennis players.

exercise speeds varying from 0° to 300° per second, to simulate the type of muscular contraction employed in a particular sport. A major advantage is safety: in recovery from injury a joint may not tolerate the compression, traction, or torsion effects of external weights, though it may be perfectly safe when responding to the inbuilt accommodative effects of the dynamometer, particularly at the higher speeds.

Arising from the experience of the Sports and Fitness Assessment Unit at the London Bridge Clinic in isokinetic rehabilitation following knee or thigh muscle injury, two parameters have been found to be useful:

(i)   power per pound body weight of both the knee flexors and the knee extensors at different angular velocities—additionally fatiguability is assessed at the higher speeds;

(ii) hamstring-to-quadriceps torque ratios at different speeds.

Rehabilitative exercise concentrates on normalizing deficiencies or imbalances by reference to the normal leg and the type of sport played (Fig. 12.5). Allowances are made for the dominant and non-dominant legs. Isokinetic training is described further in Chapter 11.

Whatever the arguments for or against the use of certain types of exercise such as isokinetics in rehabilitation, it should be recognized that muscle activity of this type is *not physiological*,

and that the graded reintroduction of specific sports training at an appropriate stage is an important step in rehabilitation.

Manipulation

Manipulative techniques are used in a variety of circumstances, though some old-established concepts require critical reassessment. Normal joint mobility is lost in the majority of acute injuries. The mobilization techniques already described may be successful in restoring mobility, though specific indications exist for the use of procedures which utilize a greater degree of thrust.

Peripheral joints. Manipulation may readjust the position of an intra-articular fragment, namely a loose body or a meniscal tear. The techniques involve a combination of distraction and rotational movements of the affected joint. The reader may learn the techniques of manipulation of the knee and elbow, for instance, by reference to Cyriax's *Textbook of orthopaedic medicine*. A joint may be 'unlocked' by a manipulative procedure, though, since the offending loose or torn fragment is still present in the joint, the ultimate management is referral for surgical removal. A patient may learn the knack of self-releasing a locked joint, in which case the history alone provides the physician with a suspicion of intra-articular derangement. Other manipulative techniques used for mobilizing joints which are 'dysfunctional'—that is, have lost their normal range of motion due to neurophysio-

(a)   (b)

Fɪɢ. 12.6 (a) The position of the patient and physician are demonstrated in assessment of joint play in the cervical spine. (b) A commonly used position of facet locking prior to manipulation is demonstrated.

FIG. 12.7 The position of the patient and physician are demonstrated for
(a) thoracic joint manipulation and
(b) segmental manipulation of the lumbar spinal joints.

(a)

(b)

FIG.12.8 The position of the patient and physician are demonstrated for manipulation of the sacroiliac joint.

logical disturbance or capsular contracture—are described by Mennell (1960) and Maitland (1986).

Spinal manipulation. There is much debate over the nature of the spinal lesion that is responsive to manipulation. The author's belief is that sacroiliac dysfunction and facet (apophyseal) joint dysfunction in the cervical, thoracic, and lumbar spine are the manipulable lesions. In any event, as long as appropriate criteria of suitability for treatment by manipulation have been established (see Chapter 5) the standard manipulative procedures (Figs 12.6–12.8) are safe and effective, if only on empirical grounds. Since a variety of techniques are available, the reader is advised to pursue his interest by attending courses and symposia run by the British Institute of Musculoskeletal Medicine, the Society of Orthopaedic Medicine, or the London College of Osteopathic Medicine. Referral of a patient to a suitably qualified physiotherapist or osteopath is the alternative approach.

Relative contraindications to manipulation in the cervical and lumbar spines are nuclear disc protrusions. They may be suspected by the presence of radicular symptoms (root pain, paraesthesiae, and numbness), dural signs, and articular signs. Positive neurological signs (motor weakness or altered reflexes) are confirmatory evidence. Under these circumstances sustained daily traction or (in the case of sciatica) epidural injections should be employed. A suspicion of vertebrobasilar insufficiency is a contraindication to the use of cervical manipulation by the inexperienced manipulator. An absolute contraindication is the inability to diagnose a benign mechanical lesion.

A suitable manipulation schedule is to review the patient every two to three days, reassess, and remanipulate until resolution of the signs—that is, until establishment of normal joint mobility. Once mobility is restored a suitable range of exercises is prescribed to strengthen the abdominal and pelvic muscles in lumbar or sacroiliac disorders, and the neck muscles in cervical disorders. This is particularly important when the patient intends to return to vigorous exercise, such as rugby football.

Spinal traction. The indication for spinal traction is the diagnosis of nuclear disc protrusion (HNP). There is radiological evidence from epidurographic studies that the size of a disc protrusion is reduced by a suitable distracting force in the long axis of the spine. Daily sustained traction is applied using one of a number of commercially available traction couches (see Fig. 5.16, p. 90). A skilled therapist adjusts the level of traction according to the site of the lesion and the weight of the patient. It may be applied for between fifteen and thirty minutes to a maximum of 25 lb to the neck, and 140 lb (for a well-built male) to the lumbar region. Daily reassessment of symptoms and signs is made, though improvement may not be detected until half-way through an average course of ten treatments. However, treatment should be continued until the signs have resolved or until no further benefit is gained (fifteen sessions may be required).

Injection techniques

The indications for and techniques of localized injections, usually for the purpose of infiltration of steroids and/or local anaesthetic, must be understood by the practising sports physician. The indications may be as follows.

1. **Diagnostic** using local anaesthetic—for example, infiltration of the subacromial space for the detection of subacromial bursitis, or epidural anaesthesia with 0.5 per cent procaine to diagnose lumbar nerve root irritation in a patient with posterior thigh pain of undetermined origin. With increasing experience it becomes less necessary to confirm diagnosis by these methods. The addition of local anaesthetic to a steroid suspension during treatment is largely to demonstrate to the patient that immediate improvement reflects accurate localization.

2. **Therapeutic**. The rationale is the accurate introduction of anti-inflammatory drugs into inflamed tissues.

(i) *Local anaesthetic* alone is occasionally effective, although the desired effect is often enhanced by the addition of steroid. Lignocaine 1 per cent, for instance, may be used in injection of trigger points which are secondary to spinal joint dysfunction. The effect of the injection may be due as much to the needling of the tissues as to the chemical effect of the lignocaine. It may have a similar effect to that of the vapocoolant spray developed by Travell (Travell and Simons 1983), or the use of subcutaneous salicylate injections developed by Fox (1981). Reflex inhibition of the pain impulse may occur. Melzack and Wall (1965) consider this and other concepts in their 'gate theory' of pain control.

(ii) *Steroid injections.* The advantages and disadvantages of the use of injectable steroids should be fully appreciated. Unfortunately the general public have become suspicious of their use, for a number of reasons. First, they are often assumed to be in the same mould as anabolic steroids, known universally to be involved in drug abuse in sport. Many patients are acquainted with the fact that high dosage of steroids—for example, used for collagen diseases or for cerebral oedema—causes side-effects including 'moon face'. Lastly patients sometimes believe, often quite rightly if steroids are used indiscriminately in the absence of an appropriate rehabilitation programme, that an injection may simply ameliorate the symptoms without establishing a cure.

The advantage of a localized injection of steroid is the rapid anti-inflammatory response that is gained: in some instances it may be quite dramatic. Conditions such as medial coronary ligament sprain of the knee, even if present for several months, resolve within a few days of treatment by injection. Other conditions such as subacromial bursitis are difficult to treat by other means because of their anatomical position.

The disadvantages are the side-effects which may occur with overdosage. The effect on collagen is such that subcutaneous seepage may give rise to the typical mauve-coloured discoloration and thinning of the skin overlying a lesion. This is cosmetically undesirable, and often indicates poor technique and/or overdosage. Repeated injections rarely give rise to systemic side-effects, such as weight gain or peptic ulceration, though a metabolic effect may be seen in diabetics, in whom there can be a temporary increase in insulin requirement. There may be a disturbance of the menstrual cycle in susceptible females in the form of intermenstrual bleeding. To a large extent the likelihood of such side-effects is reduced by using the minimum dosage of triamcinolone hexacetonide (or equivalent) according to the following guidelines.

Soft tissue, for example ligament or teno-osseous junction	10 mg
Intra-articular	10–20 mg depending upon size of joint—for example, 20 mg for shoulder or knee joint, 10 mg for acromioclavicular joint
Epidural	20–40 mg

Normally 10 mg of triamcinolone or methyl prednisolone is all that is required—this is one-quarter the dose that may be commercially available in a 1 ml ampoule. Injections that need to be repeated should preferably be of the lower dosages. One further major disadvantage of injectible steroid is the weakening effect on collagen, particularly tendons. There is **no indication for injecting into a weightbearing tendon**—for example, the Achilles tendon. Although there is controversy over whether rupture may be caused by intratendinous injection, the argument should become a theoretical one: the sheath or paratenon only should be injected. The minimal pressure needed to inject into a tendon sheath is quite different from the force required to inject into the tendon.

A summary of the indications is as follows.

1. *Intrabursal*—for example, for subacromial bursitis, postcalcaneal bursitis, and anserine bursitis. A dramatic response may be expected in acute conditions, and early relief from months of discomfort in chronic conditions in which adhesions and fibrosis are features.

2. *Intrasynovial* (a) When used in tenosynovitis—for example, de Quervain's tenosynovitis or tenosynovitis of the foot dorsiflexors—the response may be dramatic. When used for primary Achilles paratendinitis the response is equally dramatic: when paratendinitis is secondary to significant pathology of the tendon additional therapeutic modalities are needed.

(b) Intra-articular (IA) injections have tended to fall into some disrepute as a result of the concern over the possible degradative effect on articular cartilage. Although discretion is advocated in the use of IA injection of the weightbearing joints of the lower limb, nevertheless a 'one-off' injection may be extremely useful. There should be evidence of the persistence of synovitis (for example, discomfort, dysfunction, synovial thickening, and restriction of joint movements in the capsular pattern) beyond what may reasonably be expected after trauma. Chondral or osteochondral injury should be excluded. Synovitis of the elbow, after jarring or overuse, may require two or three injections. Interphalangeal joint injuries may give rise to prolonged discomfort and stiffness, which are often helped by one intra-articular injection. There is hardly a synovial joint in the body that does not occasionally merit IA injection: numerous examples are given in the text. The shoulder joint is worthy of further consideration: both adhesive capsulitis and post-traumatic capsulitis respond to IA injections, which should be repeated at one- to three-weekly intervals until the pain settles (at least until the patient is comfortable at night). Graded stretching exercises may then be instituted on resolution of the inflammatory phase.

3. *Intraligamentous.* Some ligament sprains, for example, coronary ligament sprains of the knee, respond dramatically. Without localized injection or friction massage they may linger for months. Degenerative joints are more prone to ligament sprain. The knee is one example; the acromioclavicular joint is another. A localized intraligamentous injection at the acromioclavicular joint may be combined with an IA injection.

Discomfort that persists for an inordinate length of time after partial ligamentous disruption, for example at the femoral attachment of the MCL of the knee and the lateral collateral ligament of the ankle, may be helped by localized infiltration.

4. *Intratendinous.* As previously indicated, injections into the substance of tendons, particularly weightbearing tendons, are eschewed. No indication exists, and there is a risk of steroid-induced rupture. However, lesions at teno-osseous junctions (enthesopathies) may be injected. Examples of such conditions are lateral and medial epicondylitis, patella apicitis, chronic adductor tendon strain in the groin, and insertional tendinitis of the supraspinatus tendon. Care is taken to rehabilitate the involved musculature, and sufficient time is allowed after the injection to establish sound healing. Steroid injections should not be given purely for pain relief to allow competitive sport to be undertaken.

Precautions

(i) An aseptic technique using disposable syringes and needles should be used at all times. An injection is withheld in the presence of local skin sepsis.

(ii) Single-dose ampoules of steroid and local anaesthetic are preferable.

FIG. 12.9 (a) Injection of the left glenohumeral joint by the posterior approach is demonstrated. (b) The posterior aspect of the shoulder. The examiner's thumb palpates the spine of the scapula as it angulates forwards to become the acromion.

(a)

(b)

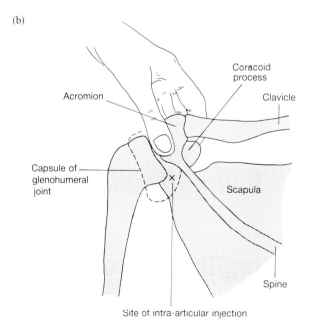

(iii) Skin preparation with chlorhexidine in 5 per cent spirit or a Mediswab is satisfactory. If a 'marker' is required the use of a pen or the impression made by a thumb-nail prior to swabbing is ideal.

(iv) The minimum dosage of steroid is used.

(v) Patients are warned that occasionally, particularly in the treatment of enthesopathies, pain may be exacerbated for up to forty-eight hours.

(vi) Care should be taken to explain to patients the nature of the treatment and the need to rest the injury for a week or so after the injection.

The more common injection techniques are now outlined.

The shoulder

The *shoulder joint* is entered most easily and with most certainty posteriorly: there is no preferred indication for an anterior or lateral approach. The patient lies prone (or sits if this position is too painful) with the affected arm internally rotated across the abdomen. The index finger of the examiner's non-dominant hand palpates the coracoid process, and the thumb the spine of the scapula as it angulates forwards by 90° to become the acromion. The needle pierces the skin 1 cm inferior to the thumb and is directed anteriorly towards the index finger (Fig. 12.9). After penetrating the infraspinatus the resistance of the capsule is felt, and then a loss of resistance as the joint cavity is entered; impingement against bone or articular cartilage is felt.

The following materials are required:

5 ml syringe
2 inch 21 G needle
20 mg triamcinolone hexacetonide in 1 ml
4 ml 1 per cent lignocaine.

The *subacromial bursa* is approached most easily in the sitting patient from the posterolateral aspect of the shoulder. The needle pierces the skin immediately posterior to the head of the humerus and inferior to the acromion (Fig. 12.10) and is directed anteromedially. A loss of resistance is felt when the bursa is entered, and the injection is made easily. If 5 ml or more is injected bulging is noted over the anterior aspect of the subacromial space.

The following materials are required:

5–10 ml syringe
1½ inch 21 G needle
20 mg triamcinolone hexacetonide in 1 ml
4–9 ml 1 per cent lignocaine.

The *supraspinatus insertion* is approached from the anterior aspect of the shoulder. The patient is seated with his arm medially rotated behind his back (Fig. 12.11) so that the greater tuberosity is rotated anteriorly. The supraspinatus tendon may be palpated through the deltoid muscle and the tenderness (of insertional tendinitis) identified. The injection may be made either at right angles to the skin, or by inclining the needle downwards and backwards from a more superior approach.

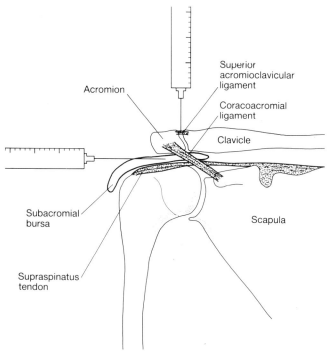

Fig. 12.10 (a) The subacromial bursa may be injected via a posterolateral approach. (b) Injection techniques for the acromoclavicular joint and subacromial bursa.

FIG. 12.11 The supraspinatus tendon insertion is injected with the patient sitting with arm internally rotated.

The following materials are required:

2 ml syringe
1 inch 23 G needle
10 mg triamcinolone hexacetonide in 1 ml
1 ml 1 per cent lignocaine.

The *infraspinatus tendon* is approached from the posterior aspect of the shoulder when the patient lies prone, resting on his elbows with the forearms externally rotated (Fig. 12.12). The infraspinatus may be palpated immediately inferior to the posterior margin of the acromion. It is usually this site—the musculotendinous junction—that is affected in infraspinatus tendinitis. A direct approach at right angles to the skin is made.

The following materials are required:

2 ml syringe
1 inch 23 G needle
10 mg triamcinolone hexacetonide in 1 ml
1 ml 1 per cent lignocaine.

The *subscapularis tendon* is approached from the anteromedial aspect of the shoulder when the patient is seated with his arm hanging loosely by his side (Fig. 12.13). In the presence of subscapularis tendinitis the affected tendinous insertion into the lesser tuberosity is found to be tender, and may be injected from a direct anterior approach.

The following materials are required:

2 ml syringe
1 inch 23 G (or 1$\frac{1}{2}$ inch 21 G) needle
10 mg triamcinolone hexacetonide in 1 ml
1 ml 1 per cent lignocaine.

The *biceps brachii tendon* may be palpated in the bicipital groove when the patient's arm hangs loosely by his side, or when the arm is supported in external rotation. The injection is made (Fig. 12.14) almost parallel to the tendon—that is, into the tendon sheath—and the resistance to the injection is minimal.

The following materials are required:

2 ml syringe
1 inch 23 G needle
10 mg triamcinolone hexacetonide in 1 ml
1 ml 1 per cent lignocaine.

The *acromioclavicular joint* may be injected from a superior approach. If identification of the joint is difficult, the joint surfaces may be palpated when stress is applied concomitantly to sublux the joint by applying a distracting force to the upper

FIG. 12.12 The position of the patient is demonstrated for injection of the infraspinatus (at the musculotendinous junction).

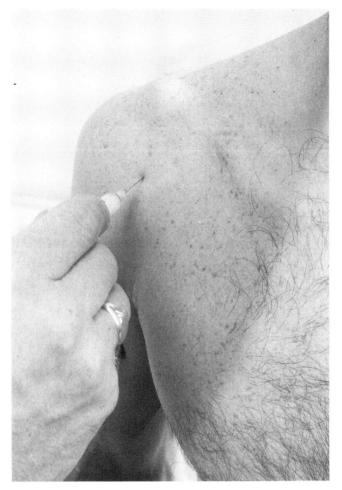

FIG. 12.13 The patient sits with his arm by his side during injection of the subscapularis tendon.

FIG. 12.14 The biceps brachii tendon sheath may be injected in the bicipital groove.

arm. The superior acromioclavicular ligament is infiltrated and then penetrated for intra-articular injection. The direction of the needle is downwards, and slightly forwards and medially, to accommodate the continuous joint surfaces which are often disposed obliquely (Figs. 12.10 and 12.15).

The following materials are required:

2 ml syringe
1 inch 23 G needle
10 mg triamcinolone hexacetonide in 1 ml
1 ml 1 per cent lignocaine

The elbow, forearm, and wrist

The *common extensor* and *common flexor* origins from the relevant epicondyles are identified by digital palpation in the treatment of epicondylitis. From one puncture site droplets are infiltrated into the teno-osseous junction (Fig. 12.16). In the treatment of enthesopathies injections are made into the tendinous attachment down to the underlying bone. The patient rests his elbow in a comfortable position on the examination couch.

The following materials are required:

2 ml syringe
1 inch 23 G needle
10 mg triamcinolone hexacetonide in 1 ml
1 ml 1 per cent lignocaine

The *elbow joint* is approached most easily from the posterolateral aspect (between the radial head and the lateral epicondyle). The patient lies prone with the affected forearm fully supinated. The gap between the radial head (inferiorly) and the posterior margin of the lateral epicondyle (superiorly) is palpated. The needle is inserted (Fig. 12.17) in an anteromedial direction into the joint cavity. If an effusion is present, this should be aspirated initially using a syringe of larger capacity.

The following materials are required:

2 ml syringe
1 inch 23 G needle
20 mg triamcinolone hexacetonide in 1 ml
1 ml 1 per cent lignocaine

Tenosynovitis of the tendons of the short extensor and long abductor of the thumb may occur in the mid-forearm or overlying the radial styloid (Fig. 12.18). In the forearm a 21 G needle is introduced into the swollen tendon sheath at an angle that is close to parallel. A 23 G needle is used at the radial styloid with a similar technique.

The following materials are required:

2 ml syringe
1 inch 23 G or $1\frac{1}{2}$ inch 21 G needle
10 mg triamcinolone hexacetonide in 1 ml
1 ml 1 per cent lignocaine

FIG. 12.15 The acromioclavicular joint is injected when the physician stands behind the patient.

The *carpal tunnel* is approached at an angle of 45° to the skin. The needle is inserted at the distal wrist crease midway between the pisiform (medially) and the scaphoid tubercle (laterally) (Fig. 12.19). If the palmaris longus tendon is present, the injection should be made on its ulnar side. A loss of resistance is felt after needle penetration to a depth of between 1.0 and 1.5 cm.

The following materials are required:

2 ml syringe
1 inch 23 G needle
10 mg triamcinolone hexacetonide in 1 ml
1 ml 1 per cent lignocaine.

The hip

The *hip joint.* An injection (or aspiration) may occasionally be required for which the anterior route is entirely safe. Needle entry is made from a point 3 cm lateral to the femoral artery and 2–3 cm inferior to the inguinal ligament (Fig. 12.20). The approach is anterior–posterior. Alternatively a lateral route may be used, when the needle penetrates in a medial, and slightly superior and anterior, direction from a point adjacent to the superior margin of the greater troachanter.

The following materials are required:

5 ml syringe
2 inch 21 G needle (or $3\frac{1}{2}$ inch 20 G spinal needle for lateral approach)

20 mg triamcinolone hexacetonide in 1 ml
4 ml 1 per cent lignocaine.

Trochanteric bursitis is identified by tenderness that is localized to the superolateral aspect of the greater trochanter. A direct approach is used and the injection is made over an area of approximately 2 cm².

The following materials are required:

10 ml syringe
2 inch 21 G needle
10 mg triamcinolone hexacetonide in 1 ml
9 ml 1 per cent lignocaine.

The knee

Iliotibial tract bursitis is identified by tenderness that is localized to the lateral epicondyle of the femur or the portion of the iliotibial tract that is immediately adjacent to this (see Fig. 7.3, p. 116). Infiltration is made down to the underlying periosteum.

The following materials are required:

2 ml syringe
1 inch 23 G needle
10 mg triamcinolone hexacetonide in 1 ml
1 ml 1 per cent lignocaine.

The *knee joint* may be approached superiorly, inferiorly, medially, or laterally, though it is recommended that one approach is used regularly to gain experience. The author favours the medial approach. With the patient supine and the patella stabilized by digital pressure to its lateral border, the needle is inserted in the gap between the patella (at its medial midpoint) and the femur (Fig. 12.21). The direction of penetration is horizontally and posteriorly; loss of resistance indicates that the joint cavity has been entered. An effusion should be aspirated (using a 20–50 ml syringe) prior to steroid injection.

The following materials are required:

5 ml syringe (50 ml for aspiration)
2 inch 21 G needle (20 G for aspiration)
20 mg triamcinolone hexacetonide in 1 ml
4 ml 1 per cent lignocaine.

Coronary (meniscotibial) ligament sprains are identified by localized tenderness and induration. Needle penetration is tangential to the joint line and the injection is made (using firm pressure) over approximately 2 cm (Fig. 12.22).

The following materials are required:

2 ml syringe
1 inch 23 G needle
10 mg triamcinolone hexacetonide in 1 ml
1 ml 1 per cent lignocaine.

The ankle region

The *ankle joint* is approached anteriorly with the patient lying supine. The skin is pierced between the tendons of tibialis anterior (medially) and extensor hallucis longus laterally (Fig. 12.23). The needle is directed posteriorly and superiorly (to accommodate the convex articular surface of the talus). An effusion should be aspirated initially.

The following materials are required:

5 ml syringe
$1\frac{1}{2}$ inch 21 G needle
20 mg triamcinolone hexacetonide in 1 ml
4 ml 1 per cent lignocaine.

(a)

(b)

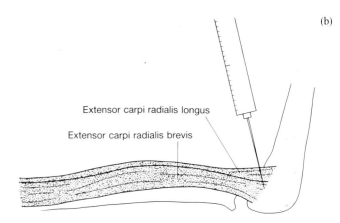

Extensor carpi radialis longus

Extensor carpi radialis brevis

FIG. 12.16 (a) The patient sits with his elbow supported in 90° flexion prior to injection of lateral epicondylitis. (b) Injection of lateral epicondylitis ('tennis elbow').

FIG. 12.17 The elbow joint may be injected from a posterolateral approach when the patient lies prone with his forearm supinated.

The *Achilles paratenon* is approached posteriorly with the patient lying prone. Injections are made parallel to the tendon, both medially and laterally. Once attached to the syringe, the needle inside its guard may be bent to 20° close to its base (Fig. 12.24) to facilitate the direction of penetration.

The following materials are required:

5 ml syringe
2 × 2 inch 21 G needle
10 mg triamcinolone hexacetonide in 1 ml
4 ml 1 per cent lignocaine.

The *subtalar joint* may be approached most easily from the medial side. The sustentaculum tali is identified below the

FIG. 12.18 The injection site for de Quervain's tenosynovitis of the long abductor and short extensor of the thumb is shown.

Abductor pollicis longus and Extensor pollicis brevis

medial malleolus and the needle is inserted above its superior margin and directed laterally (Fig. 12.25). Alternatively, the sinus tarsi may be approached laterally via the hollow that is felt antero-inferior to the lateral malleolus, or the posterior subtalar joint penetrated from a posterolateral approach.

The following materials are required:

2 ml syringe
1 inch 23 G needle
10 mg triamcinolone hexacetonide in 1 ml
1 ml 1 per cent lignocaine.

Plantar fasciitis is identified by localized tenderness over the medial tubercle of the calcaneus: the patient lies prone for ease of access. The injection may be made either by penetration of the needle at right angles to the lesion or from a more medial approach (Fig. 12.26). Infiltration is made at the fibro-osseous junction: firm pressure is required.

The following materials are required:

2 ml syringe
1 inch 23 G needle
10 mg triamcinolone hexacetonide in 1 ml
1 ml 1 per cent lignocaine.

FIG. 12.19 The injection site (at the level of the distal wrist crease) for the carpal tunnel is demonstrated.

Femoral artery

Inguinal ligament

Femoral sheath

Femoral canal   Femoral vein

FIG. 12.20 The injection sites for the hip joint are demonstrated.

FIG. 12.21 The medial approach for intra-articular injection of the knee joint is demonstrated.

FIG. 12.22 An approach tangential to the joint line is made for injection of a medial coronary ligament sprain of the knee.

FIG. 12.23 An anterior approach for intra-articular injection of the ankle joint is demonstrated.

FIG. 12.24 (a) A bent needle is useful to inject the Achilles paratenon. (b) Injection of the Achilles paratenon.

FIG. 12.25 The subtalar joint may be injected from a medial approach above the sustentaculum tali.

FIG. 12.26 Plantar fasciitis may be injected from inferior or medial approaches: (a) inferior; (b) medial.

The spine

A *caudal epidural* injection (for back pain and/or sciatica) is given via the sacral hiatus (Fig. 12.27). The patient lies prone and the sacral hiatus is identified by palpation of the depression between the sacral cornua. Local anaesthesia to the skin and subcutaneous tissues as far as the hiatus is induced initially. The epidural needle pierces the skin at an angle of approximately 45° and penetrates the ligament overlying the hiatus, whereupon a loss of resistance is felt. Attempted aspiration excludes the penetration of an epidural vein or the dura mater (which normally terminates at the level of S2). The injection is given slowly over ten minutes, taking account of the severity of any reproduction of the patient's symptoms. A period of recumbency of ten to thirty minutes following the procedure allows early lightheadedness, when resuming the upright position, to dissipate rapidly.

Rarely, the patient reacts 'adversely' to a caudal epidural approach if the above precautions are taken. Nevertheless, the procedure should be carried out with adequate nursing help and with resuscitation facilities available, in view of the occasional reported case of hypersensitivity to local anaesthetic.

The following materials are required:

2 ml syringe, 23 G needle, and 2 ml 1 per cent lignocaine for skin anaesthesia
24–50 ml syringe
2 inch 21 G needle (or $3\frac{1}{2}$ inch 20 G needle for obese patients)
20–50 ml 0.5 per cent procaine HCl
± 20–40 mg triamcinolone hexacetonide.

The *lumbar facet (apophyseal) joints* which are most commonly injected are L4/5 and L5/S1. The patient lies prone and the relevant facet joint position is identified by dropping an imaginary line down (anteriorly) from the level of the relevant spinous process (for example, L4 spinous process for the L4/5 facet joint) 3 cm from the midline. When the typical resistance offered by capsule and ligament to the needle is met the injection is given with only moderate pressure. Infiltration of the posterior aspect(s) of the joint(s) is made. Commonly, bilateral injections are required.

Alternatively, an oblique approach (from a skin position approximately 6 cm from the midline, as demonstrated in Fig. 12.28) may be used. Certainty of entry into the facet joint capsule is only possible with fluoroscopic screening and contrast media. Such screening greatly facilitates accurate injection, though in the author's experience it is often unnecessary for therapeutic efficacy in facet joint syndromes. The oblique approach, in a slightly more caudal direction, is used for L4/5 or L5/S1 sinuvertebral nerve-block injections.

The following materials are required:

5 ml syringe
2 inch 21 G needle
20 mg triamcinolone hexacetonide in 1ml
4 ml 1 per cent lignocaine
(for oblique approach: $3\frac{1}{2}$ inch 20 G (spinal) needle + 2 ml syringe, 23 G needle, and 2 ml 1 per cent lignocaine for skin anaesthesia).

The *sacroiliac joint* is approached from the midline (or within 1-2 cm of the midline) at the level of the L4/5 interspinous ligament. The direction of the needle is anteriorly, inferiorly, and laterally. The correct angle is essential, and the full length of a 3 inch needle is often required.

The following materials are required:

2 ml syringe, 23 G needle, and 2 ml 1 per cent lignocaine (for skin anaesthesia)
5 ml syringe
$3\frac{1}{2}$ inch 20 G (spinal) needle
20 mg triamcinolone hexacetonide in 1 ml
4 ml 1 per cent lignocaine.

Sclerosant injections are given to the low lumbar and sacroiliac ligaments in patients with lumbar and/or sacroiliac instability. Prior sedation, for example with intravenous midazolam, is recommended. From one puncture site between the L4 and L5

FIG. 12.27 A caudal epidural injection is given via the sacral hiatus.

FIG. 12.28 The oblique approach for the right L4/5 facet (posterior apophyseal) joint is demonstrated. A similar approach, in a slightly more caudal direction, may be used for L4/5 or L5/S1 sinuvertebral nerve-block injections.

spinous processes the following ligaments are injected at their ligamento-osseous junction:

L4/5 supraspinous and interspinous ligaments
L5/S1 interspinous ligaments
L4/5 capsular ligaments
L5/S1 capsular ligaments
iliolumbar ligaments
sacroiliac interosseous ligaments
posterior sacroiliac ligaments
sacrotuberous ligaments

The following materials are required:

2 ml syringe, 23 G needle, 23 G butterfly IV set, and 2 ml midazolam
10 ml syringe
$3\frac{1}{2}$ inch 20 G (spinal) needle
5.0 ml P2G (Boots plc)
5.0 ml 2 per cent lignocaine.

References

Akeson, W. H., Amiel, D., and LaViolette, D. (1967). Connective tissue response to immobility. *Clin. Orthop.*, **51**, 183–97.

Bassett, F. H., Beck, J. L., and Weiker, G. (1980). A modified cast brace: its use in nonoperative and postoperative management of serious knee ligament injuries. *Am. J. Sports Med.*, **8**(2), 63–7.

Calabrese, L. H. and Rooney, T. W. (1986). The use of non-steroidal anti-inflammatory drugs in sports. *Physician Sportsmed.*, **14**(2), 89–97.

Cyriax, J. and Russell, G. (1984). *Textbook of orthopaedic medicine*, Vol. 2, *Treatment* (11th edn). Baillière Tindall, London.

Drez, D., Faust, D. C., and Evans, J. P. (1981). Cryotherapy and nerve palsy. *Am J. Sports Med.*, **9**(4), 256–7.

Dyson, M. and Pond, J. B. (1970). The effects of pulsed ultrasound on tissue regeneration. *Physiotherapy*, **59**, 284–7.

Dyson, M. (1987). Mechanisms involved in therapeutic ultrasound. *Physiotheraphy*, **73**, 116–20.

Finsterbush, A. and Friedman, B. (1973). Early changes in an immobilised rabbit knee joint. *Clin. Orthop*, **92**, 305–19.

Fox, W. W. (1981). *Arthritis: is your suffering really necessary*. Sheldon Press, London.

Gieck, J. H. and Saliba, E. N. (1987). Application of modalities in overuse syndromes. *Clin. Sports Med.*, **6**(2), 459–61.

Grimby, J., Gustafsson, E., Petersen, L., and Renstrøm, P. (1980). Quadriceps function and training after knee ligament surgery. *Med. Sci. Sports*, **12**, 70–5.

Haggmark, T. and Eriksson, E. (1979). Cylinder or mobile cast brace after knee ligament surgery. *Am. J. Sports Med.*, **7**(1), 48–56.

Hutson, M. A. (1986). A double-blind study comparing ibuprofen 1800 mg or 2400 mg daily and placebo in sports injuries. *J. Int. Med. Res.*, **14**(3), 142–7.

Hutson, M. A. and Jackson, J. P. (1982). Injuries to the lateral ligament of the ankle: assessment and treatment. *Br. J. Sports Med.*, **16**(4), 245–9.

Laros, G. S., Tipton, C. M., and Cooper, R. R. (1971). Influence of physical activity on ligament insertions in knees of dogs. *J. Bone Jt. Surg.*, **53A**, 275–86.

Lewit, K. (1985). *Manipulative therapy in rehabilitation of the motor system*. Butterworth, London.

Maitland, G. D. (1986). *Vertebral manipulation* (5th edn). Butterworth, London.

Melzack, R. and Wall, P. D. (1965). Pain mechanisms: a new theory. *Science*, **150**, 971–9.

Mennell, J. McM. (1960). *Back pain*. Little, Brown, Boston, MA.

Mooney, V. (1974). Cast bracing. *Clin. Orthop.*, **102**, 159–66.

Mooney, V. and Ferguson, A. B. (1966). The influence of immobilisation and motion on the formation of fibrocartilage in the repair granuloma after joint resection in the rabbit. *J. Bone Jt. Surg.*, **48A**, 1145–55.

Sloan, J. P., Hain, R., and Pownall, R. (1989). Clinical benefits of early cold therapy in accident and emergency following ankle sprain. Arch. Emerg. Med., **6**, 1–6.

Stoddard, A. (1980). *Manual of osteopathic technique* (3rd edn). Hutchinson, London.

Travell, J. and Simons, D. G. (1983). *Myofascial pain and dysfunction— trigger points manual*. Williams and Wilkins, Baltimore, MD.

Viidik, A. (1967). Effect of training on the tensile strength of isolated rabbit tendons. *Scand. J. Plast. Reconstr. Surg.*, **1**, 141–7.

Zohn, D. A. and Mennell, J. McM. (1976). *Diagnosis and physical treatment of musculoskeletal pain*. Little, Brown, Boston, MA.

13 First aid in sport

M. A. HUTSON

A sports physician will often be prevailed upon to lecture to groups of paramedics, first-aiders, trainers, and coaches on the initial management of acute injury (first aid) in sport. As far as is practically convenient it should be considered an obligation to accept the teaching responsibilities, inherent in the physician's role as medical adviser, to sports groups and associations. These responsibilities should also extend to the provision of advice to sports clubs on the adequacy of first-aid facilities which are available to sports participants (and in the case of large stadia to spectators also). The reader is referred to the *First Aid Manual* prepared by the St. John Ambulance Association for a comprehensive guide to the first-aiders management of injury. It is a useful reference work for the physician when faced with the need to structure a series of lectures on this topic. As far as the application to sport is concerned, the following guidelines may be found to be useful for teaching purposes:

Principles of first aid in sport

The responsibilities of the attendant are determined by the general principles of first aid:

(i) maintain life;
(ii) reduce the likelihood of more extensive injury;
(iii) promote recovery.

These actions are dependent upon the recognition of the nature of the injury (at least as far as is possible by non-qualified personnel).

Injury recognition

Musculoskeletal injury may be classified by reference to the type of anatomical structure involved. Management depends on the initial assessment, which should be made by inspection and gentle handling of the casualty.

Osseous—a fracture is suspected by the presence of
- pain
- swelling
- distortion (deformity)
- dysfunction

The more experienced first-aider will be able to distinguish between the temporary 'numbing' effect of direct trauma to exposed bone (for example, the shin), which causes periosteal bruising, and the disabling effect of the tibial fracture. Pain and soft tissue swelling are often poor guides to diagnosis when com-

pared with the resultant dysfunction. Once a general appraisal of the situation has been made, a determination of whether the injured player is able to move the limb is the most important step. If voluntary movement has become completely inhibited there is a significant risk of substantial structural injury. Patients with a fracture do not squirm or roll around in apparent agony—they lie still. This is an indication for the most careful degree of handling, more particularly if spinal injury is suspected. The integrity of the spinal cord may be gauged by the patient's response to questioning on loss of sensation or muscle function.

Joint (i): a *dislocation* also gives rise to distortion and dysfunction. Differentiation from (or complication by) a fracture is not discernible by a first-aider (and often not by a physician) until an X-ray has been taken. It is necessary to stress the value of neurovascular assessment—for example, the subject's comments on skin sensation, and the observation of abnormal skin colour or absent arterial pulsation—in the presence of severe distortion. Examples should be given of neurovascular complications from elbow dislocations and spinal fracture/dislocations.

Joint (ii): a *ligament sprain or tear* may be suspected by the nature of the stress or wrench applied to a joint. Thus medial knee pain in a rugby player following a valgus force during a tackle is likely to be due to injury to the medial collateral ligament: it should be within the capacity of the average first-aider to understand the principle of ligament injury by indirect force. Pain may be substantial, and early swelling is a possibility. Dysfunction following a ligament injury is usually less profound than with a fracture: even in the presence of substantial ligament tears, for instance to the knee, players involved in team sports may attempt to carry on playing for a while, and indeed may be encouraged to do so by an unsuspecting trainer if the initial assessment has failed to establish the true nature of the injury. Within five or ten minutes, however, it becomes obvious to the player, his attendants, and his manager that all is not well, so that a further careful examination in the treatment room is required.

Experienced first-aiders may be able to detect instability by stress-tests or examination of the limb at the time of injury, though this should not be expected of them. The importance of gentle stress tests for ligament function should be emphasized by the physician. All too often it is apparent to the medical officer observing from a distance that a trainer's only assessment of knee function following an injury on the pitch is the range of passive flexion and extension (which offers very limited information on injury to the soft tissues, though it may give some confidence to both the player and his examiner).

Muscle/tendon: a tear or rupture may be suspected as a result of a history of sudden pain and dysfunction in a limb when there is no evidence of direct trauma. There is often little in the way of alternative diagnosis—for example, in acute hamstring tears in sprinters. Muscle contusion due to direct trauma may be common in times of war and during other acts of violence, particularly when crushing injuries are caused by falling masonry: shock and renal failure may ensue if muscle trauma is extensive. Such situations are uncommon in sport; nevertheless a medical officer or first-aider may be required to assist in the management of severe injuries sustained by victims of spectator tragedies (for instance, in the case of crush injuries at Hillsborough and at the Heysel Stadium, and the severe burns resulting from the fire at the Bradford City Football Club). In less serious incidents, in which direct trauma is involved, first-aiders may not appreciate that muscle, as well as skin and subcutaneous tissues, may be contused—for example, in the charley horse injury to the quadriceps femoris. When muscle is torn, movement is usually hampered and strength impaired, though there is rarely any initial evidence of swelling.

Neurovascular: involvement of the neurological or vascular systems in sports injuries is often a result of a complicated fracture or dislocation. Any suspicion of a spinal fracture or cord pressure affects the subsequent management. As advised in Chapter 2 (Ocular injuries), the first-aider may remove an easily accessible foreign body from the surface of the eye using a sterile cotton-wool swab, though he should apply a taped hard eye-shield on suspicion of a penetrating injury.

The initial assessment of a patient collapsed either as a result of pain or for some other reason should be performed *prior* to his transportation elsewhere. Therefore, the sports event should either be discontinued permanently (for example, in motor-racing pile ups) or temporarily suspended while injured persons are cared for. Resuscitation must commence 'on the spot'. Examples which may be given are the initiation of resuscitative therapy for a drowned victim while he is still in the water (not waiting until *terra firma* is reached) and CPR (cardiopulmonary resuscitation) for any patient who collapses on the field of play. Initial management of severe musculoskeletal injury should also commence at the site of injury—for instance, on-site splinting for suspected fractures.

Initial management

Cardiopulmonary resuscitation (CPR)

The main threats to life result from asphyxia, cardiac arrest, and circulatory collapse (usually due to haemorrhage). Management may be taught by attention to the ABC of resuscitation (Fig. 13.1):

A = airway
B = breathing
C = circulation.

Urgent action is required in the presence of cyanosis resulting from respiratory embarrassment. Apart from inhalation of water in swimming accidents, the usual cause of asphyxia in sports accidents is mechanical obstruction. (The tragic events at Hillsborough in 1989 revealed the devastating effects of mechanical obstruction to breathing resulting from the crush of bodies on the terraces.) An unconscious casualty lying in the supine position may 'swallow his tongue'—that is, be asphyxiated by posterior prolapse of the tongue. Strangulation by external sources such as harnesses may occur. Relief of obstruction, manual protraction of the jaw, and the establishment of the 'coma' position may be all that is required. If respiration fails the casualty is laid in the supine position and mouth-to-mouth resuscitation is begun.

Cardiac arrest is detected by the first-aider by an absent carotid pulse. External cardiac massage is commenced immediately.

External haemorrhage should be controlled by direct pressure, and not by the use of tourniquets. The likelihood of circulatory failure may be reduced by elevation of the legs, reassurance, and gentle handling of the patient.

First-aiders should be taught to *monitor* and *record* such vital signs as pupil size and reactivity, respiratory rate, and pulse rate and strength when dealing with head and/or spinal injury.

Stabilization

Mechanical support is required for certain joint and bone injuries, and may be taught by qualified St. John Ambulance instructors. An adequate description of the technical aspects of the application of triangular bandages, roll bandages, splints, and slings is available in the St. John *First Aid Manual*. Familiarity should be gained in respect of the siting of stretchers, their types, and their indications for use.

Reduction of anxiety by reassurance (as far as possible) of the casualty is the most important aspect of the early management stage. The casualty's confidence will be gained by the first-aider's competence. Even if the injury is severe, the positive attitude of the management team helps to allay further injury and reduce shock. Analgesia is not offered at this time: a clinical assessment by a physician is clearly necessary for injuries other than trivial trauma.

Continuation of play

A casualty should not be allowed to try out an injury on the field of play unless the examiner is satisfied that the condition is relatively minor. The determined attempts of a player to continue to participate in a game when clearly he is unfit to do so, for instance with a locked knee or flail arm, or when concussed, should be met with equal resistance. The senseless approach of (albeit, the minority of) sportsmen that a player should continue to play in pain should be discouraged. If in doubt the first-aider should arrange for suitable transportation and a medical opinion rather than take risks with injuries.

When a serious injury has been sustained, particularly out of doors in the winter months, an adequate body temperature should be maintained; for this purpose blankets should be available. The use of modern heat-retaining blankets and 'space suits' has become commonplace in endurance events, when sudden reduction in muscle activity may give rise to hypothermia. Although physiological disturbances are not considered in this text, the usefulness of such thermoregulatory mechanisms has a relevance to musculoskeletal injury also.

A patient with a suspected spinal injury should not be moved until an appropriate number of trained helpers are available. One assistant supports the neck while the body is moved without change of position. The technique of log-roll, in which

THE Ⓐ Ⓑ Ⓒ OF RESUSCITATION

Read the diagram in columns from left to right, and follow the black or grey lines, according to the patient's condition

APPROACH

DANGER

Establish there is no danger to yourself or the patient. For instance the patient may be unconscious due to electric shock or gas leak, so check the relevant supply.

IS THE PATIENT CONSCIOUS?
(Establish by gentle shaking & shouting)

No — Yes

PLACE IN RECOVERY POSITION
OBSERVE Ⓐ Ⓑ Ⓒ
CONTROL EXTERNAL BLEEDING

1. Establish there is no danger to yourself or the casualty. For instance the patient may be unconscious due to electric shock or gas leak, so check the relevant supply.
2. Establish consciousness of the casualty by shouting 'WAKE-UP' loudly 2-3 times and shaking the shoulder gently, remembering the possibility of a neck or other upper body injury.
3. Place casualty in recovery position.

Ⓐ AIRWAY

OPEN AIRWAY

1. Place patient on back
2. Clear mouth of obstructions
3. Tilt head to open airway
4. Support jaw & CALL FOR HELP

Tilt head
and Support jaw

IF THE CASUALTY IS UNCONSCIOUS
1. Open Airway
Inspect the casualty's mouth and throat. Remove blood, vomit, loose teeth or broken dentures. Leave a well fitting full dentures in place as it will assist in expired air respiration if this is necessary.
2. If there is any doubt whether the casualty is breathing adequately, tilt the head and support the jaw as shown in the diagram. This will open the airway. At this joint check again to see if the casualty is breathing (see B Breathing).

Ⓑ BREATHING

IS PATIENT BREATHING?

No — Yes

PLACE IN RECOVERY POSITION
OBSERVE Ⓐ Ⓑ Ⓒ &
CONTROL EXTERNAL BLEEDING

TWO SLOW FULL BREATHS

ARE BREATHS EASY TO GET IN?
Yes — No

HAS BREATHING RETURNED?
Yes — No

CHECK FOR AIRWAY OBSTRUCTION RELIEVE AND TRY AGAIN

CONTINUE RESUSCITATION

1. Look, listen and feel for breathing.
2. Kneel beside casualty, tilt his head back and raise the chin upwards thus opening the airway. Remember to clear the mouth of any obstructions and commence Expired Air Respiration. Open casualty's mouth and pinch his nose. Open your mouth, take a breath, seal his mouth with yours and breathe firmly into it. Breathe just firmly enough to raise the casualty's chest. Remove your mouth and allow his chest to fall.
3. As soon as the casualty's breathing returns place him in the recovery position. Vomiting often occurs when breathing returns and placing the casualty in the recovery position will prevent him from choking if vomiting does occur.
4. If there are no signs of life after two breaths, check if there is a pulse (see C Circulation).

Ⓒ CIRCULATION

IS THERE A PULSE?

No — Yes

CONTINUE EXPIRED AIR RESPIRATION
Return of Breathing

PLACE IN RECOVERY POSITION
OBSERVE A B C & CONTROL EXTERNAL BLEEDING

RETURN OF PULSE

COMMENCE CHEST COMPRESSION and CONTINUE EXPIRED AIR RESPIRATION
Check pulse after 1 min & then every 3 mins
Single Person 15:2
Two-Person 5:1

1. Check for the presence of the Carotid pulse in the neck.
2. To commence External Chest Compression (E.C.C.) place the casualty flat on his back. Apply interlocked hands two finger breadths above the lower end of the breastbone and commence chest compression. Keep your hands on the chest at all times, this will minimise chest damage.
3. The rates for E.C.C. are as follows: *Working alone:* 15 Cardiac compressions (rate approximately 80 compressions per minute) followed by 2 inflations. *With assistance:* 5 Cardiac compressions (rate 60 compressions per minute) followed by 1 inflation.
4. If spontaneous pulse does not return, prepare to continue E.C.C. until skilled help arrives.
5. External bleeding should be controlled by direct pressure over the wound, using a clean dressing such as a handkerchief. When a pulse is detected, elevation of both lower legs on a suitable support will reduce the severity of shock.

Fig. 13.1

the spine is kept perfectly straight, should be familiar to a trained first-aider.

Promotion of recovery

Once the first-aider is satisfied that an injury is relatively minor, a coolant spray may be applied to the skin overlying soft tissue trauma. Although of temporary benefit only, the reassurance that is implied in this 'therapeutic' action may have great effect. Dowsing of the head and the back of the neck with cold water is time honoured, and appears to have a stimulant effect! If a player is able to continue, review of the injury on the completion of the game should be made in a well-lit treatment or first-aid room.

The principles of the early stages of treatment of soft tissue injuries are incorporated in 'RICE':

R = rest
I = ice
C = compression
E = elevation.

This phase of first-aid management merges with the inflammatory phase of healing. It is important to stress that during the first forty-eight hours after injury the priority, other than for a thorough assessment, is for a period of rest in which there is minimal activity of the injured area.

Bleeding, whether internal or external, should be controlled in preparation for the subsequent physiological vasodilation of the healing phase. The use of elevation, by a sling for the upper limb and by recumbency with limb elevation for the lower limb, is important for comfort, reduction of further bleeding, and reduction of tissue pressure from oedema. This is especially relevant to injuries below the knee, when gravitational oedema and bruising may cause prolonged or severe inflammatory responses. Suitable strapping techniques help to control both periarticular and intra-articular swelling. For added protection the use of wool and crepe is time-honoured, particularly in the form of the Robert Jones bandage for knee joint injuries. The use of strapping should not be a substitute for an adequate period of rest. In particular, players injured in those team sports which are traditionally associated with after match drinking should be discouraged from persuing these social activities by standing 'propped up' at a bar.

The use of ice or one of the proprietary cold applications which are universally available is hardly ever contraindicated once the casualty has been assessed and stabilized in the relatively comfortable surroundings of the treatment or first-aid room. Twenty minutes of ice application, repeated every three hours or so, is considered to be helpful by most authorities. Care should be taken to avoid ice-burns by wrapping ice in a thin damp cloth or plastic bag, or by the application of massage techniques. In view of the occasional reports of nerve damage, ice compression should be avoided over exposed nerves, such as the common peroneal nerve at the head of the fibula.

Conclusion

Facilities for early diagnosis and first-aid management at sports clubs and arenas vary widely. A treatment room should be available, and equipped with a refrigerator for ice or cold compresses, and an adequate supply of bandages and gauze swabs. A stretcher in good working order should be readily available. For the equipment to be used with maximum effectiveness, it is necessary for as many club members as possible to have attended a first-aid course, augmented by training in management of sports injuries. A baseline of knowledge of those injuries that tend to be frequently encountered in individual sports should be provided.

Posters demonstrating CPR techniques should be prominently displayed. From time to time CPR drills should be organized by the medical officer; if necessary the help of certified teachers from the St. John Ambulance Association should be enlisted. Suitable equipment such as a Brook airway and Ambu bag should be maintained in an easily accessible area.

References

First Aid Manual—the authorised manual of the St. John Ambulance Association and Brigade, St. Andrews Ambulance Association, and the British Red Cross Society (1982). Dorling Kindersley, London.

Epilogue: whither sports injury services?

M. A. HUTSON

Discussion of the need for sports injury services and the responsibility for provision of services within the UK has taken place amongst interested parties, and no doubt will continue to take place for the foreseeable future. However, despite varying views as to responsibility, the following facts are inescapable.

1. Sport will continue to be played (and despite outbreaks of crowd hooliganism in recent years it may even continue to receive governmental blessing); therefore sports injuries will continue to occur.

2. Despite recent changes in the way in which health care is provided and funded, it seems very unlikely that appropriate funding will become available in the foreseeable future to support a separate specialty or subspecialty of 'Sports Medicine' within the National Health Service in the UK. Hence patients with injuries sustained in sport will continue to swell the workload of the general practitioner and the junior traumatologist. The author can illustrate this view by quoting from a letter to the British Medical Journal (Hutson 1987):

> An appreciable proportion of attendances at hospital accident departments, particularly at weekends, result from acute musculoskeletal injuries caused by sport. The numbers stretch the resources of junior emergency staff to a level at which their primary concern is to define whether (using conventional orthopaedic priorities) an injury requires referral to a fracture clinic. Patients with overuse injuries peculiar to sport also present to general practitioners, whose difficulties are often due to a lack of knowledge of biomechanics and techniques related to particular sports; decision-making and advice in consequence become arbitrary.
>
> The only satisfactory remedy ultimately lies in an improved level of tuition in musculoskeletal examination techniques for medical students and an improved level of postgraduate education in recognizing and managing soft-tissue injuries. Such training would allow the doctor of first contact—the general practitioner and traumatologist—to cope adequately with most of the problems (however and wherever occurred) as part of primary health-care. The future generalist sports physician must inevitably come therefore from the ranks of general practice, and orthopaedic (physical) medical teaching needs to be an obligatory part of the general practitioner's vocational training scheme. Appropriate postgraduate education in sports medicine would then lead to the establishment of a satisfactory career structure for doctors in this specialty. With some two million sports injuries occurring every year this may well be inevitable.
>
> Regrettably, there continues to be a body of opinion within the medical profession which considers sports injuries as self-imposed and therefore deserving of private treatment only. Soft-tissue trauma, however, may give rise to as much morbidity and loss of time from work as fractures, which have historically been accorded priority in orthopaedic practice. There is no point in attempting to gloss over the absence of fundamental training, but first there needs to be a radical revision of medical opinion in line with rising consumer demand in favour of accepting the need for the development of orthopaedic and sports medicine within the general framework of medicine in the United Kingdom.

As a final comment, the self-imposed or self-inflicted injury philosophy appears to be largely a medical argument. Will the National Lottery, by releasing funds to regional centres of excellence supported by the Sports Council, enable the development of sports medicine? Perhaps the more vocal element of the sporting community will be the final arbiter, by its support for, and hopefully its demand for, an appropriate level of service provision.

References

Hutson, M. A. (1987). Why sports injury clinics? *Br. Med. J.*, **295**, 1210.

INDEX

Page numbers in **bold** indicate main discussions.

ABC of resuscitation   21, 23, 226, 227
abdominal muscles
   strengthening exercises   **189**, 190
   use in lifting   80
abductor pollicis longus injection   216, 219
Achilles paratendinitis   9, 157
Achilles paratenon injection   157, **218**, 221
Achilles tendon
   insertional tendinitis   158
   overuse injuries   **156–8**
   postcalcaneal bursitis   158
   retrocalcaneal bursitis   158
   rupture   8, **139**, 157, 171
   tendinitis   156–7
acromioclavicular (AC) joint   **47–8**
   anatomy/biomechanics   31, 32
   assessment   38, 47–8
   injection   48, 214, **215–16**, 217
   osteoarthritis   48
   osteolysis   40
   painful arc   41
   treatment   48
adductor longus   105
   myositis ossificans   106
   rupture   105–6, 143–4
   strain   105, 106
   tendon, ectopic ossification   106
adductors, thigh   105
   acute injuries   105–6, 143–4
   chronic strain   106
   stretching exercises   199
   tendinitis   106
adolescents
   pelvic injuries   111, 112
   traction osteochondroses   12
   see also children
aerobic exercise   196–7
aerobic fitness   **195**, 196
Aircast inflatable stirrup brace   136
alkaline phosphatase, plasma   167
American football   33, 81, 98, 183, 184
amnesia   21
anaerobic fitness   195
anaerobic threshold (AT)   195
ankle
   acute injuries   **131–9**
   anatomy/biomechanics   131–2
   anterior impingement syndrome   155–6
   arthrography   134, 178–9
   avulsion fractures   133, 137, 172
   brace   136
   cast-bracing   136, 204
   eversion injury   133, **137–8**
   examination summary   139
   exercises   136–7

injections   137, **217–19**, 220–1
instability   134, 135–6
inversion injury   **132–7**
   assessment   132–5
   management   135–7
joint   131
   capsular pattern   131
   capsulitis   137
   haemarthrosis   134, 138
   injection   137, **217**, 220
   lateral ligamentous complex   132, 133
   osteoarthritis   156
ligament injuries   132–8
overuse injuries   **155–62**
posterior impingement syndrome   159
sprained   131, 134, 135
strapping   135
varus   163
weak, syndrome of   131, 132, 135, 136–7
ankylosing spondylitis   82, 86, 93, 107, 167
anserine bursitis   149
anterior apprehension test, shoulder   42–3
anterior cruciate ligament (ACL)
   anatomy/biomechanics   115, 116
   assessment of injury   119–20
   avulsion fracture of inferior attachment   197
   chronic instability   121–2, 123–4
   management of injury   120–2
   surgical management   120–1, **122–4**
   tears   117, **118–24**, 125
anterior drawer sign
   ankle   133, 134, 135
   knee   120
anterior inferior iliac spine (AIIS), apophyseal
      injuries   111, 112, 141–2
anterior interosseous nerve compression   57
anterior stress test, ankle   132–3, 134
anterior superior iliac spine (ASIS), apophyseal
      injuries   111, 112
anterior talofibular ligament   132, 133
   assessment   132–3
   rupture   133, 134, 135–6
   sprain   132, 133, 134, 135
antinuclear factor (ANF)   167
Apley test   126
apophyses
   fracture separation   12, 13, 197
   anterior inferior iliac spine (AIIS)   111,
      112, 141–2
      anterior superior iliac spine (ASIS)   111,
         112
      iliac crest   111, 112
      ischial tuberosity   12, 13, 111, 112, 143
      lesser trochanter   111, 112
   traction osteochondroses   12, 197

apprehension tests
   anterior, shoulder instability   42–3
   patella instability   117
arch
   strain   161
   transverse, inadequacy   161
arthrography   178
   ankle   134, 178–9
   knee   123, 126, 178
   shoulder   180
arthroscopy
   knee, see knee, arthroscopy
   shoulder   46
asphyxia   226
aspiration, joint   **167**
assessment   **1–3**, 14–15
   of function   2
autogenous grafts, knee instability   122,
      123–4
autonomic dysreflexia   101
avulsion fractures   **171–3**

back pain, low (LBP)   84–6, 222
   see also lumbar spine
badminton   25, 53
Bankart lesion   44, 177, 180
baseball pitchers
   elbow problems   53, 54, 197
   shoulder problems   33, 35, 46
beat knee   150
Bennett's fracture   60, **73**
biceps brachii
   anatomy/biomechanics   32, 51
   distal insertional lesions   54
   examination   39, 40
   lesions   51
   superior labrum detachment   34
   tendinitis   39, 45
   tendon sheath injection   215, 216
biceps femoris tendon   116
   avulsion   143
   tendinitis   150
bicycle maintenance   147, **187**
biomechanics   **188–91**
biopsy   168
bleeding, see haemorrhage/bleeding
blindness   27
blood pressure, in head injuries   23
bone   **12**
   radioisotope scans   3, 148, 152, **177**
   tumours   154, 175, 176
   see also fractures
boutonnière injury   74–6
'boxer's fracture'   60

boxing
  brain injuries   18, 180, 181
  eye injuries   26
  hand injuries   60, 73
brachioradialis lesions   54
brain
  acceleration injury   17–18
  bridging vessel disruption   18
  cavitation   18–19
  contre-coup injury   18–19
  CT scanning   180, 181
  deformation injury   17
  injury   **17–19**, 94
  penetrating injury   17
  shear   18
  shift   17, 21
  swelling   17, 19
'breast-stroker's knee'   148
British Standards Institute (BSI)   20, 183
Broca lesion   44
bunions   161
bursa   12
bursitis   12, 213
buttock, sign of   109

calcaneocuboid ligament sprain   137
calcaneofibular ligament   132, 133
  assessment   133–4
  rupture   132, 133, 134, 135–6, 178
calcification, ectopic   8, 176
  flexor tendons of wrist   9, 55
  medial collateral ligament of knee   118, 148–9
  rotator cuff (supraspinatus)   35, 40, 45
  see also myositis ossificans
calcium, plasma   167
calf
  compartments   151, 152
  muscle injury   **144**
capitate   62
capsular pattern   10
capsulitis   9
cardiac arrest   226
cardiopulmonary resuscitation (CPR)   19, 23, **226**, 227, 228
carpal instability   **65–7**
carpal tunnel
  injection   56, 217, 219
  syndrome   55–6
carpo-metacarpal joints
  dislocations and fracture-dislocations   65
  sprain-impaction   73
carpus
  dislocations/fracture-dislocations   65–7
  fractures   62–5
cartilage   **12**
cast-bracing   10, **203–4**
  ankle   136, 204
  knee   118, 120–1, 203–4
cast immobilization
  in Achilles tendon rupture   139
  in patella dislocation   117
  in quadriceps contusion   141
cataracts   27
catheterization, urinary   101
caudal epidural injection   222

cavoid foot   163, 164
cavum pellucidum   180, 181
cerebral blood flow
  auto-regulation   19
  control measures   19
cerebrospinal fluid (CSF), post-traumatic leakage   19
cervical spine
  biomechanics/anatomy   79
  'burner'/'stinger' injury   81
  capsular pattern   82
  disc prolapse   81, 82
  examination   **82**, 93
  facet dysfunction   81, 82
  injuries   **81–2**, 94, 97–8
  joint play   82, 210
  manipulation   82, 210, 212
  neural tension test   82
  patho-anatomy   81–2
  shoulder dysfunction and   33, **49**
  spondylitis   82
  whiplash injury   81–2
charley horse injury   141
children
  elbow injuries   52
  epiphyseal fractures   12, 72, 171, 197
  head injuries   23
  injury prevention   **197–200**
  overuse injuries   164, 197
chondral injuries   12, **176**
chondromalacia patellae   145, **146**
choroid rupture   27
Clarke's sign   117
classification of injuries   5–6
clothing, protective   184
'cocktail party' syndrome   86
Codman exercises   45
cold applications   **204–5**, 228
collagen
  immobilization effects   10
  in wound healing   5
collateral ligaments of knee, see lateral collateral ligament; medial collateral ligament
Colles' fracture   58, **62**
communications   24
community fitness   196–7
compartment syndrome, chronic   **151–2**, 153
computerized tomography (CT)   24, **180–1**
coning (of brain)   17
conjoined tendon strain   108
consciousness, assessment of   21, 22, 23
coolant spray   228
cool down   8, 197
coronary artery disease   196
coronary (meniscotibial) ligaments   115
  injection   217, 220
  sprain   126, **127**, 148
costochondral joints   79, 84
costovertebral joints   83
creatine phosphokinase (CPK; CK), serum   167, 191
cricket   183
  back injuries   85
  eye injuries   27
  hand injuries   71
  shoulder problems   33, 35

cruciate ligaments, see anterior cruciate ligament; posterior cruciate ligament
cryotherapy   **204–5**, 228
cuboid syndrome   161
cyclists
  handlebar neuropathy   56, 57
  injury prevention   186, 187
  knee problems   146, 147, 148, 150

dancers
  ankle/foot problems   155–6, 159, 161
  injury prevention   186, 187, 188, 197
  trochanteric bursitis   110
dangerous play   184, 185
darts   27
dead leg   141
deep peroneal nerve compression   154
deltoid ligament rupture   133, 137, 138
deltoid muscle   32, 33
de Quervain's tenosynovitis   55, 216, 219
diathermy, short-wave   205
digits, see finger(s)
diplopia   27
disability, in spinal cord injuries   99
disabled, sport for   99, 100
disc, intervertebral, see intervertebral disc
dislocations   9, 12, **177**
  recognition   225
  recurrent   177
distal tibiofibular ligament lesions   137, 138
divers   57, 58, 94, 187
DNA binding   167

eccentric exercise   192, 208–9
effleurage   206
elbow
  acute injury   **52**
  anatomy/biomechanics   51–2
  examination summary   58–9
  fractures around   52
  haemarthrosis   52
  impingement syndromes   52
  injections   53, **216–17**, 218
  medial joint injuries   53
  mobilization exercises   207
  muscle lesions   53–4
  nerve entrapment   53, 55–7
  osteoarthritis   **54**, 55
  osteochondritis dissecans   54
  overuse injury   **52–7**
  radiology   172
elevation of limbs   228
employment, in spinal cord injuries   99
endurance training   192, 195, 196–7
enophthalmos   27
enthesitis   8
enthesopathies   8, 9
  injection techniques   213, 216
epicondylitis
  lateral (tennis elbow)   **53**, 216, 218
  medial (golfer's elbow)   53
epidural injection, caudal   222
epilepsy, post-traumatic   **19–20**, 24
epiphyseal fractures   12, 72, 171, 197

equipment
    first aid   228
    protective   20, 28, **183–4**
erythrocyte sedimentation rate (ESR)   167
evoked potentials   96, 98
excessive lateral pressure syndrome (ELPS),
    patella   146, 147
exercise(s)
    cool down   8, 197
    eccentric   192, 208–9
    flexibility   **192–4**, 198–201, 207
    health benefits   196
    isokinetic   192, 193, **209–10**
    isometric   207, 208
    isotonic   192, 207–8
    mobilization   **206–7**
    prescription   196–7
    strengthening   191–2, **207–10**
    stretching   162–3, 186, 191, **194**,
      198–201
    warm-up   7–8, 196
    see also training
extensor pollicis brevis injection   216, 219
extensors of wrist, common origin   53, 216,
    218
extensor tenosynovitis (foot)   156
external rotation/recurvatum test, knee
    instability   124
extradural haematoma   17, 19, 180
eye guards (goggles)   28, 183–4
eye injuries, *see* ocular injuries
eye-shields   28
Eysenck's Personality Questionnaire   196

facet joints (zygo-apophyseal joints)   79
    arthrosis   86, 92
    cervical dysfunction   81, 82
    injections   222, 223
    lumbar dysfunction   85, 86, 91, 92
    thoracic dysfunction   83
fat, body   194
fatigue index   195
femoral anteversion   104, 188
femoral hernia   108
femoral stretch test (FST)   91, 142
femur
    lesser trochanter apophyseal injury   111,
      112
    stress fractures   107, 148
fibula
    lateral malleolus, avulsion fracture   137
    oblique fracture   133, 137, 138
    stress fractures   151, 152–3
field athletes   159, 187–8
finger(s)
    avulsion fractures   172–3
    boutonnière injury   74–6
    examination   59
    fractures   68–72
    joint injuries   **73–6**
    mallet   75, **76**
    rotational deformity   68, 69
    splints   68, 70
    trigger   55
    X-rays   62
Finkelstein's test   55, 59

first aid   **225–8**
    in eye injuries   28, 226
    injury recognition   225–6
    principles   225
    in spinal injuries   **97**, 225, 226–8
fishhooks   27
Fitch catch test   88
fitness
    aerobic   195
    anaerobic   195
    assessment   **194–6**
    community   196–7
    inadequate   7
    physiological   194–6
    psychological   196
flat foot   163
flexibility   10
    assessment   194–5
    exercises   **192–4**, 198–201, 207
    overuse injuries and   162–3, 186
flexor digitorum profundus (FDP) tendon
    rupture   76
flexor hallucis longus tendinitis   159
flexors of wrist, common origin   53, 216
flexor tendons (hand and wrist)
    calcific tendinitis   9, 55
    stenosing tenovaginitis   55
foot
    accessory ossicles   173
    acute injuries   **131–9**
    anatomy/biomechanics   131–2, 190–1
    avulsion fractures   172
    biomechanical abnormalities   162, 163–4
    cavoid   163, 164
    examination summary   139
    extensor tenosynovitis   156
    overuse injuries   **155–62**
    see also forefoot; rearfoot
'footballer's ankle'   155
football (soccer)   185
    ankle/foot problems   155–6, 159
    eye injuries   25
    pelvic/thigh injuries   105, 106, 107
footwear, *see* shoes
forearm
    anatomy/biomechanics   51–2
    examination summary   58–9
    injections   **216–17**
    nerve entrapment   55–7
    overuse injury   **52–7**
    tenosynovitis   **54–5**, 216, 219
forefoot
    biomechanics   132
    pain   **161**
    valgus   162
    varus   162, 163, 164
fractures   2, 6, 12
    avulsion   **171–3**
    diagnosis   225
    epiphyseal   12, 72, 171, 197
    greenstick   170, 171
    osteochondral   12, **176**, 177
    plain film radiography   169–71
    sesamoid   176
    stress, *see* stress fractures
Freiberg's disease   161
frozen hip   108

frozen shoulder (adhesive capsulitis)   41, 180,
    213

gait   87
Galeazzi fracture-dislocation   51
gamekeeper's thumb   73
ganglia   58
gastrocnemius
    stretching   201
    tears   143, 144
genu valgus   147
Gilmore's groin   108
Glasgow coma scale   22, 23
glaucoma, secondary   26
glenohumeral joint
    anatomy   31
    capsulitis, *see* shoulder, capsulitis
    dislocation   33, 34–6, 42–4, 177
    injection   213, 214
    subluxation   33, 42–3, 44
gluteal bursitis   105, **109**
glutei   104–5
    insertional tendinitis   105
    stretch   200
    tears   106
goggles (eye guards)   28, 183–4
golfers   27, 55, 65, 85
golfer's elbow   53
granulation tissue   5
greenstick fractures   170, 171
groin
    Gilmore's   108
    pain   103, 106, 108
    strain   105, 106
growth factors   164, 197
guns, sporting   26, 60
gymnasts
    injury prevention   184, 197
    spinal problems   83, 86, 95
    upper limb problems   54, 58

haemarthrosis   9–10, 167
    ankle   134, 138
    elbow   52
    first metatarsophalangeal joint   161
    knee   **116–17**, 118, 120
haematological tests   167
haematoma
    extradural   17, 19, 180
    intracranial   19
    intramuscular   8, 181
    subdural   18, 19, 180
    subungual   71–2
haemoglobin (Hb)   167
haemorrhage/bleeding
    first aid   226, 228
    into optic nerve sheath   27
    intraocular   26
    subarachnoid   180
Haglund deformity   158
hallux rigidus   161
hallux valgus   161
hamate, fractured hook of   60, 61, 64, **65**
hamstrings
    acute injury   **142–3**

hamtrings—*cont.*
  chronic strain, of origin   110, 111
  exercises   121, 122
  stretching   200
  syndrome   110–11
  tendinitis of medial   149
hand
  assessment of injuries   60–2
  biomechanics   51–2
  causes of injury   60
  examination   60–1
  flexor tenovaginitis, stenosing   55
  fractures   **67–73**
    reduction   68
    rehabilitation   71
    retention   68–71
  injuries   **60–76**
  safe (Edinburgh) position   68, 70
  see also finger(s); thumb
'handlebar neuropathy'   56, 57
head injuries   **17–29**
  associated injuries   22–3, 94
  basic assessment   21
  communications and   24
  CT scan   24, 180
  intracranial   17–24
  management   20, **23–4**
  mechanisms   17–19
  prevention   20
  risk status   21–2
  secondary complications   19
  severity   21
  tertiary lesions   19–20
  vital signs   21
  see also ocular injuries
head protection   20, 28, 183
healing   4–5
heart rate, maximal   196
heat, therapeutic   205, 206
heel
  pad contusion   160
  pain   158–9
  raise   144, 157
  see also plantar fasciitis
helmets, protective   20, 28, 183
hernia
  femoral/inguinal   108
  muscle   151, 152, 153
'hiatal signs', in head injury   21
Hill-Sachs lesion   44
hip joint
  anatomy/biomechanics   80, 103, **104–5**
  capsular pattern   104, 109
  disorders   108–9
  examination   91, 112
  flexibility exercises   199–200
  'frozen'   108
  injections   **217**, 219
  osteoarthritis   109
  synovitis   108–9
history, clinical   2
hockey   106
Hoffa's disease   127
hook of hamate fractures   60, 61, 64, **65**
horse-riders   94–5, 106, 183
housemaid's knee   150
housing, in spinal cord injuries   99

humero-ulnar joint   51
humerus
  fracture separation of lesser tuberosity   12, 13
  see also olecranon
hydrocephalus   18, **19**
hyperextension test, one-legged   88, 89
hypermobility   **10–11**, 194
hyphaema   25, 26, 27

ice application   204–5, 228
ice hockey   27–8, 73
iliac crest, apophyseal injuries   111, 112
iliopsoas, *see* psoas
iliotibial tract (band)   116
  bursitis   105, 217
  injection   217
  stretching exercises   199
  syndrome   149
illegal play   184, 185
immobilization   7, 10, 203
  hand   68, 70
  see also cast immobilization
impingement
  anterior ankle   155–6
  elbow   52
  posterior ankle   159
  shoulder, *see* shoulder, impingement
inflammation
  acute   **4**
  chronic   4
  in overuse injury   6
infraorbital nerve injury   27
infrapatellar bursitis   150
infraspinatus   31, 32
  examination   37, 39, 40
  injection   215
  tears   39
  tendinitis   39, 45
inguinal hernia   108
injections   **212–23**
  diagnostic   212
  intra-articular (IA)   213
  intrabursal   213
  intraligamentous   213
  intrasynovial   213
  precautions   213–14
  therapeutic   212–13
insoles   163–4
intercostal muscle strain   83, 84
interferential therapy   206
intermetatarsal joints   132
intermittent claudication   154
interphalangeal joints
  distal (DIP), injuries   75, **76**
  foot   132
  proximal (PIP)   **74–6**
    boutonnière injury   74–6
    dislocation   74
    fractures   71
    sprains   74
    tears of collateral ligament   74
intersection syndrome   55
intervertebral disc
  biomechanics/anatomy   79
  prolapse   12, 180, 212

cervical   81, 82
lumbar   84–5, 90, 91
thoracic   83, 84
intracompartment pressure monitoring (ICPM)   152, 153
intracranial pressure, raised   17, 19
inversion stress test, ankle   133–4
investigations   3, **167–81**
iris sphincter tears   26
ischial bursitis   110
ischial tuberosity
  apophyseal injuries   12, 13, 111, 112, 143
  avulsion fracture   172
isokinetic dynamometers   121, 192, 193, 195–6, 209
isokinetic exercises   192, 193, **209–10**
isometric exercises   207, 208
isotonic exercises   192, 207–8

javelin throwers   1, 159, 187–8
jerk test, knee injuries   119, 120
Jobe relocation test   43
joint   **10–12**
  aspiration   **167**
  assessment of function   2
  capsular pattern   10
  degenerative disease, *see* osteoarthritis
  effusions   9–10, 167, 172
  flexibility, *see* flexibility
  hypermobility   **10–11**, 194
  hypomobility   11
  injections into   213
  laxity   10, 194
  in ligament injuries   9–10
  loose bodies   12, 15, 127, 210
  manipulation   210–12
  mobilization exercises   207
  radiological investigations   171, **178–80**
  stability   9
  subluxation   12
  see also capsulitis; dislocations; haemarthrosis; synovitis; *specific joints*
'jumper's knee'   145, 150

kicking   105, 141
Kienböck's disease   65
knee   **115–28**
  acute injuries   **115–28**
  anatomy/biomechanics   115–16
  anterior pain   145–8
  arthrography   123, 126, 178
  arthroscopy   115, **127**, 128, 147
    diagnostic   120, 123, 126
    therapeutic   123, 127
  aspiration   117, 128
  avulsion fractures   173
  brace   122, 204, 205
  cast-bracing   118, 120–1, 203–4
  examination summary   127–8
  flexors, *see* hamstrings
  haemarthrosis   **116–17**, 118, 120
  injections   127, 148, **217**, 220
  instability   116, 125
    assessment   119–20, 124–5
    management   120–4, 125

lateral ligamentous complex 116
ligament injuries **117–25**, 127
lipohaemarthrosis 172
locking 126, 127
loose body 127
magnetic resonance imaging 120, 123, 178, 179
malalignment 147, 188
menisci, *see* menisci, knee
osteoarthritis 125, 148
osteochondritis dissecans 127, 177
overuse injuries **145–50**
pseudolocking 119
quadriceps expansion/patella tendon tear 117
radiology 128, 171–2
strengthening exercises 121, 190, **207**, 208, 209
synovial plicae 115, 148
traumatic synovitis 118, 119, 126
see also patella
kyphosis 84
kyphus 84

Lachman's test 119
'lame brain' jockey 18, 20
lasers 206
lateral collateral ligament (LCL) (knee)
anatomy/biomechanics 115–16
injury **125**
lateral cutaneous nerve of thigh entrapment 109
lateral epicondylitis (tennis elbow) **53**, 216, 218
lateral ligamentous complex
ankle 132, 133
knee 116
lateral malleolus, avulsion fracture 137
latex test 167
latissimus dorsi 33
tears 38
Lido isokinetic dynamometer 193, 195–6
lifting 79–80
ligament **9–10**
injections into 213
injuries 9–10, 225
injury classification 9
prostheses 123
see also specific ligaments
lipohaemarthrosis 172
'Little Leaguer's elbow' 53, 54
local anaesthetic injection 212
loose bodies 12, 15, 210
knee 127
lower limb
muscle injuries **141–4**
neurological examination 91
overuse injuries **145–64**
lumbago 84, 87
lumbar-pelvic rhythm 79
lumbar spine
acute injury 84–5
biomechanics/anatomy 79–80
canal stenosis 85–6, 93, 153
chronic ligamentous insufficiency 86, 92–3
chronic/relapsing injury 85–6

disc prolapse 84–5, 90, 91
examination 87–91, 93
facet dysfunction 85, 86, 91, 92
herniation of nucleus pulposus (HNP) 84, 88, 91
injection techniques 91, 92, 93, **222–3**
injuries **84–93**, 94
epidemiology 84–6
management 91–3
instability 85, 91–2
manipulation 211, 212
patho-anatomy 84–6
lumbosacral angle 79, 80
lumbosacral stress test 89, 90–1
lunate 62
avascular necrosis 65
dislocation 61, 63, **65**

McMurray test 126
magnetic resonance imaging (MRI) 178
in knee injuries 120, 123, 178, 179
in spinal injuries 96, 98, 180
mallet finger 75, **76**
management **3–4**, 15
manipulation **210–12**
peripheral joints 210–12
spinal 82, 84, 210, 211, **212**
martial arts 183, 185
massage **206**
deep friction 206
medial calcaneal nerve entrapment 161
medial capsular ligament (knee) 115
medial collateral ligament (MCL) (knee)
anatomy/biomechanics 115, 116
chronic sprain 148–9
ectopic calcification 118, 148–9
grade I injury (sprain) 118
grade II injury (partial tear) 118
grade III injury (complete tear) 118
injuries **117–18**, 120
medial epicondylitis (golfer's elbow) **53**
medial malleolus, fracture 133, 137
medial plantar nerve entrapment 161
medial retinaculitis 148
medial tibial syndrome 151, 152, 153
median nerve entrapments 55–6
menisci, knee 115
cyst of lateral 149–50
radiology 178, 179
tears 12, 123, **125–7**, 210
assessment 126
bucket-handle 125, 126
management 126–7
parrot beak 125, 126
peripheral 126–7
meniscotibial ligaments, *see* coronary ligaments
meralgia paraesthetica 109
metacarpal fractures **72–3**
metacarpophalangeal joint injuries **73**, 74
metatarsal (MT)
fifth, avulsion fracture of base 137
osteochondritis 161
stress fracture 161, 174
metatarsalgia **161**
metatarsophalangeal joints (MTP) 132
bunions 161

first
hallux rigidus 161
trauma 161
mid-carpal joint 61, 62
midtarsal joint 132, 191
Mill's manoeuvre 53
miserable malalignment syndrome 147
mobilization
cervical spine 82
exercises **206–7**
in knee injuries 118
in ligament injuries 10
Monteggia fracture–dislocation 51
Morton's interdigital neuroma 161
motor evoked potentials 96, 98
motor signs, in head injury 21
mouth guards 184
MRI, *see* magnetic resonance imaging
multi-gym exercises 44, 208
muscle **6–8**
balance 162–3
contusion 8, 226
fibre types 6–7, 141, 192
functional assessment 8
haematoma 8, 181
hernia 151, 152, 153
imbalance 7, 163, 196
injuries 7–8
elbow 53–4
lower limb **141–4**
recognition 226
mobilization exercises 207
pull/strain 7
strength/power measurement 195–6
stretch–shorten cycle 7
tears/rupture 7, 8
see also specific muscles
musculotendinous unit 6
myositis ossificans 6–7, 8, **176**
in adductor longus 106
in quadriceps femoris 141, 176

National Athletic Injury/Illness Reporting System (NAIRS) 25
navicular, stress fracture 160
neck, *see* cervical spine
Neer's anterior acromioplasty and decompression 46, 47
nerve **14**
nerve entrapment 14
in ankle and foot 161
in pelvis/thigh 109
in upper limb 53, **55–7**
see also specific nerves
neural tension test
cervical spine 82
lumbar spine 88–90
neurological examination 21, 97
neurovascular injuries 226
Nideffer's Test of Attention and Interpersonal Style 196
non-steroidal anti-inflammatory drugs (NSAIDs) 204

Ober's test 110

ocular injuries **25–9**
  contusion   26–7
  economics and prevention   27–8
  first-aid management   28, 226
  incidence   25–6
  mechanisms   26–7
  perforating   27, 28
  preparticipation screening   28–9
  in specific sports   27
olecranon
  bursitis   54
  fractures   52
  impingement   52
  stress fractures   52
ophthalmia, sympathetic   27
optic nerve sheath, bleeding into   27
orbital 'blow-out fractures'   27
orthotic appliances (orthoses)   164, 187
os calcis, stress fractures   158–9
Osgood–Schlatter's disease   3, 12, **150**, 197
os naviculare   161
os supranaviculare   173
osteitis pubis   106–7
osteoarthritis (OA)   10
  acromioclavicular (A–C) joint   48
  ankle   156
  elbow   **54**, 55
  hip   109
  knee   125, 148
  patellofemoral joint   146
  sternoclavicular joint   49
  wrist   58
osteochondral fractures   12, **176**, 177
  talus   **138**, 176
osteochondritis dissecans   12, **177**, 197
  elbow   54
  knee   127, 177
  metatarsal   161
osteochondroses, traction   12, 197
osteoid osteoma   175, 176
osteophytes
  in ankle impingement   155
  in shoulder impingement   34, 35
osteoporosis   196
osteosarcoma   175
os tibialis externa   173
os trigonum   159
overuse injuries   **6**
  aetiological factors   14, **161–4**
  in children   164, 197
  elbow and forearm   **52–7**
  lower limb   **145–64**
  pelvic region   **106–11**
  shoulder   **33–40**
  technical factors in   **186–8**
  upper limb   **51–9**
  wrist   **58**
oxygen consumption, maximal (max. VO_2)
    195, 196

pain
  central, in spinal cord injuries   101
  transmission in spine   80–1
painful arc syndrome, shoulder   34, 38–9,
    41–2
  acromioclavicular (A–C)   41

capsulitis   41
  composite   41–2
  subacromial   41
  treatment   45–7
parachuting   185
paraplegia   94, 98–101
paratendinitis   9, 213
patella
  alta   146, 147, 177
  anatomy/biomechanics   116, 145–6
  apicitis   150
  apprehension test   117
  bipartite   146
  dislocation   **117**
  excessive lateral pressure syndrome (ELPS)
      146, 147
  hypoplasia   146
  osteochondral fractures   176, 177
  recurrent subluxation/dislocation   146,
      147, 177
  stress fractures   146, 147
  supports/taping   148
patella (quadriceps) tendon   116
  cystic lesions   150
  in knee reconstruction   122, 123, 124
  partial tears   150
  tears   **117**, 171–2
  tendinitis   148, **150**
patellofemoral joint   **145–8**
  anatomy/biomechanics   116, **145–6**
  assessment   147
  dysfunction   117, **146–8**
  management of problems   147–8
  osteoarthritis   146
patellofemoral stress syndrome   **146–7**
pectoralis major   33
  insertional tendinitis   34
  weakness   38
Pelligrini–Steida syndrome   148–9
pelvic tilt   84, 87, 88
pelvis   **103–13**
  acute injuries   105–6
  anatomy/biomechanics   103–5
  avulsion fractures   172
  clicking/clonking   103
  examination summary   112–13
  overuse injuries   106–11
  stress fractures   107
  torsion (distortion)   103
perilunar dislocation   65, 66
  trans-scaphoid   65
peroneal tendons   133
  assessment   134
  subluxation   137
  tendinitis   159
peroneal tenography   134–5, 179
pes anserinus
  bursitis   149
  tendon, in knee reconstruction   123–4
pes cavus   188
pes planus   163, 188
phalangeal fractures   **71–2**
  comminuted   72
  epiphyseal   72
  fingertip   71
  involving joints   71–2
  shaft   72

Phalen's test   56, 59
phonophoresis   206
phosphate, plasma   167
physical treatment   3
physique   194
Piedallu sign   112
piriformis   103
  syndrome   110
pisiform, racket player's   65
pivot shift test   119
plantar fasciitis   159–60
  injection   219, 221
play
  continuation after injury   226–8
  illegal   184, 185
plica syndrome, synovial   115, **148**
plyometrics   192
popliteal entrapment syndrome   153–4
popliteus
  tendinitis   149
  tendon   116
post-contraction relaxation   194
posterior cruciate ligament (PCL)
  anatomy/biomechanics   115, 116
  tears   **124–5**
posterior drawer test, knee   120, 124
posterior interosseous nerve entrapment   53
posterior stress test, shoulder   43, 44
posterior talofibular ligament, rupture   132
posterior tibial nerve entrapment   161
post-traumatic encephalopathy   18, 20
post-traumatic epilepsy   **19–20**, 24
posture   87
pre-participation screening   28–9, **185–6**
prepatellar bursitis   150
pressure sores   97
prevention of injuries   20, 27–8, **183–200**
  biomechanics   188–91
  in children   197–200
  community fitness   196–7
  fitness assessment   194–6
  medical responsibilities   183
  overuse injuries   186–8
  pre-participation screening   185–6
  protective equipment   20, 28, **183–4**
  rules of game   184–5
  sports arena design   184
  training factors   191–4
pronator teres   52
  enthesitis of origin   53
  lesions   53–4
proprioceptive neuromuscular facilitation
    (PNF)   194
proprioceptive reflex   9
prosthetic ligaments   123
protective equipment   20, 28, **183–4**
proteins, plasma   167
psoas (iliopsoas)   103, 104
  acute strain   106
  bursitis   108
  stretch   199
psychological fitness   196
psychological support, in spinal cord injuries
    98–9
pubic symphysis
  anatomy/biomechanics   103–4
  instability   107

pubic symphysitis   106–7
'punch-drunkeness' of boxers   18, 20

Q-angle   116, 145–6, 147, 188
quadriceps femoris   116
    contusion   141
    exercises   121, **190**, 201, 207
    expansion tears   **117**
    haematoma   141
    injury   **141–2**
    myositis ossificans   141, 176
    tendon, *see* patella tendon

racket player's pisiform   65
racket sports
    elbow problems   53
    eye injuries   25, 27, 28
    forearm problems   55
    injury prevention   186, **187**
    shoulder problems   45–6
radial nerve lesions   53, **57**
radiculography   180
radiocarpal joint   61, 62
radiography, plain film (X-rays)   **169–77**
    in ankle injuries   134, 138
    in hand and wrist injuries   61–2, 64
    in knee injuries   117, 118, 120, 128,
        171–2
    in pelvic injuries   107
    in shoulder instability   43–4
    in spinal injuries   97
radiohumeral joint   51
radioisotope bone scans   3, 148, 152, **177**
radiological investigations   **169–81**
radio–ulnar joints
    inferior   51, 58
    superior   51
radius
    distal fractures   62
    fractures   51, 52
    stress fracture of distal epiphysis   57, **58**
rearfoot
    valgus   190
    varus   163, 190–1
recovery index   195
rectus femoris   104
    tears   3, 4, **141**
reflexes, in spinal injuries   97
rehabilitation   3, **203–23**
    hand fractures   71
    in spinal cord injuries   98–101
    stages   203
relaxation, post-contraction   194
repetitive strain injury   55
rest (therapeutic)   **203**, 228
resuscitation   226
    ABC sequence   21, 23, 226, 227
    cardiopulmonary (CPR)   19, 23, **226**, 227,
        228
retina
    bruising   27
    detachment   26, 28–9
    tears (dialysis)   26
reverse pivot shift test   124–5
rheumatoid factor   167

ribs   79
    'sprung'   83, 84
    stress fractures   83
RICE principles   141, **228**
'rider's thigh'   106
Ringman's shoulder   34
road traffic accidents   94
rotator cuff
    anatomy   31
    assessment   38–9
    calcific tendinitis   35, 40, 45
    degenerative changes   34, 35
    impingement, *see* shoulder, impingement
    injections   45, **214–15**
    radiology   179–80
    strengthening exercises   44, 207
    tears   34, 38, 45–7
    treatment of problems   **45–7**
rowers   55, 83, 85, 187
rugby football
    hand injuries   60, 76
    injury prevention   184–5, 200
    knee injuries   117
    spinal injuries   81, 95, 97, 98
rules of the game   184–5
runners   3, 189, 191
    ankle/foot problems   156, 158–9, 161
    knee problems   146, 148, 149
    overuse injuries of lower limb   162–4, 186
    pelvic/thigh problems   109, 110
    shin pain   151, 152–3
    see also sprinters
'runner's knee'   145, 147
running   1
    biomechanics   **190–1**
    surface   14, **162**
running-gait cycle   191

sacroiliac joints (SIJ)
    acute dysfunction   85, 103
    anatomy/biomechanics   103, 104
    examination   88, 91, 93, 112
    injections   222–3
    injuries   **84–93**
    management of injuries   91
    manipulation   211
    stress   107–8
sacroiliac mobility test   88, 91
sacroiliitis   86, 93, 107, 108
sag sign   124
scaphoid   62
    fractures   61, **62–4**
    non-union   64
    plaster   64
scapula
    'snapping'   32, 49
    winging   38
scapulothoracic bursitis   49
scapulothoracic joint   31–2, **48–9**
    assessment   48–9
    treatment   49
Scheuermann's disease   82–3, 197
Schmorl's nodes   83
Schober test   87–8
sciatica   84, 85–6, 91, 153
    assessment   87, 90

caudal epidural injection   222
    hamstring syndrome and   111
    unexplained   93
sclerosant injections   92, 93, 222–3
scoliosis   83, 84
    sciatic   83, 87, 88
screening, pre-participation   28–9, **185–6**
serological tests   165
sesamoid fractures   176
sesamoiditis   161
Sever's disease (apophysitis)   12, **157–8**, 197
sexuality, in spinal cord injuries   99
shin pain ('splints')   145, **151–4**
    clinical presentation   151–2
    differential diagnosis   153–4
    investigations   152
    management   152–3
    pathophysiology   151
shoes   **186–7**
    adjusting biomechanics   157, 163–4
    inadequate   164, 186
shoulder   **31–50**
    anatomy/biomechanics   31–3
    arthrography   180
    assessment   36–42
    capsular pattern   36–8
    capsulitis   36, 38, 213
        adhesive (frozen shoulder)   41, 180, 213
        painful arc   41
    dislocation   33, 34–6, 42–4, 177, 180
    examination   **36–40**, 49–50
    flexibility exercises   45, 198
    impingement   **34**
        assessment   36, 41, 42
        injection test   38–9
        signs   39, 40
        treatment   **45–7**
    injections   213, **214–16**, 217
    instability   33, **34–6**, 42
        anterior   42–3, 44
        assessment   42–4
        investigations   43–4
        multidirectional   44
        posterior   43, 44
        treatment   44
    investigations   40, **179–80**
    joint, *see* glenohumeral joint
    management of injuries   40–2
    mobilization exercises   207
    muscle balance assessment   38
    neck problems and   33, **49**
    non-capsular pattern   38
    overuse syndromes   33–40
    pain   41–2
    painful arc syndrome   34, 38–9, 41–2,
        45–7
    repetitive propulsive/explosive stress   33–4
    sport technique changes   45–6
    'sprained'   35
    strengthening exercises   44, **45**, 46, 47
    surgery   44, 46–7
    see also rotator cuff
Sinding-Larsen-Johannson syndrome   150
single photon emission computed tomography
    (SPECT)   91
sinuvertebral nerve   80, 81, 223
skier's thumb   73

skiing
   hand injuries   73
   injury prevention   184, 185, 188
   knee injuries   117
skull fractures   17, 20
slump test   88–90
Smith's fracture   62
snuff box, anatomical   61
soccer, *see* football
soft tissue injuries   **6–14**
   acute inflammatory phase   4
   healing   4–5
   plain film radiography   171–2
   promotion of recovery   228
   recognition   225–6
soleus stretching   201
somatosensory evoked potentials   96, 98
spasticity   99–100, 101
spinal cord injuries   **94–102**
   aetiology   94–5
   assessment/early management   97
   complete   96, 99
   education/prevention of complications   101
   immediate care   **97**, 225, 226–8
   incidence   94
   incomplete   96, 99
   investigations   97–8
   pathology   95–6
   rehabilitation   98–101
spinal injuries   **79–102**, 94, 97–8
   associated injuries   22–3, 94
   instability   101
   magnetic resonance imaging   96, 98, 180
   radiological investigations   180–1
   soft tissue   **79–93**
   see also spinal cord injuries
spinal injury centres   98–9
spinal shock   95, 97
spine
   biomechanics/anatomy   79–81
   canal stenosis   85–6, 93, 153
   injections   **222–3**
   manipulation   82, 84, 210, 211, **212**
   traction   90, 91, **212**
   see also cervical, thoracic, lumbar
spondylolisthesis   88, 91, 92
spondylolysis   80, 85, 86, 197
   assessment   88, 89
   management   91
spondylosis   81
sports arena design   184
sports injury services   229
sports technique   45–6, **187–8**
sprains   9, 10, 225
sprinters   143, 162–3, 189, 191
squash   184, 186
   elbow problems   53
   eye injuries   25, 26, 27, 28
Stack splint   76
sternoclavicular joint   31, 32, **49**
   assessment   49
   treatment   49
sternocostal joints   79
steroid injections   212–13
straight leg raising (SLR)   89, 90–1
strapping techniques   135, 228
strengthening exercises   191–2, **207–10**

stress fractures   12, 14
   in children   197
   distal radial epiphysis   57, **58**
   femur   107, 148
   metatarsals   161, 174
   navicular   160
   olecranon   52
   os calcis   158–9
   pars interarticularis, *see* spondylolysis
   patella   146, 147
   puboischial rami   107
   radioisotope bone scans   148, 152, 177
   ribs   83
   tibia (and fibula)   149, 151, 152–3, 174, 175
   X-rays   **173–5**
stretchers   97, 228
stretching
   ballistic   194
   exercises   162–3, 186, 191, **194**, 198–201
   passive   194
styloiditis radii   55
subacromial bursa   32
   injection   45, 214
subacromial bursitis   34, 38, 39, 45
subacromial decompression surgery   46, 47
subacromial impingement, *see* shoulder, impingement
subacromial joint   31, 32
   painful arc   41
subarachnoid haemorrhage   180
subdural haematoma   18, 19, 180
subluxation   12
subscapularis   31, 32
   examination   39, 40
   tendinitis   45
   tendon injection   215, 216
subtalar joint (STJ)
   anatomy/biomechanics   131–2, 190–1
   biomechanical abnormalities   162, 163
   capsulitis   137
   injections   137, **218–19**, 221
   instability   137
   neutral position   190, 191
subungual haematoma   71–2
sulcus sign, shoulder   43
superficial peroneal nerve entrapment   154
supraspinatus   31, 32
   injection   214–15
   tendinitis   38, 40, 45
   test   38
swimmers
   injury prevention   186, 187, 197
   knee problems   148
   shoulder problems   33–4, 44, 45
'swimmer's impingement'   34
sympathetic ophthalmia   27
synovial plica syndrome   115, **148**
synovitis   10, 213
   traumatic   9
syringomyelia (syrinx formation)   95, 101

talar compression syndrome   159
talar tilt   134, 135, 138
talocalcanean joint, *see* subtalar joint
talocrural joint, *see* ankle, joint

talus   131
   osteochondral injury   **138**, 176
tarsal tunnel syndrome   161
tarsometatarsal joints   132
tarsus
   degenerative changes   161
   overuse injuries   **160–1**
technique, sports   45–6, **187–8**
teeth, protection   184
temperature, body   226
tendinitis   2, 8
   calcific   8, 9
tendinopathies   8–9
tendo-Achilles, *see* Achilles tendon
tendon   **8–9**
   diagnostic ultrasound   181
   grafts for knee reconstruction   122, 123–4
   injections into   213
   magnetic resonance imaging   180
   recognition of injuries   226
tennis   186
   elbow problems   53
   playing techniques   1, 2, 3, 4
   shoulder problems   33, 46
tennis elbow (lateral epicondylitis)   **53**, 216, 218
tennis leg   144
tenodesis, lateral knee   123
tenosynovitis   8–9, 213
tensor fascia lata   105
teres minor   31, 32
terrain, running   14, **162**
Terry-Thomas sign   65, 67
tetraplegia   94, 101
'theatre-goer's' syndrome   86
Thompson's squeeze test   139, 157
thoracic spine
   biomechanics/anatomy   79
   disc prolapse   83, 84
   examination   **84**, 93
   injuries   **82–4**, 94
   joint dysfunction   83, 84
   manipulation   84, 211, 212
   patho-anatomy   82–3
   sprains   83
throwing
   elbow problems   52, 53
   median nerve compression   55
   shoulder problems   **33–4**, 45–6
thumb
   Bennett's fracture   60, **73**
   examination   59
   fractures   68, 73
   gamekeeper's   73
   joint injuries   73, 74
   skier's   73
   trigger   55
   ulnar digital nerve compression   57
tibia
   medial malleolus, fracture   133, 137
   stress fractures   149, 151, 152–3, 174, 175
tibialis posterior tendinitis   159
tibiofemoral joint   115–16
tibiofibular joint
   inferior   131
   superior, injury to   **125**

tibiofibular ligament, rupture 133
Tinel's test 56, 59, 154
tissue typing 167
traction, spinal 90, 91, **212**
training **191–4**
 common sense 191
 endurance 192, 195, 196–7
 errors 146, 162, 164
 flexibility 192–4
 progressive resistance 192
 schedules 14, **191**
 strength 191–2
 variable resistance 192
 see also exercise(s)
trans-scaphoid perilunar dislocation 65
transverse arch (forefoot), inadequacy 161
trauma **5–6**
 continuation of play 226–7
 direct 5–6
 indirect 5, 6
 initial management 226–7
 recognition 225–6
 stabilization 226
 upper limb 51
treatment **203–23**
 first aid 228
 modalities 204–23
triangular cartilage disruption 58
triceps brachii
 anatomy 51
 tendinitis of long head 34
triceps surae injury 144
trigger finger/thumb 55
trochanteric bursitis 110
 injections 110, 217

trunk, flexibility exercises 198
ulna
 distal fractures **62**
 proximal fractures 51
ulnar nerve compression 56–7
ultrasound
 diagnostic **181**
 therapy **205–6**
unconsciousness 17, 21, 23–4
upper limb **51–76**
 anatomy/biomechanics 51–2
 examination summary 58–9
 nerve entrapment 53, **55–7**
 neural tension test 82
 neurological assessment 82
 overuse injuries **51–9**
 radicular pain 82
 trauma 51
 see also elbow; forearm; hand; wrist
uric acid, plasma 167
urinalysis 168
urinary catheterization 101

varus stress test 10, 125
vastus medialis (obliquus) (VMO) 116
 strengthening exercises 148, 190, 207
 wasting 146, 147
ventilation, in head injury 19
vital signs 21

war games 27
warm down (cool down) 8, 197
warm-up exercises 7–8, 196

water-skiing 106, 184
weight-lifters 40, 55, 80, 150
weight-training 80, 150, 187
wheelchair sports 99, 100
whiplash 81–2
white cell count (WBC) 167
Wingate test 195
wobble board 137
wound healing 4–5
wrist
 assessment of injuries 60–2
 biomechanics 51–2
 causes of injury 60
 chronic ligament sprains 58
 degenerative lesions 58
 examination 58–9, 60–1
 fractures around **62–5**
 injections **216–17**
 injuries **60–76**
 joint injuries **65–7**
 nerve entrapment 55–7
 overuse injury **58**
 perilunar dislocation 65, 66
 sprain 67
 trans-scaphoid perilunar dislocation 65

X-rays, *see* radiography, plain film

zygo-apophyseal joints, *see* facet joints